OXFORD MEDICAL PUBLICATIONS

PAEDIATRIC DENTISTRY

Paediatric Dentistry

Edited by

Richard R. Welbury

*Consultant in Paediatric Dentistry and Honorary Senior
Clinical Lecturer, Newcastle upon Tyne Dental Hospital and School,
Royal Victoria Infirmary, and Associated Hospitals Trust*

Oxford   New York   Tokyo
OXFORD UNIVERSITY PRESS
1997

Oxford University Press, Great Clarendon Street, Oxford OX2 6DP

Oxford   New York

Athens   Auckland   Bangkok   Bogota   Bombay   Buenos Aires
Calcutta   Cape Town   Dar es Salaam   Delhi   Florence   Hong Kong
Istanbul   Karachi   Kuala Lumpur   Madras   Madrid   Melbourne
Mexico City   Nairobi   Paris   Singapore   Taipei   Tokyo   Toronto

and associated companies in
Berlin   Ibadan

Oxford is a trade mark of Oxford University Press

Published in the United States
by Oxford University Press Inc., New York

A catalogue record for this book is available
from the British Library

Library of Congress Cataloging in Publication Data
(applied for)
ISBN 0 19 262631 0 (h/b)
(0 19 262630 2 pbk)

Typeset by Expo Holdings,
Printed in Hong Kong

CONTENTS

CONTRIBUTORS

A. S. Blinkhorn   Professor of Oral Health
University of Manchester

N. E. Carter   Department of Child Dental Health
Newcastle upon Tyne Dental Hospital and School
R.V.I. and Associated Hospitals Trust

P. H. Gordon   Department of Child Dental Health
University of Newcastle upon Tyne

N. M. Kilpatrick   Department of Paediatric Dentistry
University of Sydney

P. A. Heasman   Department of Restorative Dentistry
University of Newcastle upon Tyne

J. G. Meechan   Department of Oral Surgery
University of Newcastle upon Tyne

J. J. Murray   Professor of Child Dental Health
University of Newcastle upon Tyne

J. H. Nunn   Department of Child Dental Health
University of Newcastle upon Tyne

J. Page   Specialist Dental Practitioner
Tunbridge Wells, Kent

A. J. Rugg-Gunn   Professor of Preventive Dentistry
University of Newcastle upon Tyne

G. J. Roberts   Professor of Children's Dentistry
Great Ormond Street Hospital, London
Eastman Dental Institute and Institute of Child Health
London

L. Shaw   Department of Children's Dentistry and Orthodontics
Birmingham Children's Hospital
University of Birmingham Dental Hospital and School

R. R. Welbury   Department of Child Dental Health
Newcastle upon Tyne Dental Hospital and School
R.V.I. and Associated Hospitals Trust

J. M. Whitworth   Department of Restorative Dentistry
University of Newcastle upon Tyne

G. B. Winter   Emeritus Professor of Children's Dentistry
Eastman Dental Institute and the Institute of Child
Health, London

PREFACE

The child and adolescent deserves the best of care in all the different disciplines of dentistry. I was delighted to be given the opportunity of trying to draw together all the different aspects of paediatric dentistry and am most grateful to my colleagues for agreeing to contribute the various chapters which make up the book. We have tried to cover as much ground as possible within the obvious publishing restrictions and the finished product will inevitably reflect the editor's perceptions of where current needs and deficiencies exist. The sudden increase in both erosive tooth surface loss and cosmetic awareness in our younger patients made their inclusion in Chapter 8 important, where previously they have not achieved such prominence in paediatric texts. Similarly periodontal disease (Chapter 10), oral pathology and oral surgery (Chapter 14) and disability (Chapter 16) are as deserving of detailed inclusion in a 'paediatric' as much as in any 'general' text.

The book was written with undergraduate dental students in mind but we hope it will also be useful to those engaged in postgraduate studies and to general dental practitioners. Exhaustive references are deliberately not given but suggested 'further reading' lists are included to help expedite further enquiry and learning.

I hope we have shown in *Paediatric Dentistry* that the early years of life are the time to get it right for the child and adolescent and there is no reason why our young patients should be denied correct and appropriate care.

R. R. W.

Newcastle upon Tyne
April 1996

ACKNOWLEDGEMENTS

I would like to thank the staff of Oxford University Press, for encouraging me to develop *Paediatric Dentistry* and for their help and guidance with the many queries along the way.

Finally, I thank all the contributors and their secretaries for their help, and most especially Denise Kingsbury who has been responsible for most of the secretarial work involved.

1 Craniofacial growth and development

1 Craniofacial growth and development

P. H. GORDON

1.1 INTRODUCTION

This chapter describes, in general terms, the postnatal growth of the craniofacial skeleton and the occlusal development of the primary and permanent dentitions. There is a great deal of individual variation in the process of growth and in the final form of the craniofacial structures; this chapter presents a simplified, or rather idealized, account of craniofacial growth and occlusal development, then goes on to discuss the effect of individual variation in producing departures from this idealized pattern.

Figure 1.1 illustrates the typical changes that take place in the stature of an individual during growth and the extent of normal variation. A chart such as this will present an overall view of the process of growth and will help to detect instances in which growth is not proceeding in the usual manner, but it disguises the fact that the various tissues of the body grow at different rates at different ages, which is illustrated in Fig. 1.2. Neural tissues reach their maximum growth rate at a relatively early age, while the maximum rate for general skeletal growth occurs later. The maximum growth rate for lymphoid tissue occupies an intermediate position.

1.2 GENERAL PRINCIPLES OF CRANIOFACIAL GROWTH

One way of assessing the changes that take place during craniofacial growth is to superimpose tracings of two lateral skull radiographs, taken of the same person, but at different ages. The two radiographs can be compared, as shown in Fig. 1.3 and the changes that have taken place during growth can be examined. One potential difficulty with this approach is that the various bones of the skull grow at different rates at different ages, and there is no single central point about which growth occurs in a radial fashion — there is no valid, fixed radiographic landmark on which to superimpose the films. One convention is to superimpose the tracings of the radiographs on the outline of the sella turcica, using the line from sella to the frontonasal suture to orientate the films. If this method of superimposition is used, then it appears that the cranium expands in a more or less radial fashion to accommodate the brain and the facial skeleton then grows downwards and forwards, away from the cranial base.

The growth of the cranium is linked to the growth of the brain and so the calvarial bones increase in size at an earlier age than the bones of the face, whose growth is linked to that of the musculoskeletal system. Of course, the centre of the sella turcica and the frontonasal suture are not fixed points and are themselves subject to changes in the course of growth, but the growth of the bones in the anterior cranial fossa is largely complete by the age of 5 years and

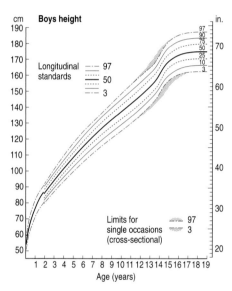

Fig. 1.1 Growth and development record.

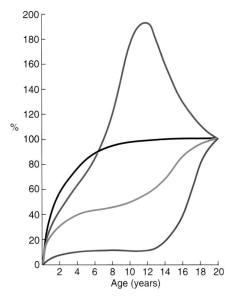

Fig. 1.2 Postnatal growth of various tissues expressed as a percentage of total gain from birth to maturity. Lymphoid type: green; neural type: black; general type: red; genital type: blue. (Redrawn from Scammon, R. E. (1930) The measurements of the body in childhood. In *Measurement of Man* (Ed. J. A. Harris, C. M. Jackson, D. G. Paterson, and R. E. Scammon, University of Minnesota Press Minneapolis.)

while there is a certain amount of remodelling, the area between the sella and the frontonasal suture provides relatively stable landmarks for superimposition, from that age onwards.

Bones grow at their edges. Unlike soft tissues such as, for example, the liver, the calcified structure of bone prevents growth by means of the generalized division of cells producing expansion of the organ as a whole. Alteration in the size and shape of bones takes place by deposition and resorption of material on the external and internal surfaces of the bone, by proliferation of cartilage and its replacement by bone, and by growth at the sutures. These different mechanisms all come into play at various stages in the growth of different regions of the craniofacial skeleton.

A long bone, such as the femur, increases in length by proliferation of cartilage at the epiphyses and its replacement by bone. The head of the femur and its shaft are pushed apart by the expanding cartilage, which is then replaced with bone and this process is sufficiently forceful to counteract the compressive force exerted by the weight of the owner of the bone. There are not many sites in the craniofacial skeleton at which growth proceeds by this mechanism. Proliferation of cartilage in the nasal septum may be responsible in part for the downward and forward translation of the maxilla, and the spheno-occipital synchondrosis in the floor of the middle cranial fossa provides a mechanism for some increase in anteroposterior length of the cranial base. These epiphyses and synchondroses are capable of pushing bones apart and acting as primary growth centres rather than providing a mechanism whereby bones can respond or react to growth in other areas.

Sutures, on the other hand, form bone when subjected to traction. In the case of the calvarial bones, the suture systems form new bone and enable the bones to

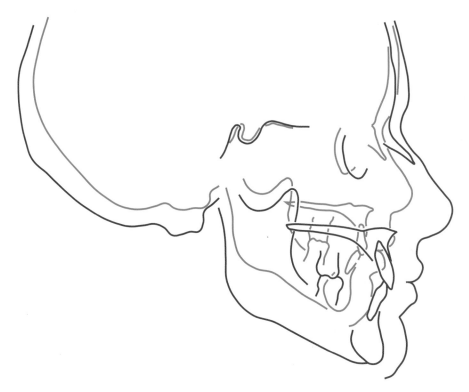

Fig. 1.3 Lateral skull radiographs of the same subject, taken at ages 6 and 18 years, superimposed on the Sella–Nasion line, registered on Sella.

stay in contact with each other when the expansion of the growing brain would otherwise move the bones apart. The suture systems allow the bones to respond to growth in neighbouring soft tissue; the suture systems that lie between the maxilla and the cranial base allow the downward and forward translation of the maxilla in response to growth of the soft tissues of the face. It is not proliferation of the vascular connective tissue in the sutures that pushes the bones apart, the whole arrangement of the connective tissue in a suture seems designed to enable the suture to respond to a tensile force.

Surface deposition and resorption are very important mechanisms that allow for the translation and remodelling of bone. Deposition and resorption go hand in hand, seldom does one occur without the other. Deposition of bone on one aspect of a cortical plate of bone, accompanied by resorption on the other aspect allows for translation of bones — that is to say a change in their relative positions — and resorption and deposition occurring on the same aspect of a bone allow for changes in shape. Change in the size of a bone will involve both mechanisms. Surface deposition and resorption of bone are functions of the periosteum or 'osteogenic membrane' that covers its surface.

The mechanisms that control the process of facial growth are not completely understood. It is likely that there is a genetic component in the control mechanism; after all, children tend to resemble their parents in facial appearance. Apart from that, the growth of the bony skeleton is influenced by signals received from its growing soft tissue integument and, probably, vice versa.

1.2.1 Cranial growth

At birth, the cranium has reached some 60–65 per cent of its adult longitudinal dimension and about 90 per cent by the age of 5 years. The calvarial bones are carried away from each other by the expanding brain, and respond by forming new bone in the sutures that separate the bones of the vault of the skull. The six fontanelles that are present at birth reduce in size, the largest — the anterior fontanelle — closes at about 1 year of age and the last to close — the posterolateral fontanelle — closes at about 18 months. The calvarial bones undergo a process of remodelling with areas of bone deposition and resorption altering the contour of the bones as the volume of the brain cavity increases.

The cranial base is also growing to accommodate the changes in the size and shape of the brain, but the process is different to that seen in the calvarial bones. There is considerable lateral growth of the cranial base as the cerebral hemispheres expand, but less increase in anteroposterior dimension. No sutures are present to allow for expansion of the deeper compartments of the cranial base, a process that takes place by surface deposition and extensive remodelling. In addition, there are three synchondroses in the mid-ventral floor of the cranial base that allow for increase in anteroposterior dimension. These are the spheno-occipital synchondrosis (the most important of the three), the intersphenoid synchondrosis and the spheno-ethmoidal synchondrosis. Growth in the spheno-occipital synchondrosis does not cease until about the age of 15 years in boys, rather earlier in girls and it closes at about the age of 20. The pattern and the timing of growth in the cranial base is intermediate between the neural type of growth that characterizes the growth of the calvarial bones and the musculoskeletal pattern of growth exhibited by the facial skeleton.

The shape of the cranial fossae is much more complex than the relatively smooth form of the bones of the vault of the skull. The partitions which separate the cranial fossae are formed by surface deposition and subsequent remodelling, the final size and shape of the compartments being determined by the size of the lobes of the brain.

1.2.2 Nasomaxillary growth

The nasomaxillary complex grows downwards and forwards relative to the cranial base. Unlike the growth of the cranium, which occurs in conjunction with the growth of the brain at a relatively early age, being almost complete by the age of 5 years, the nasomaxillary complex grows fastest at about the time of the pubertal growth spurt, in conjunction with the general growth of the musculoskeletal system. There are two mechanisms which might account for the downward and forward growth of the maxilla. One is proliferation of cartilage in the nasal septum which could provide a force to actively push the maxilla in this direction. Another factor is the 'functional matrix' of the soft tissue environment of the maxilla. As the soft tissue grows, the maxilla is translated downward and forward. In any event, the sutures positioned between the maxilla and the cranial base respond by producing new bone, which is formed both on the maxillary and the cranial aspects of the suture system.

As the maxilla moves downwards and forwards, new bone is created by surface deposition in the area of the maxillary tuberosity, while the anterior aspect of the maxilla is remodelled not by surface apposition, as might be expected in a bone that is growing forwards, but by a process of resorption. The downward and forward movement of the maxilla is effected by a translation of the bone accompanied by surface deposition on the posterior aspect of the maxilla, rather than by surface apposition on the anterior aspect of the bone.

As bone is deposited on the external aspect of the maxilla in the region of the tuberosity, it is also resorbed from the internal aspect of the bone in this area, thereby enlarging the maxillary sinus. As the bone is translated downwards, the nasal cavities and the maxillary sinus expand by a process of bone resorption at the floor of the nose and the sinus, together with bone deposition on the palatal aspect of the maxilla.

1.2.3 Mandibular growth

Growth of the mandible, like that of the maxilla, is co-ordinated with the pattern of general musculoskeletal growth, growing at its fastest rate at about the time of the pubertal growth spurt. Growth of the mandible has to be co-ordinated with the downward and forward growth of the maxilla. This task is made more complicated by the fact that the mandibular condyles articulate in the glenoid fossa, which lies behind the spheno-occipital synchondrosis, while the maxilla lies in front of it; therefore, growth of the mandible has to keep pace not just with the translation of the maxilla, but also with growth in the cranial base.

Taking the anterior cranial fossa as a stable reference area it appears that the mandible, like the maxilla, grows downwards and forwards. As is the case with the maxilla, this downwards and forwards growth is not achieved by deposition of bone on the anterior aspect of the mandible; it is achieved by translation of the bone, accompanied by growth in the region of the ramus and the mandibular condyle, as illustrated in Fig. 1.4. Bone is deposited on the posterior aspects of the ramus and the coronoid processes and resorbed from the anterior aspect of the ramus. At the same time the condylar cartilage is contributing to growth of the mandibular condyle. Although there are similarities between the condylar cartilage and the epiphysis of a long bone — both grow by proliferation of cartilage and its replacement by bone — it is likely that the condylar cartilage operates as a reactive growth site, responding to translation of the mandible rather than causing it. It is not proliferation of the condylar cartilage that pushes the mandible downwards and forwards.

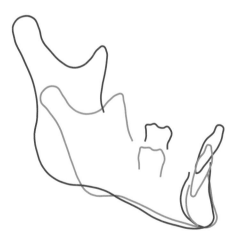

Fig. 1.4 Growth of the mandible occurs mainly in the region of the ramus and the mandibular condyle.

As the ramus of the mandible grows upwards and backwards, the anterior aspect of the ramus undergoes resorption and becomes remodelled into the body of the mandible. This process involves resorption on the lateral aspect of the bone and deposition on the lingual aspect, which forms new bone in correct alignment with the body of the mandible and helps maintain an appropriate intercondylar width. Growth of the mandibular ramus and condyle has to keep pace with changes in the position of the maxilla, in both vertical and horizontal directions and with growth in the middle cranial fossa. It is easy for a small discrepancy to arise, for example, in the amount of vertical growth of the mandibular ramus, resulting in a rotation of the body of the mandible and a corresponding tilt of the occlusal plane.

1.2.4 Regulation of craniofacial growth

It is generally accepted that musculoskeletal growth proceeds at least partly under genetic control, but there is still some uncertainty as to how this control is exercised. If it was exercised at the level of the bone itself, if the final size and shape were programmed directly into the bone, then control would be exercised at the level of the sutures and the periosteum. This seems unlikely, as a suture is designed to respond to traction rather than to produce an increase in size by pushing bones apart.

If control was exercised at the level of cartilage, then the final size and shape of a bone would be determined by the amount of activity in the cartilages associated with the bone. The nasal septum may well play a part in controlling the translation of the maxilla, pushing it downwards and forwards, away from the cranial base. The synchondroses in the cranial base resemble the epiphyses that play an important part in the formation of the long bones. Though their inaccessiblity makes them difficult to study, they probably determine the amount of anteroposterior growth in the cranial base. The cartilage in the mandibular condyle appears to be a secondary growth site, allowing growth of the condyle, rather than initiating such growth.

A third possibility is that the final size and shape of a bone is determined by the 'functional matrix' of its soft tissue environment. It is easy to accept that the size and shape of the cranium could be determined by the size and shape of the brain, or that the developing eyeball and its associated muscles determine the growth of the orbit. In the context of the face, it would be growth of the soft tissues of the face and the muscles of mastication that brought about the translation of the maxilla and the mandible, the cartilage of the nasal septum and the suture systems between the facial bones and the cranial base would simply provide a mechanism whereby this could be achieved.

This third possibility seems to be the main way in which growth of the facial skeleton and growth of the cranium is regulated. The cartilage in the cranial base is important in determining its final size and shape and the cartilage in the nasal septum may play some part in initiating the downward and forward translation of the maxilla; however, the growth of the brain, the soft tissues of the face, and the muscles of mastication seems to be the main factor regulating the growth of the craniofacial skeleton.

1.2.5 Normal variation

There is always variation between individuals. Variation in the pattern of facial growth is only to be expected and there are a number of compensatory mechanisms that operate to minimize the impact of such variation. Variation in the position or size of one structure is often compensated by corresponding change in

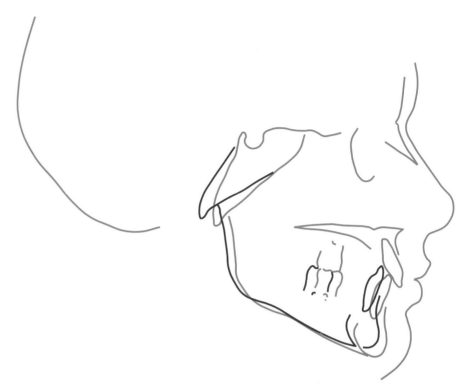

Fig. 1.5 A small change in the angle between the anterior cranial fossa and the middle cranial fossa can produce a class II skeletal relationship, with the resulting class II malocclusion of the teeth.

another. The process of growth is constantly creating imbalances as related structures grow and develop at different rates, but the overall direction of growth is towards some position of overall balance or harmony.

Anteroposterior discrepancies can arise during facial growth on account of the position of a bone, or as the result of an imbalance in the sizes of bones, or can arise from a mixture of both. A class II skeletal pattern can be caused by insufficient growth in a backwards direction of the ramus of the mandible; alternatively, a class II skeletal pattern can be the result of a forward tilt of the middle cranial fossa, as illustrated in Fig. 1.5. This change in angulation results in the maxilla having a more anterior position, relative to the glenoid fossa than would otherwise have been the case. The normal-sized mandible, occluding in the glenoid fossa, now has a class II relationship to the normal-sized maxilla. In a similar way, a converse alteration in the pattern of growth — excessive backwards growth of the ramus of the mandible, a more vertical tilt of the middle cranial fossa — can produce a class III skeletal relationship, with the accompanying dental malocclusion.

Vertical growth in the nasomaxillary region has to be matched with vertical growth of the mandibular ramus. Imbalances here will have the effect of producing a mandibular rotation. If there is an excess of vertical maxillary growth, which is not matched by vertical growth of the ramus, then the effect will be to produce a downwards and backwards rotation of the mandible. This downwards and backwards rotation will, in turn, produce an anteroposterior discrepancy, with a tendency towards a class II relationship.

Horizontal and vertical discrepancies tend to be accompanied by dento-alveolar compensations. In the case of a class III skeletal pattern, the upper incisor teeth are frequently proclined and the lower incisor teeth retroclined, as illustrated in

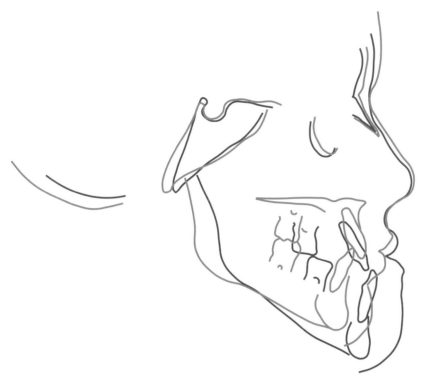

Fig. 1.6 Dento-alveolar compensation of a class III skeletal relationship, with proclination of the upper incisor teeth and retroclination of the lower.

Fig. 1.6. These compensations are almost certainly brought about by muscular activity in the soft tissue integument affecting the position of the teeth and they minimize what may otherwise have been a large reversed incisor overjet. In the case of class II skeletal patterns, the dento-alveolar compensation can take two forms. If the lips function in front of the upper incisor teeth, then these are generally retroclined, with the effect that the incisor overjet is virtually normal. If, however, the lower lip functions behind the upper incisors, then these teeth are usually proclined, and the lower incisors retroclined, to make way for the lip. This results in an increased incisor overjet.

Downward and backward mandibular rotations tend to be accompanied by a vertical drifting of the premolar, canine, and incisor teeth, to compensate for an arrangement that would otherwise have produced an anterior open bite. This vertical drifting should be distinguished from over-eruption, which would produce a lengthening of the clinical crowns of the teeth.

1.2.6 Modification of the pattern of facial growth

Attempts to modify the pattern of facial growth have met with a certain amount of success. Orthodontic appliances have been designed that hold the mandible postured downwards and forwards. This moves the condyle out of the glenoid fossa and encourages upwards and backwards growth of the mandibular ramus. At the same time, the stretched muscles of mastication exert an upwards and backwards force (through the appliance) to the maxilla, which tends to inhibit its downwards and forwards growth. The effect on the growing face is to help correct a developing class II skeletal pattern. If this developing class II skeletal pattern is being caused not so much by underdevelopment of the mandible (which seems to be the more common cause), but by excessive forwards growth of the maxilla, then an appliance may be used simply to exert an upwards and backwards force on the maxilla, without involving the mandible and help, in that way, to influence the course of facial growth.

These appliances apply forces to the developing maxilla and mandible via the teeth — the appliances are attached to the teeth — and work partly by inducing a dento-alveolar compensation for the underlying skeletal discrepancy. This process is sometimes referred to as 'orthodontic camouflage'. There is likely to be some restraint of the downwards and forwards growth of the maxilla, but the appliances seem to have only a minimal effect on the eventual size of the mandible. The so-called 'myofunctional appliances', that derive their impetus from the muscles of mastication, are used most often to help correct class II mal-occlusions. The appliances work by maintaining a forward and downwards pos-turing of the mandible and while it is possible to use myofunctional–functional appliances to correct a developing class III malocclusion, they are less often used in this context, as it is difficult to obtain the necessary backwards posturing of the mandible. In addition, the dento-alveolar compensations that these appli-ances tend to produce are often already present in untreated class III occlusions.

1.3   TOOTH DEVELOPMENT

Teeth start to form during the fifth week of embryonic life and the process of tooth formation continues until the roots of the third permanent molars are com-pleted at about the age of 20 years. The stages of tooth formation are the same whether the tooth is of the primary or the permanent dentition, although, obvi-ously, the teeth develop at different times. The tooth germs develop from the dental lamina, a sheet of epithelial cells which develops, itself, from the primary epithelial band. This is a layer of thickened epithelium which forms around the mouth in the area soon to be occupied by the upper and lower jaws. The primary epithelial band quickly organizes into two discrete epithelial ingrowths — the vestibular lamina and the dental lamina. The vestibular lamina grows down into the underlying ectomesenchyme, the epithelial cells enlarge and then break down, thereby forming the cleft which becomes the sulcus between the cheeks and the alveolar processes.

The dental lamina forms a series of epithelial buds that grow outward into the surrounding connective tissue. These buds represent the first stage in the devel-opment of the tooth germs of the primary dentition. The epithelial bud continues to grow and becomes associated with a condensation of mesenchymal cells to form a tooth germ at the cap stage of development. The epithelial bud develops into the enamel organ, the condensation of mesenchymal cells will constitute the dental papilla and comes to extend around the enamel organ to form the dental follicle. The cells at the margin of the epithelial bud continue to proliferate and grow to enfold the mesenchymal cells of the dental follicle, producing a tooth germ at the bell stage of development. Around this time — the transition from cap stage to bell stage — a process of histodifferentiation produces the recognizable structures of the enamel organ, with its external and internal enamel epithelia, stratum intermedium, and stellate reticulum.

Further proliferation of the cells of the dental lamina, at a point adjacent to each primary tooth germ, but on its lingual aspect, produces the tooth germ of the permanent successor. The tooth germs of the permanent molar teeth, which have no primary precursors are formed by distal extension of the dental lamina, which tunnels backwards as the jaws lengthen posteriorly.

The cells of the inner enamel epithelium lengthen to a columnar shape, with the cell nuclei occupying the portion of the cell beside the stratum intermedium, away from the dental papilla. The cells of the dental papilla adjacent to the internal enamel epithelium, also elongate to a columnar form, with their nuclei aligned away from the enamel organ and towards the centre of the dental papilla. These columnar cells of the dental papilla differentiate into odontoblasts, the cells which form dentine. Dentine formation, which is induced by the cells of the internal enamel epithelium, always precedes enamel formation. Although dentine is formed by the odontoblasts of the dental papilla, the process is initiated by the epithelial cells of the enamel organ. Once dentine formation begins, the cells of the internal enamel epithelium differentiate into ameloblasts, and commence the formation of enamel. Dentine and enamel formation occurs initially in the region of the cusp tips and incisal edges of the teeth, then continues towards the cervical margin of their crowns.

Differentiation of odontoblasts and the formation of dentine is induced by the cells of the internal enamel epithelium. A similar process is involved in the production of dentine to form the roots of teeth. The epithelial cells at the cervical loop of the enamel organ proliferate and migrate in an apical direction to form a tubular epithelial sheath around the dental papilla. These epithelial cells — the root sheath of Hertwig — induce the formation of odontoblasts from the cells of the dental papilla and the production of dentine to form the roots of the teeth, a process which is not complete until 3–5 years after the eruption of the crown of the tooth.

The stages of tooth development are the same for both primary and permanent teeth, although progression through the stages occurs at different times and at varying rates for the different teeth. Tables 1.1 and 1.2 summarize the chronology of tooth development for the two dentitions.

1.4 TOOTH ERUPTION

There are several possible explanations to account for the phenomenon of tooth eruption. Some possibilities are more likely than others to play a part in the process and some earlier theories have been largely discounted. Extrusion of pulp tissue through the apical foramen, arising from growth of dentine and proliferation of cells in the pulp has been suggested as a mechanism for providing a force that could be responsible for bringing about the eruption of teeth. The effect of

Table 1.1 The chronology of the development of the primary dentition

Stage of development	Central incisor		Lateral incisor		Canine		First molar		Second molar		Time
	Max	Mand	Max	Mand	Max	Mand	Max	Mand	Max	Mand	
Hard tissue formation begins	13–16	13–16	14.7–16.5	14.7–16.5	15–18	16–18	14.5–17	14.5–17	16–23.5	17–19.5	Weeks after ovulation
Crown formation complete	1.5	2.5	2.5	3	9	8–9	6	5–6	11	8–11	Months after birth
Beginning of eruption	8–12	6–10	9–13	10–16	16–22	17–23	13–19	14–18	25–33	23–31	Months after birth
Completion of root formation	33	33	33	30	43	43	37	34	47	42	Months after birth

(Adapted from Schroeder, 1991.)

Table 1.2 The chronology of the development of the permanent dentition

Stage of development	Central incisor		Lateral incisor		Canine		First premolar		Second premolar		Time
	Max	Mand	Max	Mand	Max	Mand	Max	Mand	Max	Mand	
Hard tissue formation begins (histology)	3–4		10–12	3–4	4–5		18–24		24–30		Months after birth
Hard tissue formation begins (radiology)	—		—		6		19		36		Months after birth
Crown formation complete	3.3–4.1	3.4–5.4	4.4–4.9	3.1–5.9	4.5–5.8	4.0–4.7	6.3–7.0	5–6	6.6–7.2	6.1–7.1	Years of age (decimal)
Beginning of eruption	6.7–8.1	6.0–6.9	7.0–8.8	6.8–8.1	10.0–12.2	9.2–11.4	9.6–10.9	9.6–11.5	10.2–11.4	10.1–12.1	Years of age (decimal)
Completion of root formation	8.6–9.8	7.7–8.6	9.6–10.8	8.5–9.6	11.2–13.3	10.8–13.0	11.2–13.6	11.0–13.4	11.6–14.0	11.7–14.3	Years of age (decimal)

Table 1.2 *Continued*

Stage of development	First molar		Second molar		Third molar		Time
	Max	Mand	Max	Mand	Max	Mand	
Hard tissue formation begins (histology)	7–8 ao		30–36 mo		7–9 yr	8–10 yr	Months after ovulation (ao) or months (mo) and years (yr) after birth
Hard tissue formation begins (radiology)	2 mo		36–48 mo		9–10 yr		Months (mo) or years (yr) after birth
Crown formation complete	2.1–3.5	2.1–3.6	6.9–7.4	6.2–7.4	12.8–13.2	12.0–13.7	Years of age with decimal fractions
Beginning of eruption	6.1–6.7	5.9–6.9	11.9–12.8	11.2–12.2	17.0–19.0	17.0–19.0	Years of age with decimal fractions
Completion of root formation	9.3–10.8	7.8–9.8	12.9–16.2	11.0–15.7	19.5–19.6	20.0–20.8	Years of age with decimal fractions

(Adapted from Schroeder, 1991.)
Max = maxilla
Mand = Mandible

blood pressure within the pulp, or simple root lengthening have also been put forward as possible causative agents. However, observational and experimental studies of rootless teeth have shown that they erupt into a functional occlusion, so it is unlikely that these mechanisms have an important part to play in the process of eruption.

Remodelling of dento-alveolar bone has been proposed as a mechanism for tooth eruption, but its part is difficult to assess. Bone remodelling has to occur as teeth erupt and it is hard to know whether the remodelling is a cause of tooth eruption or whether it is simply in response to the eruption of the teeth. Tooth eruption may occur in response to activity within the periodontal ligament, where contraction of fibroblasts could be capable of elevating the tooth root, but it is most likely that agents responsible for tooth eruption lie within the dental follicle itself, rather than the tooth. The connective tissue of the dental follicle is a rich source of factors that are responsible for the local mediation of bone deposition and resorption and it seems probable that the dental follicle has a major part to play in the process of tooth eruption.

1.5 OCCLUSAL DEVELOPMENT

1.5.1 The primary dentition

The first tooth to erupt is usually the lower central incisor. Occasionally, this tooth is present at birth, but the average age for its eruption is about 7 or 8 months, although there is, inevitably, some individual variation. The other incisor teeth follow soon after, with the upper central incisors erupting at about

10 months followed by the upper lateral incisors at about 11 months and the lower lateral incisors at about 13 months. At about the age of 16 months the first primary molars put in an appearance, followed by the primary canine teeth at about 19 months. The second primary molars erupt at about 27–29 months, with the lower teeth usually erupting before the upper. While the eruption sequence — the order in which the teeth erupt — is usually as described above, there is considerable variation in the actual age at which the teeth erupt. In any event there is almost a continuous process of tooth eruption between the ages of 7 and 29 months.

There are some occlusal features that occur relatively frequently in the established primary dentition.

1. The incisor teeth tend to be spaced. The permanent incisor teeth have to fit into the same space as their primary predecessors. The permanent incisors are larger teeth than the primary incisors and if the primary teeth are not spaced, then the permanent teeth will be crowded. Crowding of the permanent incisor teeth is a relatively common occurrence, but the crowding is seldom so severe that there is no spacing of the primary incisors.
2. The so-called 'anthropoid' spaces between the upper lateral incisor and the canine and between the lower canine and the first primary molar are particularly common.
3. In the case of a class I occlusion, the mesiobuccal cusp of the primary second molar occludes in the mesiobuccal groove of the lower second molar, a situation analogous to the class I occlusion of first permanent molars. However, the lower second primary molar is much longer, mesiodistally, than the upper second molar and the class I occlusion of the mesiobuccal cusp of the upper means that the distal surfaces of the teeth are in the same vertical plane.

The incisor relationship tends more towards edge-to-edge than is the case with permanent teeth (although with increasing wear of the primary teeth there may be a postural element in this) and the upper incisors tend to be more upright. There is sometimes an anterior open bite, associated with a sucking habit and there may be cross-bites of the buccal segment teeth, but in general, the teeth in the primary dentition tend to be well aligned and while there may be some anteroposterior, lateral, or vertical discrepancy, these deviations are seldom so marked that they give rise to comment.

1.5.2 The mixed dentition

The primary dentition erupts more or less continuously over a 2 year period. The permanent dentition, however, erupts in two stages as first the incisor teeth and the first permanent molars erupt, then the other teeth in the buccal segments. The lower central incisor and the first permanent molars erupt at about the age of 6 years. The upper central incisor and the lower lateral incisor erupt at about the age of 7 and the upper lateral incisor at about the age of 8 years. As with the primary teeth, while some variation in the timing of tooth eruption is only to be expected, this eruption sequence should not vary. In particular, the upper central incisor should erupt before the upper lateral incisor. If the upper lateral incisor erupts before the central then, almost certainly, there is something impeding the eruption of the central incisor, for example: a supernumerary tooth, or dilaceration of the root of the central incisor.

The lower canine and the first premolar teeth are the next to erupt, at about the age of 10, followed by the upper canine and the second premolar teeth at about the age of 11 and the second molar teeth at about the age of 12. Third molar teeth start to erupt from about the age of 16 onwards, but the eruption of third molars is very variable; not uncommonly, these teeth are impacted against their neighbours and fail to erupt at all.

The upper central incisors are more proclined than their primary counterparts. This allows some forward repositioning of the mandible when the first permanent molars erupt in a cusp-to-cusp relationship with their opponents. The distal surfaces of the second primary molars tend to be in the same vertical plane, so the first permanent molars, erupting behind them, tend to adopt a class II occlusal relationship. The forward repositioning of the mandible allows the establishment of a class I intercuspal position. The primary teeth in the buccal segments have a larger combined mesiodistal width than do the permanent teeth which replace them. This means that, provided the primary teeth are shed in the ordinary way, there should not be any problem with lack of space for the permanent teeth in the buccal segments of the dental arch. The 'leeway space' as it is sometimes called — the amount by which the combined size of the primary canine and molar teeth exceeds the combined mesiodistal widths of the permanent canine and premolar teeth — amounts to 1.5 mm in the upper arch and 2.5 mm in the lower, with its large second primary molar.

The size and shape of the anterior segments of the dento-alveolar arches do not change much following the eruption of the permanent incisor teeth; there is not much growth by deposition of bone on the labial aspect of the maxilla or mandible, these bones grow by forward and downward translation, with deposition of new bone on their posterior surfaces. If there is insufficient space to accommodate the teeth in the dental arches when the teeth erupt, then it is unlikely that the situation will improve as growth proceeds. There is a small expansion in the width of the dental arch, with deposition of bone on the lateral aspect of the maxilla and the mandible and while most of the 'leeway space' is taken up by mesial movement of the posterior teeth, it may allow for some improvement in the alignment of crowded incisors.

1.5.3 The permanent dentition

As with the primary dentition, it is possible to identify occlusal features of the established permanent dentition that occur consistently in ideal dental arches.

1. The mesiobuccal cusp of the upper first permanent molar occludes in the mesiobuccal groove of the lower first permanent molar, with the distal aspect of the upper first molar contacting the mesial aspect of the lower second molar.
2. The teeth should have a normal labiolingual inclination. In the case of the anterior teeth, the crown inclination must be sufficient to prevent over-eruption of the teeth and an increased incisor overbite. In the case of the posterior teeth, the upper teeth should have a lingual inclination, which remains constant in the premolar and molar regions, while the lower teeth have a lingual inclination which becomes more pronounced towards the back of the arch.
3. The teeth should have a normal mesiodistal angulation, with the crowns of the teeth more mesially positioned than their roots.
4. There should be no rotated teeth.
5. There should be no spacing or crowding of the teeth.
6. The occlusal plane should be flat or with only a mild curve of Spee.

Not all these features are necessary for dental health, but taken together, they provide a definition of the ideal class I occlusion.

1.6 SUMMARY

This chapter has set out to outline the pattern of normal craniofacial growth.

1. While normal variation on this pattern will produce the differences that occur between individuals, the underlying patterns of growth should not be radically different from those described here; that is, if development is to proceed in a normal fashion.

2. The growth of the brain and of the cranium is almost complete by the age of 5 years.

3. The facial skeleton grows downwards and forwards, relative to the cranial base, starting to grow rapidly at about the time of the pubertal growth spurt, and with facial growth virtually complete at about the age of 15.5 years in girls, slightly later in boys.

4. With regard to occlusal development, while the exact age at which structures form will vary from person to person, the overall pattern of tooth development and the process by which the dental occlusion becomes established should probably be much as described in this chapter.

5. The eruption sequence — the order in which the teeth erupt — is more important than the age at which they erupt, in that if there is a local problem with regard to the establishment of a normal occlusion, it is likely to become apparent, in the first instance, as a disturbance of the eruption sequence.

1.7 FURTHER READING

Enlow D. H. (1990). *Facial growth* (3rd edn). W. B. Saunders, Philadelphia. (*This is a widely recommended textbook, which deals with the subject of facial growth, very much from a clinical point of view.*)

Schroeder H. E. (1991). *Oral structural biology.* Georg Thieme Verlag, Stuttgart. (*A pocket-sized book which presents a concise review of the subject, this text is best used as a reference rather than as an introduction to the subject. The points raised in the text are well documented by references to the academic literature.*)

Ten Cate, A. R. (1994). *Oral histology – development, structure and function* (4th edn). Mosby, St Louis. (*A popular, complete, and well illustrated text, now in its 4th edition which presents the subject clearly and in a modular, well organized format.*)

2   Introduction to the dental surgery

2 Introduction to the dental surgery
A. S. BLINKHORN

2.1 INTRODUCTION

It is a common belief among many individuals that being 'good with people' is an inborn art and owes little to science or training. It is true that some individuals have a more open disposition and can relate well to others (Fig. 2.1). However, there is no logical reason why all of us shouldn't be able to put young patients at their ease and show that we are interested in their problems.

It is particularly important for dentists to learn how to help people relax, as failure to empathize and communicate, will result in disappointed patients and an unsuccessful practising career. Communicating effectively with children is of great value as 'being good with younger patients' is a practice builder and can reduce the stress involved when offering clinical care.

All undergraduate and postgraduate dental training should include a thorough understanding of how children relate to an adult world, how the dental visit should be structured, and what strategies are available to help children cope with their apprehension about dental procedures. This chapter will consider these items, beginning with a discussion on the theories of psychological development, and following this up with sections on: parents and their influence on dental treatment; dentist–patient relationships; anxious and uncooperative children, and helping anxious patients to cope with dental care.

> Effective communication, good for patients and dentists.

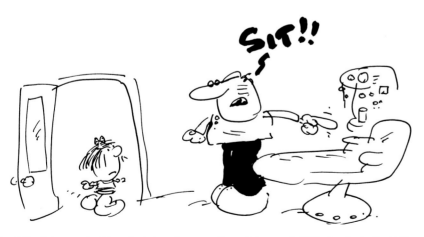

Fig. 2.1   Being good with patients is not necessarily an inborn art! (With thanks to David Myers and kind permission of Eden Bianchi Press.)

2.2   PSYCHOLOGY OF CHILD DEVELOPMENT

At one time the psychological development of children was split into a series of well defined phases, but more recently this division has been criticized and development should now be seen as a continuum. The phases of development may well differ from child to child, so a rigidly applied definition will be artificial. Nevertheless, for the sake of clarity when describing a child's psychological development from infancy into adulthood certain milestones of development should be considered.

The academic considerations about psychological development have been dominated by a number of internationally known authorities who have, for the most part, concentrated on different aspects of the systematic progression from child to adult. However, the most important theoretical perspective which now influences thinking about child development is that of attachment theory which was developed by John Bowlby, a psychoanalyst. In a series of writings over three decades, Bowlby developed his theory that child development could best be understood within the framework of patterns of interaction between the infant and primary caregiver. If there were problems in this interaction, then the child was likely to develop insecure and/or anxious patterns which would affect their ability to form stable relations with others, to develop a sense of self-worth, and to move towards independence. The other important concept to note is that development is a lifelong process, we do not switch off at 18, nor is development an even process. Development is uneven, influenced by periods of rapid bodily change.

There are many accounts of the changes accompanying development in the psychological literature; therefore, this section will present a general outline of the major 'psychological signposts' that the dental team should be aware of. As the newborn child is not a 'common' visitor to the dental surgery no specific description of newborn behaviour will be offered, instead general accounts of motor, cognitive, perceptual, and social development from birth to adolescence will be offered. It is important to understand that the thinking about child development has become less certain and simplistic in its approach; hence, dentists who make hard and fast rules about the way they offer care to children will cause stress to both their patients and themselves.

2.2.1   Motor development

A newborn child does not have an extensive range of movements, but these develop rapidly and by the age of 2 years the majority of children are capable of walking on their own. The 'motor milestones' occur in a predictable order and many of the tests used by paediatricians assess normal development in infancy in terms of motor skills. The predictability of early motor development suggests that it must be genetically programmed. Although this is true to some extent there is evidence that the environment can influence motor development. This has led to a greater interest in the early diagnosis of motor problems so that remedial intervention can be offered. A good example of intervention is the help offered to Down syndrome babies, who have slow motor development. Specific programmes which give large amounts of practise on sensory-motor tasks can greatly accelerate motor development to almost normal levels.

Motor development is really completed in infancy, the changes which follow the walking milestone are refinements rather than new skill development. Eye–hand co-ordination gradually becomes more precise and elaborate with increasing experience. The dominance of one hand emerges at an early age and is usually linked to hemisphere dominance for language processing. The left

Quality of the interaction with primary care givers

Psychological sign posts.

Motor development — environment important.

Motor development completed early in life.

hemisphere controls the right hand and the right hemisphere controls the left. The majority of right-handed people appear to be strongly left hemisphere dominant for language processings, as are nearly all left handers. Some children with motor retardation may fail to show specific right or left manual dominance and will lack good co-ordination between the hands.

Children of 6–7 years of age usually have sufficient co-ordination to brush their teeth reasonably well. Below that age many areas of the mouth will be missed and there is a tendency to swallow relatively large amounts of toothpaste, hence parental supervision is important.

2.2.2 Cognitive development

The cognitive capability of children changes radically from birth through to adulthood, and the process is divided into a number of stages for ease of description. A Swiss psychologist called Piaget formulated the 'stages view' of cognitive development on the basis of detailed observations of his own children and suggested that children pass through four broad stages of cognitive development, namely:-

Piaget and his 'stages'.

1. Sensorimotor: this stage lasts until about 2 years of age. The prime achievement is 'object permanence'. The infant can think of things as permanent; continuing to exist when out of sight, and can think of objects without having to see them directly.

2. Pre-operational thought: this runs from 2 to 7 years of age. The sensorimotor stage is further developed allowing the child to predict outcomes of behaviour. Language development facilitates these changes. The thought patterns are not well developed, being egocentric, unable to encompass another person's point of view, single-tracked, and inflexible (sums up most politicians, some dental professors, and hospital administrators). Typically, children in this age band are unable to understand that areas and volumes remain the same despite changes in position or shape.

3. Concrete operations: This is the stage of thinking from about 7 to 11 years. Children are able to apply logical reasoning, consider another person's point of view, and assess more than one aspect of a particular situation (Fig. 2.2). Thinking is rooted in concrete objects, abstract thought is not well developed.

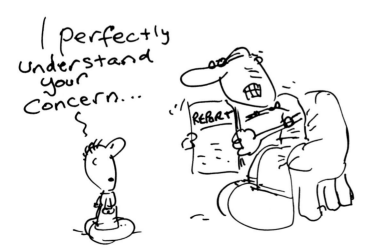

Fig. 2.2 Children aged 7–11 years are able to consider another person's point of view. (With thanks to David Myers and kind permission of Eden Bianchi Press.)

4. Formal operations: This is the last stage in the transition to adult thinking ability. It begins at about 11 years of age and results in the development of logical abstract thinking so that different possibilities for action can be considered.

Dogma bites the dust.

These stages have been highlighted because of the importance of Piaget's early work on cognitive development. However, an over-reliance on 'dogma' may well limit the development of a subject, and this was the case with cognitive development. Few scientists challenged Piaget's findings and the field of infant perception became a rather sterile area for a number of years. This changed with the work of Bowlby and research has now developed enormously and many doubts have been raised about Piaget's original interpretation of his data. He underestimated the thinking abilities of younger children and there is evidence to show that not all pre-school thinking is totally egocentric. Of just as much interest is the modern view that not all adult thinking is logical, many of us are biased and illogical. A self-evident truth when one considers the arguments raised against water fluoridation!

Are adults sensible?

There is, however, a serious point to this observation on adult illogicality. We must be prepared for parents who don't agree with our perceived wisdom (Fig. 2.3) or do not understand the basic tenets of specific programmes. Dentists will lead less stressful practising lives if they remember that not all their patients will always agree with or follow oral health advice.

So Piaget should be seen as a pioneer who really set in motion work on cognitive development, but it is now recognized that the developmental stages are not so clear-cut and many kids are smarter than we think!

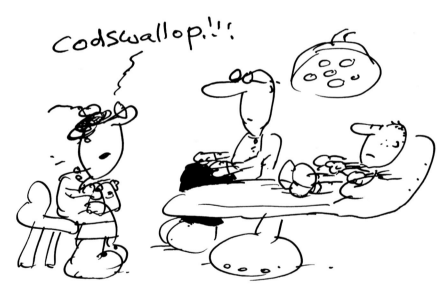

Fig. 2.3 Be prepared for parents who don't agree! (With thanks to David Myers and kind permission of Eden Bianchi Press.)

2.2.3   Perceptual development

Kids can pull the wool over our eyes!

Clearly, it is very difficult to discover what babies and infants are experiencing perceptually so much research has concentrated on eye movements. These types of studies have shown that with increasing age, scanning becomes broader and larger amounts of information are sought. Compared with adults, 6 year old children cover less of the object, fixate on details and gain less information. However,

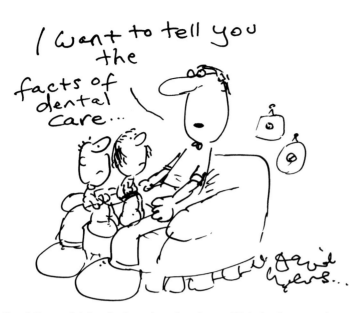

Fig. 2.4 Spend time explaining the facts about dental care. (With thanks to David Myers and kind permission of Eden Bianchi Press.)

children do develop their selective attention and by the age of 7 years can determine which messages merit attention and which can be ignored. Concentration skills also improve. Some dental advice can be offered to children of this age but given the importance of the home environment parents should be the main focus of any information given on oral health care.

Children are not vertically challenged adults!

With increasing age children become more efficient at discriminating between different visual patterns and reach adult proficiency by about 9 years of age.

The majority of perceptual development is a function of the growth of knowledge about the environment in which a child lives, hence the necessity to spend time explaining aspects of dental care to new child patients (Fig. 2.4).

2.2.4 Language development

A lack of the appropriate stimulation will retard a child's learning, particularly language. A child of 5 who can only speak in monosyllables and has no sensible sentence structure will not only be unable to communicate with others but will be unable to think about the things he/she sees and hears. Stimulation is important as language development is such a rapid process in childhood that any delay can seriously handicap a child. Newborn children show a remarkable ability to distinguish speech sounds and by the age of 5 years most children can use over 2000 or more words. Language and thought are tied together and are important in cognitive development but the complexities of the relationship between the two are not well understood.

Keep jargon to a minimum.

Dentistry has a highly specialized vocabulary and it is unlikely that many children, even adolescents, will understand our meaning if we rely on jargon. The key to successful communication is to pitch your advice and instructions at just the right level for different age groups of children. There is a risk of being patronizing if every child patient is told that 'little pixies are eating away tiny bits of your tooth and I am going to run my little engine to frighten them away to fairyland'. A streetwise 10 year old who is a 'Sonic' officionado would probably call the police if you used such language! There is no universal approach to patients and careful treatment planning and assessment are required before children or their parents are given specific written or verbal advice.

Assess patients before offering advice.

2.2.5   Social development

Until fairly recently it was believed that newborn infants were individuals who spent most of their time sleeping. However, recent research reveals that babies interact quite markedly with their environment, often initiating interactions with other humans by movement of their eyes or limbs.

Separation anxiety.

Babies tend to form specific attachments to people and are prone to separation anxiety. At about 8 months infants show a definite fear of strangers. This potential for anxiety separation remains high until about 5 years of age when separation anxiety declines quite markedly. This is consistent with studies of children in hospital which show that after the age of 5 there is less distress on entering hospital. Separation anxiety should also be considered by dentists who insist that all young children must enter the dental surgery alone. Clearly, this will cause severe anxiety to patients under 5.

Love your parents – they made you!

It has been reported that a loving early parental attachment is associated with a better social adjustment in later childhood and is a good basis for engendering trust and friendship with peers. This is important as a successful transition from home to school depends on the ability to interact with other individuals apart from parents. The home environment will play a major part in social development, but the effects of community expectations should not be underestimated. We are all products of our broad social environment, mediated to some extent by parental influences.

2.2.6   Adolescence

The waning of parental influence can be seen in the final stage of child development, adolescence. This is the end of childhood and the beginning of adulthood. It is conceptualized as a period of emotional turmoil and a time of identity formation. This view is a 'Western' creation and is culturally biased. In many societies 'terrible teenagers' do not exist; childhood ends and adult responsibilities are offered at a relatively early age.

Teenagers are not always nasty.

It is interesting to note that even in Western industrialized societies there is little real evidence to support the idea that the majority of adolescents are rebellious and non-conformist. The main change is the evolution of a different sort of parental relationship. There is increasing independency and self-sufficiency. The research does show that young people tend to be moody, are oversensitive to criticism, and feel miserable for no apparent reason but do not on the whole rebel against their parental role models.

Health an abstract concept.

There are some clear messages to dentists who wish to retain their adolescent patients; don't criticize them excessively as this may compromise their future oral health. These patients are looking for support and reassurance. Many health professionals need to rethink their assumptions about young people, as personal behaviour patterns are not really related to health issues at all. Until there are acute problems 'health *per se*' is of little relevance to adolescents being a rather abstract concept. Future orientation is low and the major issues of concern are finding employment, exploring their sexuality, and having the friendship and support of their peers.

2.3   PARENTS AND THEIR INFLUENCE ON DENTAL TREATMENT

Socialization.

Children learn from their parents the basic aspects of everyday life, this process is termed socialization and is an ongoing and gradual process. By the age of 4 children know many of the conventions current in their culture, such as male and female roles. The process of transmitting cultural information early in life is called primary socialization. In industrialized countries obtaining information on many aspects of life is gained formally in schools and colleges, rather than from the family. This is termed secondary socialization.

Interestingly, primary socialization can have a profound and lasting effect. For example, fear of dental treatment and when we first begin to clean our teeth can often be traced back to family influence. So parents can shape a child's expectations and attitudes about oral health; thus, every attempt should be made to involve them when attempting to offer dental care or change a child's health habits.

Involving parents means that the dentist must look to positive reinforcement rather than 'victim blaming'. Parents who are accused of oral neglect may well feel aggrieved or threatened. All too often children's oral health is compromised by a lack of parental knowledge so programmes have to be carefully designed to reduce any chances of making people feel guilty. Guilt often results in parents spending more time in seeking excuses for problems than trying to implement solutions.

Avoid victim blaming.

Parents who are convinced that their child has an oral health problem which can be solved tend to react in a positive way, both to their dental advisor and the preventive programme itself. It is especially helpful if the preventive strategy can include a system of positive reinforcement for the child (Fig. 2.5). Features such as brushing charts, diet sheets, gold stars for brushing well, extra pocket money for curtailing thumbsucking are all useful tips to help parents maintain a child's enthusiasm for a particular dental project.

Positive reinforcement is important.

It must be emphasized that preventive programmes must be carefully planned so as to include only one major goal at a time. Parents will be unable to cope if too much is expected of them at any one time. Programmes that involve families have much higher success rates than those which concentrate solely on the patient. Interestingly, families also have a profound influence on levels of dental anxiety among their children. Dentally anxious mothers have children who exhibit negative behaviour at the dentist. Hence, the need for dentists to look 'beyond' the child when assessing the reasons for dental anxiety.

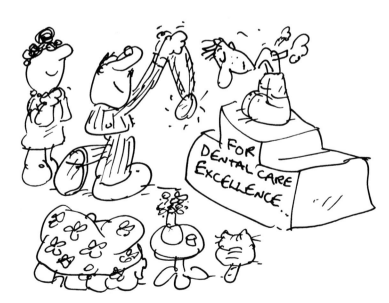

Fig. 2.5 Positive reinforcement is important. (With thanks to David Myers and kind permission of Eden Bianchi Press.)

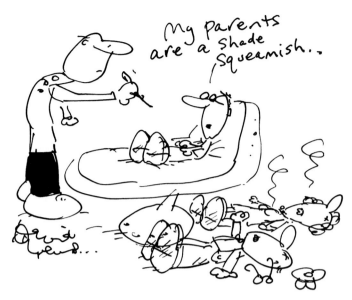

Fig. 2.6   Should we allow parents into the surgery? (With thanks to David Myers and kind permission of Eden Bianchi Press.)

Should parents join children in the surgery?

One of the great debates in paediatric dentistry centres on whether parents should be allowed in the dental surgery while their child is receiving treatment. A child's family, it could be argued, can offer emotional support during treatment. There is no doubt that within the medical field there is great support for the concept of a parent actually 'living in' while a child is hospitalized. However, the issue is not so clear-cut in dentistry (Fig. 2.6).

The first issue that must be raised is whether dentists have the ethical/moral right to bar parents from sitting in with their children when dental care is being undertaken. Clearly, parents have views and anxiety levels may be raised if parents feel their familial rights are being threatened and a child may be stressed by tension between parents and the operator.

Wright *et al.* in their comprehensive book on child management summarize the advantages of keeping parents out of the surgery as:

(1) the parent often repeats orders, creating an annoyance for both dentist and child patient (Fig. 2.7);
(2) the parents intercept orders, becoming a barrier to the development of rapport between the dentist and the child;
(3) the dentist is unable to use voice intonation in the presence of the parent because he or she is offended;
(4) the child divides attention between parent and dentist;
(5) the dentist divides attention between parent and child;
(6) dentists are probably more relaxed and comfortable when the parent remains in the reception area.

These suggestions have merit but they do have a rather authoritarian feel to them, stressing the ordering and voice intonation rather than sympathetic communication. Practical research to support parents 'in or out' of the surgery is not available to suggest whether there is a right or wrong way to handle this particular question. In the end it is a personal decision taken by the dentist in the light of parental concerns and clinical experience. As in any branch of medicine there can be no 'hard and fast' rules for dealing with the general public, an adherence to any type of dogma 'come what may' is a recipe for confrontation

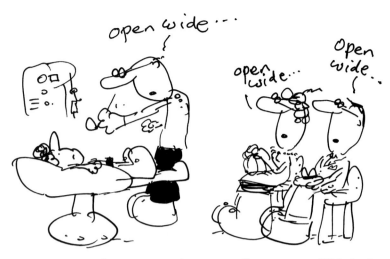

Fig. 2.7 Some parents can be very irritating by repeating all your requests. (With thanks to David Myers and kind permission of Eden Bianchi Press.)

and stress. Therefore, parents sitting in with children should be a decision taken for each individual rather than implementing a keep parents out policy.

Patients with special needs require a high degree of parental involvement in oral health care, particularly for those children with educational, behavioural, and physical difficulties. For example, toothbrushing is a complex cognitive and motor task which will tax the skills of many handicapped children. A parent will have to be taught how to monitor the efficiency of the plaque removal and intervene when necessary, to ensure the mouth is cleaned adequately. Diet is also important, so clear advice must be offered and reinforcement planned at regular intervals.

2.4 DENTIST–PATIENT RELATIONSHIP

The way a dentist interacts with patients will have a major influence on the success of any clinical or preventive care. Clearly, only broad guidelines can be presented on how to maintain an effective relationship with a patient, as all of us are unique individuals with different needs and aspirations. This is especially so in paediatric dentistry where a clinician may have to treat a frightened 3 year old at one appointment and an hour and a half later be faced with the problem of offering preventive advice on oral health to a recalcitrant 15 year old. There are, however, common research findings which highlight the key issues that will cause a dentist/patient consultation to founder or progress satisfactorily.

Each patient a unique individual.

The first question that must be considered is 'Why me — what factors did the parents take into account before making an appointment at my practice?'

The obvious answers are that your practice is closest to the bus stop, has good parking, and you are the only one open after 6.00 p.m. Surprisingly, the choice is not so simple. Most people try to find out details about different dental practices from friends and colleagues. While the technical skill of the dentist is of some concern, the most important features people look for are, gentle friendly manner, explains treatment procedures and tries to keep any pain to a minimum.

People like friendly dentists.

As with any health issue the social class background of the respondents influences attitudes and beliefs. For example, parents of high socio-economic status are more interested in professional competence and gaining information whereas parents from poorer areas want a dentist to reassure and be friendly to their child.

So which dentist parents choose to offer care to their child will depend to some extent on reports about technical skill from family and friends, but the major driving force to choice is well developed interpersonal skills. A major point to emphasize is that technical skill is usually judged in terms of caring and sympathy, a finding which adds further weight to the importance of dentists developing a good 'chairside manner'.

Explanation, 'taking the time to talk us through what our child's treatment will entail' is another factor which rates highly, and may actually influence the rate of attendance for follow-up appointments.

2.4.1 The structure of the dental consultation

In order to help students and new graduates improve their dentist/patient interaction it is possible to give an outline structure to a successful dental consultation. The proposed model consists of six stages, and is based on the work of Wanless and Holloway.

1. *Greeting.* The dentist greets the child by name. Avoid using generalized terms such as 'Hi sonny, hello sunshine', which are general rather than specific to the patient (Fig. 2.8). If parents are present then include them in the conversation, but do not forget that the child should be central to the developing relationship.

> Remember I have a name.

A greeting can be spoilt by proceeding too quickly to an instruction rather than an invitation. For example, 'Hello Sarah, jump in the chair' is rather abrupt and may prejudice an interactive relationship. The greeting should be used to put the child and parents at ease before proceeding to the next stage.

2. *Preliminary chat.* This phase has three objectives, to assess whether the patient or parents have any particular worries or concerns, to settle the patient into the clinical environment, and to assess the patient's emotional state.

> Talk and listen. Don't drill.

The following sequence represents one way of maximizing the effect of the 'preliminary chat':

(a) begin with non-dental topics. For children who have been before it is helpful to record useful information such as names of brothers/sisters, school, pets, and hobbies;

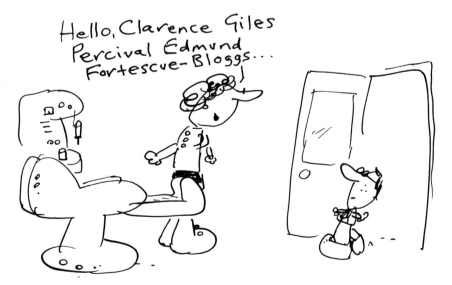

Fig. 2.8 Always greet your patient by name. (With thanks to David Myers and kind permission of Eden Bianchi Press.)

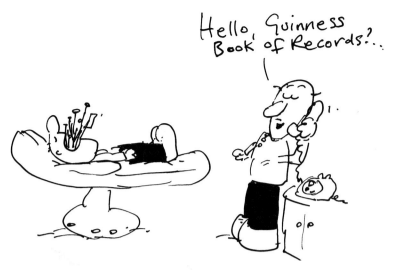

Fig. 2.9 Is your patient just a mouthful of instruments? (With thanks to David Myers and kind permission of Eden Bianchi Press.)

(b) ask an open question such as 'how are you/are you having any problems with your teeth?' Listen to the answer and probe further if necessary. All too often dentists ask questions and then ignore the answer!

By talking generally and taking note of what the child is saying you are offering a degree of control and reducing anxiety.

3. *Preliminary explanation.* In this stage the aim is to explain what the clinical or preventive objectives are in terms that parents and children will understand. This is a vital part of any visit as it establishes the credibility of the dentist as someone who knows what the ultimate goal for the treatment is, and is prepared to take the time and trouble to discuss it in non-technical language.

While not wishing to labour the point, it must be stressed that sensible information cannot be offered to the patient or parents until the clinician has a full history and a treatment plan based on adequate information. This requires a broad view of the patient and should not be totally tooth centred. It is all too easy to lose the confidence of parents and children if you find yourself making excuses for clinical decisions taken in a hurried and unscientific manner.

Full history vital.

Thus the preliminary chat sets the scene prior to actual clinical activity.

4. *Business.* The patient is now in danger of becoming a passive object who is worked on rather than being involved in the treatment. Many jokes are made about dentists who ask questions of patients who are unable to reply because of a mouthful of instruments! (Fig. 2.9). This does not mean that the visit should enter a silent phase. It is important to remain in verbal contact. Check the patient is not in pain, discuss what you are doing, use the patient's name to show a 'personal' interest, and clarify any misunderstandings.

At the end of the business stage it is helpful to summarize what has been done and offer aftercare advice. If the parent is not present in the surgery, the treatment summary is particularly important, as it is a useful way of maintaining contact with the parents.

Is your patient still alive?

5. *Health education.* Oral health is, to a large extent, dependent upon personal behaviour and as such it would be unethical for dentists not to include advice on maintaining a healthy mouth. Although offering advice to parents and patients is useful, in many instances the profession treat health education in a 'throwaway' manner. This results in both patients and dentists being disappointed.

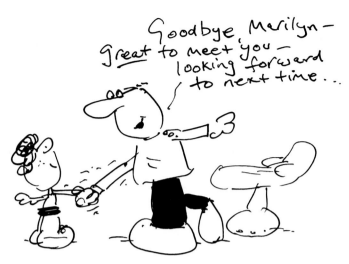

Fig. 2.10   Make sure you offer your patient a definite farewell. (With thanks to David Myers and kind permission of Eden Bianchi Press.)

Give advice as though you mean it.

The key ways to improve the value of advice sessions are as follows:

(a) make the advice specific, give a child a personal problem to solve;

(b) give simple and precise information;

(c) do not suggest goals of behaviour change which are beyond a patient's capacity to achieve;

(d) check the message has been understood and not misinterpreted;

(e) offer advice in such a way that the child and parents are not threatened or blamed;

(f) if you are trying to improve oral hygiene avoid theoretical discussions, offer a practical demonstration;

(g) at follow-up visits reinforce the advice and offer positive reinforcement.

The final part of the health education activity is goal setting. The dentist sets out in simple terms what the patient should try and achieve by the next visit. It implies a form of contract and as such helps both children and parents to gain a clearer insight into how they all can help to improve the child's oral health. Goal setting must be used sensibly. If goals are manifestly impossible then parents and child patients become disillusioned. Parents feel that the dentist does not understand their problems and complain that they are being blamed for any dental shortcomings. So always ensure that you plan goal setting carefully in a positive and friendly manner.

Set some realistic objectives.

6. *Dismissal.* This is the final part of the visit and should be clearly signposted so that everyone knows that the appointment is over. The patient should be addressed by name and a definite farewell offered (Fig. 2.10). The objective should be to ensure that wherever possible the patient and parents leave with a sense of goodwill.

Clearly, not all appointment sessions can be dissected into these six stages, however, the basic element of according the patient the maximum attention and personalizing your comments should never be forgotten.

2.5   ANXIOUS AND UNCOOPERATIVE CHILDREN

Dental anxiety should concern us as a profession because it not only prevents many potential patients from seeking care but it also causes stress to the dentists undertaking dental treatment. Indeed one of the major sources of stress for general dental practitioners is 'coping with difficult patients' (Fig. 2.11). Dentists do not want to be considered as people who inflict unnecessary anxiety on the general public. However, anxiety and dental care seem to be locked in the general folklore of many countries. In order to understand why, it is helpful to consider 'what is the nature of anxiety'.

Many definitions of anxiety have been suggested and it is a somewhat daunting task to reconcile them. However, it would seem sensible to consider the comments of Kent who reported that anxiety is 'a vague unpleasant feeling accompanied by a premonition that something undesirable is going to happen'. In other words it relates to how people feel — a subjective definition. Another point of view is that anxiety manifests itself in behaviour. If, for example a person is anxious, then she/he will act in a particular manner. A person will avoid visiting the dentist. Thus, anxiety should be seen as a multifactorial problem made up of a number of different components, all of which can exert an effect.

Anxiety must also be seen as a continuum with fear — it is almost impossible to separate the two in much of the research undertaken in the field of dentistry, where the two words are used interchangeably. One could consider that anxiety is more a general feeling of discomfort, while fear is a strong reaction to a specific event. Nevertheless it is counter-productive to search for elusive definitions as both fear and anxiety are associated with dental visiting and treatment.

From a common-sense point of view it is clear that some situations will arouse more anxiety than others. For example a fear of heights is relatively common but it is galling to note that in the United States a study by Agras, *et al.* found that visiting the dentist ranked fourth behind snakes, heights, and storms. Clearly then, anxiety about dental care is a problem that we as a profession must take seriously, especially as children remember pain and stress suffered at the dentist and carry the emotional scars into adult life. Some people may develop such a fear of dentistry that they are termed phobics. A phobia is an intense fear which is out of all proportion to the actual threat.

Research in this area suggests that the extent of anxiety a person experiences does not relate directly to dental knowledge, but is an amalgamation of personal experiences, family concerns, disease levels, and general personality traits. Such a complex situation means that it is no easy task to measure dental anxiety and pin-point aetiological agents.

Anxiety

Multifactorial.

I'm not afraid just anxious!

Dental fear — a serious issue.

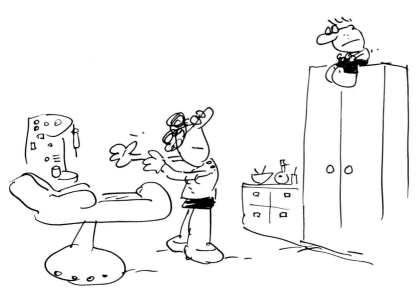

Fig. 2.11 Difficult patients can be a source of stress! (With thanks to David Myers and kind permission of Eden Bianchi Press.)

Measuring dental anxiety is problematic because it relies on subjective measures, plus the influence of the parents, the dentist's behaviour, and the reason for a visit may all exert some effect on a child's anxiety levels.

Questionnaires and rating scales are the most commonly used means by which anxiety has been quantified, although there has been some interest in physiological data such as heart rate. Some questionnaires that have been used to measure anxiety can be applied to a whole variety of situations, such as recording 'exam nerves' or fear of spiders, while others are specific to the dental situation. The most widely used dental anxiety measure is Corah's Dental Anxiety Scale, which takes the form of a questionnaire. Patients are asked to choose an answer which best sums up their feelings. The answers are scored from 1 to 5 so that a total score can be computed. A high score should alert the dental team that a particular patient is very anxious.

However, patient-administered questionnaires have a limited value in evaluating a young child's anxiety because of their poorly developed vocabulary and understanding. Therefore there has been great interest in measuring anxiety by observing behaviour. One such scale was developed by Frankl to assess the effect of a parent remaining with a child in the surgery. It consists of four ratings from definitely negative to definitely positive. It is still commonly used in paediatric dental research. Another scale which is popular with researchers is one used by Houpt, which monitors behaviour by allocating a numerical score to items such as body movement and crying.

Recent studies have used the Frankl scale to select subjects for studies and then more detailed behaviour evaluation systems are utilized to monitor the compliance with treatment. Behavioural observation research can be problematical as the presence of an observer in the surgery may upset the patient. In addition it is difficult to be totally objective when different coping strategies are being used and some bias will occur. The development of cheap lightweight video cameras has greatly helped observational research, as the patient's behaviour can be scored by a number of raters away from the surgery. Rescoring of the videos is also possible to check the reliability of the index used.

Physiological measurements such as a higher pulse rate, perspiration, and peripheral blood flow have been used to quantify children's dental anxiety. However, few physiological signs are specific to one particular emotion and the measuring techniques often provoke anxiety in the child patient, so they are rarely used.

There is as yet no standard measure of dental anxiety for children as the reproducibility and reliability of most questionnaires have not been demonstrated, plus observational and physiological indices are not well developed. This is a serious problem as the assessment of strategies to reduce anxiety is somewhat compromised by a lack of universally accepted measuring techniques.

2.6   HELPING ANXIOUS PATIENTS TO COPE WITH DENTAL CARE

A number of theories have been suggested in an effort to explain the development of anxiety. Uncertainty about what is to happen is certainly a factor, a poor past experience with a dentist could upset a patient, while others may learn anxiety responses from parents, relations, or friends.

A dentist who can alleviate anxiety or prevent it happening in the first place will always be popular with patients. Clearly, the easiest way to control anxiety is to establish an effective preventive programme so that children do not require any treatment. In addition to an effective preventive regimen it is important to establish a trusting relationship, listening to a child's specific worries and con-

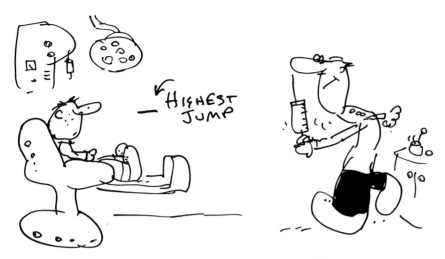

Fig. 2.12 Stab and squirt has no place in our anaesthetic technique. (With thanks to David Myers and kind permission of Eden Bianchi Press.)

cerns. Every effort must be taken to ensure that any treatment is pain free. All too often we forget that local analgesia requires time and patience. With the use of topical anaesthetic paste and slow release of the anaesthetic solution most 'injections' should be painless. There is no excuse for the 'stab and squirt method' (Fig. 2.12).

Children are not 'little adults', they are vulnerable and afraid of new surroundings so effective time management is important. Try to see young patients on time and do not stress yourself or the child by expecting to complete a clinical task in a short time on an apprehensive patient.

Despite the dental team's best efforts anxiety may persist and routine dental care is compromised. Other options will then have to be considered to help the child. An increasingly popular choice is the use of pharmacological agents; these will be discussed in Chapter 4. The alternatives to the pharmacological approach are:

(1) reducing uncertainty,
(2) modelling,
(3) cognitive approaches,
(4) relaxation,
(5) systematic desensitization.

These will be discussed in more detail.

2.6.1 Reducing uncertainty

The majority of young children have very little idea of what dental treatment involves and this will raise anxiety levels. Most children will cope if given friendly reassurance from the dentist, but some patients will need a more structured programme.

One such structured method is the tell–show–do technique. As its name implies it centres on three phases:

1. *Tell* — explanation of procedures at the right age/educational level.
2. Show — demonstrate the procedure.
3. Do — following on to undertake the task. Praise being an essential part of the exercise (Fig. 2.13).

Injections should be painless.	
Children have short attention span.	
Pharmacological alternatives.	
Tell–show–do.	

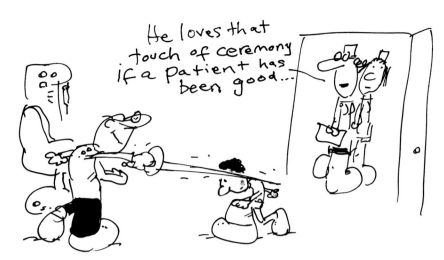

Fig. 2.13 Praise costs little, but does show you to be a caring person. (With thanks to David Myers and kind permission of Eden Bianchi Press.)

While it is a popular technique there is little experimental work to support its use.

Another technique to reduce anxiety among very worried children is to send a letter home explaining all the details of the proposed first visit so that uncertainty will be reduced. The evidence for this approach is not clear cut as parental anxiety is changed by preinformation rather than the child's.

Acclimatization programmes gradually introducing the child to dental care over a number of visits have been shown to be of value. This approach is rather time consuming and does little for the really nervous child.

More information for parents.

2.6.2   Modelling

This makes use of the fact that individuals learn much about their environment from observing the consequences of other people's behaviour. You or I might repeat an action if we see others being rewarded or if someone is punished we might well decide not to follow that behaviour. Modelling could be used to alleviate anxiety. If a child could be shown that it is possible to visit the dentist, have treatment, and then leave in a happy frame of mind (Fig. 2.14), this could reduce anxiety due to 'fear of the unknown'. A child would see behind that forbidding surgery door!

It is not necessary to use a live model, videos of co-operative patients are of value. However, the following points should be taken into consideration when setting up a programme.

Modelling reduces fear of unknown.

1. Ensure that the model is close in age to the nervous child or children involved.
2. The model should be shown entering and leaving the surgery to prove treatment has no lasting effect.
3. The dentist should be shown to be a caring person who praises the patient.

2.6.3   Cognitive approaches

Modelling helps people learn about dental treatment from watching others, but it does not take account of an individual's 'cognitions' or thoughts. People may heighten their anxiety by worrying more and more about a dental problem so

Worrying increases anxiety.

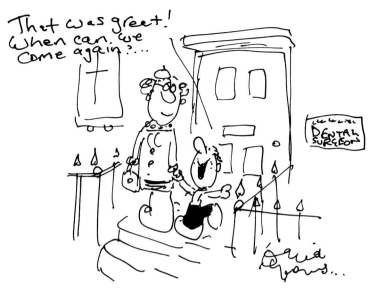

Fig. 2.14   We want our patients to leave us in a happy frame of mind. (With thanks to David Myers and kind permission of Eden Bianchi Press.)

creating a vicious reinforcing circle. Thus there has been great interest in trying to get individuals to identify and then alter their dysfunctional beliefs. There are a number of cognitive modification techniques that have been suggested and the most common ones include:

(1) asking patients to identify and make a record of their negative thoughts;

(2) helping patients to recognize their negative thoughts and suggesting more positive alternatives — 'reality based';

(3) working with a therapist to identify and change the more deep seated negative beliefs.

Cognitive therapy is useful for focused types of anxiety — hence its value in combating dental anxiety.

Another approach which could be considered a cognitive approach is distraction. This technique attempts to shift attention from the dental setting towards some other kind of situation. Distracters such as videotaped cartoons and stories have been used to help children cope with dental treatment. The results have been somewhat equivocal and the threat to switch off the video was needed to maintain co-operation.

| Distraction helps to reduce anxiety. |

2.6.4   Relaxation

Relaxation training is of value where patients report high levels of tension and consists of bringing about deep muscular relaxation. It has also been used in conjunction with biofeedback training. As the techniques require the presence of a trained therapist, the potential value in general paediatric dentistry has still to be assessed.

2.6.5   Systematic desensitization

The basic principle of this treatment consists of allowing the patient gradually to come to terms with a particular fear or set of fears by working through various levels of the feared situation, from the 'mildest' to the 'most anxiety' programme.

| Work through fears. |

This technique relies on the use of a trained therapist and in most instances a simple dentally based acclimatization programme should be tried first.

2.7 SUMMARY

1. To prevent the development of anxiety it is more important to maintain trust than concentrate on finishing a clinical task.
2. The reductions in dental caries means that children with special psychological, medical, and physical needs can be offered the oral health care they require. We are not being swamped by overwhelming clinical demand.
3. The care of children who are very anxious can be improved by using the techniques described in this chapter.
4. Preventing dental disease should always be given the same status as clinical intervention.

2.8 FURTHER READING

Agras, S., Sylvester, D., and Oliveau, D. (1969). The epidemiology of common fears and phobias. *Comprehensive Psychiatry*, **10**, 151–156. (*This paper will show you that fear of dentistry is a problem the dental profession must take seriously.*)

Blinkhorn, A. S. and Mackie, I. C. (1991). *Treatment planning for the paedodontic patient*. Quintessence, London. (*There is a comprehensive question and answer section in this book which will help you check up on your treatment planning knowledge.*)

Kent, G. G. and Blinkhorn, A. S. (1991). T*he psychology of dental care* (2nd edn). Wright, Bristol. (*This short book highlights the important psychological aspects of providing clinical care, as well as giving details of the Houpt, Frankl, and Corah dental anxiety scales.*)

Rutter, M. and Rutter, M. (1993). *Developing minds*. Penguin Books, London. (*A fascinating insight into how we develop throughout life.*)

Wanless, M. B. and Holloway, P. J. (1994). An analysis of audio-recordings of general dental practitioners' consultations with adolescent patients. *British Dental Journal*, **177**, 94–8. (*This article gives advice on how to improve communication skills in the surgery and reminds clinicians that our livelihood depends on effective communication.*)

Weinman, J. (1987). *An outline of psychology as applied to medicine* (2nd edn). pp. 132–4. Butterworth-Heineman, London. (*This book is for those students who want to take a broader view on the subject of psychology and medicine.*)

Wright, G., Starkey, P. E., Gardener, D. E., and Curzon, M. E. J. (1987). *Child management in dentistry*. Wright, Bristol. (*A detailed account of child management including advice on how to introduce different clinical techniques.*)

3 History, examination, and treatment planning

3 History, examination, and treatment planning

N. M. KILPATRICK

3.1 INTRODUCTION

This chapter attempts to give an insight into those aspects of history taking, examination, and treatment planning that differ in the paediatric patient compared with the adult patient. There are certain considerations that have to be borne in mind with young patients prior to arriving at a definitive treatment plan.

3.2 CONSENT

At the first appointment it is necessary to take a detailed history and carry out a full clinical and radiographic examination before a treatment plan can be formulated. Most children will attend the surgery accompanied by an adult, but not always a parent. It is important to establish the relationship between the child and the adult in order that a valid medical history and consent may be obtained. In the United Kingdom, for the purpose of medical and dental treatment, children attain adult status at 16 years old so that at this age a 'child' can give their own consent (and give a valid medical history). However, if a child is still living at home it is wise to discuss any proposed treatment with their parents. The Children Act of 1989 implies that a child under the age of 16 can give valid consent if they are deemed by the clinician to be mature enough to understand fully the proposed procedure. However, again it is best to consult with the parents wherever possible before carrying out any treatment other than emergency treatment. For example, it would be acceptable to reimplant an avulsed permanent incisor as an emergency in the absence of a parent; however, every effort should be made to contact a parent before proceeding to other forms of treatment. A parent's express, informed, consent is required before taking radiographs. Friends, neighbours, and other relatives cannot give valid consent.

3.3 HISTORY

Taking a good history is the key to accurate diagnosis and to appropriate treatment planning and standard forms can be used such as shown in Table 3.1. However, these forms do not replace, but rather facilitate, a good interview by acting as an *aide-mémoire*. The time spent taking a thorough history is not only useful in terms of collecting information but is also invaluable in establishing a relationship with the child and the parent.

For specific details concerning history and examination of traumatic incidents in children the reader is referred to Chapter 11.

Table 3.1   A example of a standard history form with some key relevant points

A. Social	name	*nicknames/preferred name*
	address	
	date of birth	*age*
	school	
	parental occupation	
B. Medical		
Pregnancy/neonatal	maternal health	
	details of birth	*weight, delivery*
	childhood illness	*age, severity*
Systems review	cardiac	*subacute bacterial endocarditis risk factors*
	respiratory	*asthma, hayfever*
	haematological	*anaemia, bleeding, bruising*
	gastrointestinal	*bowel habits*
	diabetes	*control*
	epilepsy	*control*
	hepatitis	
	mental or physical impairment	
Medication	regular prescriptions	*tablet, syrup, inhaler*
	recent medication	
	allergies	
Hospitalization	age and cause of admission	
	operations	
	general anaesthesia	
C. Dental		
Past history	regular or irregular attender	
	previous experiences	*prevention, restorations,*
	experience of local anaesthesia	*extractions*
	previous co-operation levels	
Home care	oral hygiene habits	*frequency of brushing*
		type and amount of toothpaste
		parental assistance
	dietary habits	*baby bottle habits*
	additional measures	*favourite snacks and drinks*
		fluoride supplements
		water fluoride levels
Reason for attendance	routine or emergency	
	presence of pain	*duration, nature, relief*
	any particular concerns	*colour, shape, position of teeth*

3.3.1   Social

Name, address, age, school, parental occupation, and number of siblings all form part of a social history. There are two aims in taking a such a history:

1. To establish communication and rapport with the child and their parent/accompanying adult. For example, calling the child by their preferred name or nickname.

2. To try and make an assessment of the social background from which the child comes. This enables one to target the preventive advice realistically and choose the most appropriate treatment plan. For example a single parent with three children, one of whom is medically compromised, is going to find it difficult to supervise toothbrushing with each child daily. It also gives one

an idea of how easy it is going to be for a parent to bring their child to the dental surgery.

3.3.2 Medical

The importance of taking a thorough medical history lies in its relevance to the safe delivery of routine dental care under both local analgesia and general anaesthesia, and in the targeting of preventive advice to children with 'special needs'. However, two other factors should be borne in mind: one is that many children with medical conditions spend a lot of time in and out of hospitals and may develop quite a negative attitude to the medical/dental professions; the second point is that these children have often already experienced considerable disruption to their schooling and further interruptions for dental appointments may not be welcomed. A thorough medical history will give the dentist a more complete understanding of total patient care.

A routine medical history should include details of the mother's health during the pregnancy and the birth as well as the child's health in the neonatal period. A brief review of all the systems should identify any particular problems. It is important to identify where and by whom the child is treated for any medical condition as it is not only polite to inform, but also often necessary to ask advice from, the child's physician prior to carrying out any active dental treatment.

3.3.3 Dental

It is important when treatment planning to try and evaluate both the child's and the parent's attitude to dental treatment. This assessment may be hard to make on the first visit to the surgery particularly if the child is in pain or has had an accident. In these instances both the child and parent may be very upset and their behaviour misleading. However, gentle questioning concerning past dental experiences can give a good indication of how well the child is likely to cope with future dental treatment. Knowledge of the attitudes and home habits will facilitate realistic planning of a patient's management. For example, the advice given to parents of a 3 year old child still having a bottle through the night should not be primarily concerned with fluoride supplements but should be targeted towards cessation of the bottle habit. Likewise, it is useful to anticipate the parent's attitude towards restoration of the primary dentition — it is unrealistic to expect all parents to attach equal importance to dental health and it is appropriate to modify a treatment plan to accommodate these differences.

Finally, it is important to establish why the child has attended your surgery in the first place. Many children do not attend in pain as an emergency and it is a good idea to ask the *child* (irrespective of their age) why they have come before addressing the same question to their parent. The two answers may be different, particularly around the early teenage years when malocclusions are becoming more obvious. It is important not to assume that the parent's attitude to their child's teeth will be mirrored by the child themselves. This factor may have considerable bearing on the potential success of any future treatment.

3.4 CLINICAL EXAMINATION

It will have become apparent during the course of the history taking how amenable to clinical examination the child is likely to be. In young children it is advisable not to try to carry out a detailed intra-oral examination immediately, but to gently introduce the child to the idea of a clinical examination. This may be achieved with the help of the parent and need not necessarily involve the child sitting in the dental chair during the first visit. However, a child may sit on the parent's knee in the dental chair and be encouraged to examine their parents' mouth or they may be given a hand mirror in which to watch their own examination. One of the difficulties encountered by clinicians treating children is to learn to distract a child while continuing to carry out a careful examination and precise treatment.

It is very important during the clinical examination to bear in mind the child as a whole. The dental practitioner may well see a child more often than any other medical professional and is, therefore, in an excellent position to notice any changes in a child's general health. Clinical examination begins as soon as the dentist meets the child when an overall impression of the child's health can be formed. Table 3.2 is an example of an examination sheet that can be used in young patients.

3.4.1 Extra-oral examination

General appearance

It is often useful to monitor a child's growth patterns. This is particularly relevant if one is concerned about abnormal dental development (delayed or advanced) and also with respect to the use of orthodontic appliances, in particular functional appliances, which rely on a current growth period in order to be

Table 3.2 An example of a standard examination sheet with some key relevant points

A. Extra-oral		
General appearance	height/weight	
	posture	
	co-ordination	
	malaise/fever	
Head and neck	skull	*asymmetry*
	hair	*quality, quantity*
	ears	*tags, hearing aids*
	eyes	*sclera*
	face	*lacerations, scars*
		bruises, swellings
	temporomandibular joint	*opening, deviation, discomfort*
B. Intra-oral		
Soft tissues	mucosa	*palate, tongue, cheeks*
	inflammation	
	swelling	*size, location, texture*
	white/red patches	
	ulcers	*number, site, size*
	frenal attachments	
Periodontal tissues	oral hygiene	*plaque, calculus*
	inflammation/bleeding	*± deposits*
	attached mucosa	*colour, stippling*
	pocketing/dehiscence	
	tooth mobility	
Occlusion	skeletal pattern	
	molar relationship	
	overjet/overbite	
	crowding	
Teeth	number	*hypodontia, supernumeraries*

effective. Percentile growth charts for both height and weight are a useful way of monitoring growth and these can be given to parents to complete.

Head and neck

It is a good idea to draw a rough sketch of a face and indicate on it the sight and extent of any lesions on the head or neck. Where feasible photographic records of anything out of the ordinary should also be taken. This is for two reasons: first, for the clinical records in order to monitor change, and secondly for medico-legal reasons particularly if any of the bruises/scars arouse suspicion of non-accidental injury (Chapter 11). This aspect of a clinical examination has to be handled with care and tact.

3.4.2 Intra-oral examination

A general impression can be obtained from a cursory look in the mouth. The standard of oral hygiene, the presence or otherwise of saliva and the colour of the mucosa all give an indication of the general status of a child's mouth. Closer examination needs to be more systematic.

Soft tissues

The condition of the oral mucosa is a good indicator of the general health of the child. The presence of inflammation, pallor, and ulceration may all be indicators of systemic disease and should be carefully noted and monitored.

Periodontal tissues

It is rare to find periodontal pocketing in the primary dentition unless there is an associated medical condition. However, the key factor to be aware of is the relationship between the degree of inflammation/bleeding and the standard of oral hygiene. If the oral hygiene is generally good with few plaque deposits and yet the gingivae bleed either spontaneously or on gentle probing further questions/investigations may be necessary. Assessment of the level of oral hygiene by a scoring system is reproducible on subsequent visits and gives a permanent record of the patient's progress.

Occlusion

A brief examination of a child's occlusion is necessary. It is important to identify areas of crowding, malaligned teeth, mandibular deviations, and factors such as thumb sucking. Malocclusions are usually dealt with in the late mixed dentition phase but some simple occlusal discrepancies are treated earlier, for example, upper incisors in cross-bite. Chapter 13 covers, in more detail, the recognition of orthodontic problems in the paediatric patient.

Teeth

It is essential to count the teeth present and to record these and any absent teeth in a full dental charting. It is very easy to overlook supernumerary or missing teeth, particularly in the lower incisor region.

The type and the distribution of any form of hypoplasia or discoloration is very relevant to the correct diagnosis of its aetiology (Chapter 9). Is the primary dentition affected as well as the permanent dentition? Does the abnormality affect all the teeth equally?

Initial diagnosis of caries can only be made after the teeth have been cleaned and dried. The lesions should be diagnosed according to whether the enamel is cavitated or not. The use of the probe in the diagnosis of dental caries should be with care — and mainly for the purpose of removing external debris from a tooth surface rather than actual probing of the enamel. The distribution of the carious lesions is important in the diagnosis of its aetiology. For example, extensive caries present on the labial surfaces of the upper primary incisors is strongly associated with a bottle feeding habit. This topic is covered in greater detail in Chapter 6.

An important and an increasingly common phenomenon particularly in adolescents is that of tooth wear or non-carious tooth surface loss. Tooth surface loss is usually obvious clinically; however, identifying its aetiology is often somewhat harder. Careful clinical examination to record the sites and extent of the tooth wear is essential. Patterns of tooth wear are often diagnostic; for example, erosive lesions on the palatal aspects of the maxillary anterior teeth may be associated with acid regurgitation. In such conditions the tongue directs the contents of the stomach forward while protecting the lower teeth. From this point of view the dentist is in a unique position to screen for such disorders. The diagnosis and management of tooth wear is covered in Chapter 9.

3.5 RADIOGRAPHIC EXAMINATION

In most cases radiographs will be a necessary part of the initial history and examination visit. However, it is important to have careful guidelines for selection criteria for dental radiography in order to avoid unnecessary exposure to ionizing radiation. Radiographs should only be taken when a diagnostic need for them has been established through prior clinical examination by a clinician. There are three general indications for taking radiographs in children:

(1) to aid the diagnosis of dental caries;
(2) to detect abnormalities in dental development;
(3) to detect bony and dental pathology.

3.5.1 Radiographic selection criteria

Table 3.3 shows guidelines that are helpful for deciding when and what radiographs to take. These guidelines are a modification of those set down by the American Dental Association in 1989.

3.5.2 Caries diagnosis

There is no doubt that the bitewing radiograph is essential in diagnosing approximal caries in both the primary and the permanent dentition. Kidd and Pitts, in 1990, reviewed 29 research studies on the value of the bitewing radiograph and concluded that clinical examination alone rarely identifies more than 50 per cent of approximal lesions compared with the number diagnosed by the additional use of bitewing radiographs. The breadth of the contact area in the primary dentition makes clinical diagnosis of approximal caries more difficult than in the permanent dentition. It is particularly important in the primary dentition to detect approximal caries early because caries progresses to the amelodentinal junction (ADJ) much more rapidly in a primary tooth than in a permanent tooth. Once caries has progressed to the ADJ in a primary tooth, pulpal involvement, pain, and sepsis are common sequelae. In the permanent dentition diagnosis of early approximal caries is equally important but does not necessarily mean that opera-

Table 3.3 Guidelines for the prescription of radiographs in children

	Child (primary dentition)	Mixed dentition	Adolescent (permanent dentition)
New patient	Bitewings (Lateral obliques)	Bitewings Orthopantomogram Occlusals/Periapicals	Bitewings Orthopantomogram
Recall patient Clinical caries: high caries risk No clinical caries: low caries risk For growth and development	6–12 monthly Bitewings 12–24 monthly Bitewings Not usually indicated unless specific problem	6–12 monthly Bitewings 12–24 monthly Bitewings Additional Orthopantomogram if: considering extractions due to caries, i.e. whether to balance or compensate; planning active orthodontic treatment; monitoring a developmental anomaly	12 monthly Bitewings 24–36 monthly Bitewings An Orthopantomogram about 18 years old to assess the position of unerupted third molars

tive treatment is mandatory. Preventive treatment aimed at delaying or arresting lesion progression can be initiated and the lesion monitored. If such treatment is successful operative treatment may be avoided.

The diagnosis of occlusal caries in the permanent dentition is a greater problem as there is no universally accepted diagnostic method for detecting early lesions. Clinical examination of a clean, dry tooth is probably the most reliable method of diagnosing occlusal caries, although often the best one can hope to obtain is a diagnosis of a 'doubtful fissure'. The management of such 'suspicious fissures' is covered in Chapter 7. However, the use of bitewing radiographs in the detection of occult (hidden) dentinal occlusal caries is well recognized. These lesions are often concealed beneath intact enamel and the visual changes may be sufficiently subtle so as to be missed on clinical examination. Radiographically, such lesions are characterized by large, diffuse, dark, radiolucent areas of dentine positioned centrally under the occlusal fissure. It is because such lesions exist that bitewing radiographs should be taken routinely prior to the placement of fissure sealants in order to prevent sealing over caries.

The role of the orthopantogram (OPT) in the diagnosis of caries is minor as the sensitivity of an OPT to detect caries is very low. In some children it may not be feasible to get good bitewing radiographs due to lack of patient co-operation. In these cases lateral oblique (bimolar) views can provide useful information concerning both approximal carious lesions and dental development.

Other methods of diagnosing caries are currently being evaluated and may be more widely adopted in the future; such as fibre-optic transillumination, electrical resistance measurements, and caries detecting dyes (see section 3.9, Further reading).

3.5.3 Abnormalities in dental development

The routine use of panoramic radiographs in adult patients may be questioned but in the child and adolescent they are an important screening tool. All children at about the age of 8 or 9 years should undergo a full panoramic radiographic examination in order to identify disturbances in the development of the dentition in terms of the number, position or form of the teeth. By this age it is possible to identify the developing second premolars and third molars and to locate the maxillary canines. Precise location of maxillary canines can then be achieved using the intra-oral parallax technique. If there are other clinical factors that indicate abnormalities in the maxillary incisor region then an upper anterior occlusal is a useful view of this area. Sequential panoramic radiographs are rarely indicated unless monitoring an anomaly, reviewing progress after surgical intervention or as part of an orthodontic treatment plan.

3.5.4   Detection of bony or dental pathology

The most appropriate radiograph to detect pathology will vary according to the situation, but in general periapical radiographs of individual teeth are the best. It is also advisable in all cases of trauma to the face to take a full panoramic view to check for bony fractures (Chapter 11). More rarely in children there are cases of specific periodontal conditions such as increased mobility or pocketing, and in these cases the use of selected periapical radiographs in addition to a panoramic view is valuable. Full mouth periapical surveys are rarely indicated in young patients.

3.6   SPECIAL INVESTIGATIONS

In addition to routine clinical and radiographic examination other special investigations can provide information that may influence treatment planning. Vitality testing is essential following trauma to the permanent dentition but is less useful in the primary dentition. Ethyl chloride, hot gutta percha, and electric pulp testing machines may all be used in children. It is important to remember that some children may not fully understand what is expected of them and false positive responses are not uncommon. Ensuring that the teeth are adequately dried and isolated minimizes the risk of sensations via the periodontal tissues and repeating the tests two or three times to check the response may obtain a more accurate diagnosis.

Blood tests rarely form part of a routine examination; however, when specifically indicated, samples of blood may be taken for haematological, biochemical, bacteriological, and virological investigations. It is very important with children that blood is taken sympathetically by someone experienced in venepuncture and collected in the appropriate bottles/medium. Prior discussion with the relevant laboratory staff is advisable.

3.7   TREATMENT PLANNING

Having obtained a full history, undertaken complete clinical examination, and carried out the necessary special investigations the clinician is armed with all the information required to draw up an appropriate treatment plan. It is not feasible to describe a precise treatment plan but rather to describe the principles of treatment planning in the child patient. The dental surgeon has two main objectives when caring for young patients: (a) that the child gains adulthood in a state of good dental health, and (b) that the child develops a positive attitude to dental care.

Bearing these two objectives in mind, treatment planning for the young patient may differ slightly from that of adult patients. A degree of compromise may be necessary in order to develop and earn a child's trust and to motivate the parents towards prevention. The role of behaviour modification in allowing the clinician to accomplish a treatment plan is discussed in Chapter 2.

3.7.1 Principles of treatment planning

These are outlined in Fig. 3.1.

Management of pain

While this is a priority of any treatment plan it is important to have the long-term treatment plan in mind before embarking on a single item of treatment. This is particularly true if extractions (and general anaesthesia) are to be involved. For example a child with an abscess associated with a non-vital first

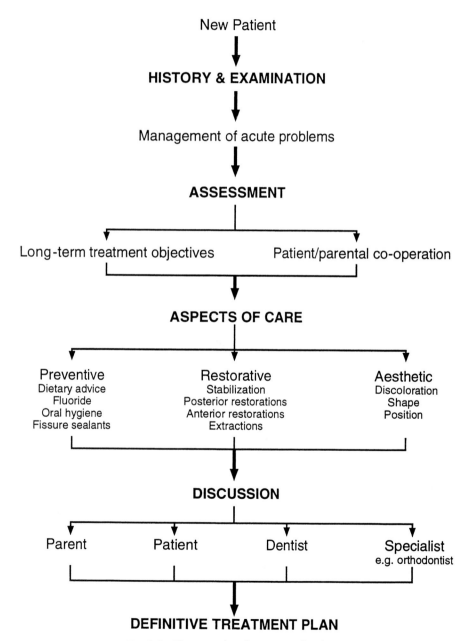

Fig. 3.1   The principles of treatment planning.

primary molar may well have extensive caries in other primary teeth, which may also require extraction. Likewise, a child with gross caries in one first permanent molar may benefit from the loss of all first permanent molars (Chapter 13).

In cases of traumatic injuries it is usually necessary to carry out immediate treatment, for example temporary dressings, pulp extirpation, or splinting in order to relieve pain and to reduce the risks of loss of vitality and root resorption. Such patients are usually seen as emergencies and treated immediately and a subsequent appointment is made to formulate a long-term treatment plan.

Long-term treatment planning

It is a good idea to have a long-term treatment plan drawn up for all patients, in the full knowledge that this may need to be modified. The implications of any treatment plan should be discussed with the parent; for example, the advantages and disadvantages of restoring as opposed to extracting primary teeth.

Before a complete treatment plan can be drawn up it is important to make an overall assessment of the general attitude of the child and the parents to dental care. There is nothing to be gained from an extensive 'textbook' course of treatment if the patient has no motivation. This is particularly true of orthodontic treatment planning; however, it can also be applied to restorative care. If there is little interest from the parent in conserving primary teeth it is more than likely that a treatment plan involving several appointments for restorations will not be completed. It is also very difficult to make an assessment on the likely attitude of a particular patient/parent to dental care when the first appointment involves pain. Delaying the final treatment planning until the acute problems have resolved is very worthwhile.

Preventive care

The provision of preventive dental care is possibly the most important aspect of treatment planning for the young patient (Chapter 6). The advice given to parent and child should be realistic and should be carefully tailored to each individual case. The principles of dietary advice, fluoride supplements, and oral hygiene measures cannot be applied in the same fashion to all children. Preventive care is an ongoing part of any child's dental care, constantly being reinforced and modified as the child develops and their perceptions change.

Restorative care

Having established the co-operation of the child and their parent it is important to make realistic decisions concerning restorative care. This involves careful consideration of the advisability of restoring an individual tooth. Is the tooth restorable? Is the tooth about to exfoliate? The initial aim should be to halt the active carious process by stabilizing as many of the carious lesions as possible. It may be necessary to temporize by placing quadrant dressings and then returning, at later visits, to carry out the definitive restoration (Chapters 7 and 8).

Aesthetic considerations

It is usual when treatment planning for adults to place aesthetic considerations low on the list of priorities. However, it is important to bear in mind that peer group pressure can be extremely strong in children. Children can suffer from a great deal of teasing as a consequence of the appearance of their teeth and it may be important to address the aesthetic problems sooner rather than later. It may not be possible to treat all aesthetic problems immediately; for example an increased overjet in a 6 year old child. However, discoloured or stained incisors can often be easily and successfully treated (Chapter 9). Such active intervention can be very useful in gaining the confidence and respect of both child and parent.

3.8 SUMMARY

Treatment planning in the child patient should not only cater for the immediate needs of the child but should have the vision and planning to allow that child to gain adulthood with a healthy mouth and positive attitude towards dental care. Perfect (careful) planning prevents poor performance (compliance) and should be positive, personal, and practical.

3.9 FURTHER READING

Blinkhorn, A. S. and Mackie, I. C. (1992). *Practical treatment planning for the paedodontic patient*. Quintessence, London. (*A useful, easily read book covering all aspects of treatment planning in young patients.*)

Holt, R. (1994) The preschool child: practical treatment planning. *Dental Update*, **21**, 339–43. (*A summary of the issues relating particularly to the under 5 year old child.*)

Kidd, E. A. M. and Pitts, N. M. (1990) A reappraisal of the value of the bitewing radiograph in the diagnosis of posterior approximal caries. *British Dental Journal*, **169**, 195–200. (*An overview on the controversies involved in the use of the bitewing radiograph.*)

Pitts, N. B. (1991a). The diagnosis of dental caries: 1. Diagnostic methods for assessing buccal, lingual and occlusal surfaces. *Dental Update*, **18**, 393–6.

Pitts, N. B. (1991b). The diagnosis of dental caries: 2. The detection of approximal, root surface and recurrent lesions. *Dental Update*, **18**, 436–42.

Pitts, N. B. (1992). The diagnosis of dental caries: 3. Rational and overview of present and possible future techniques. *Dental Update*, **19**, 32–42. (*Three papers that comprehensively cover the issues relating to caries diagnosis, with abundant references.*)

Ricketts, D. N. J., Kidd, E. A. M., and Wilson, R. F. (1995). A re-evaluation of electrical resistance measurements for the diagnosis of occlusal caries. *British Dental Journal*, **178**, 11–15. (*Sound study comparing conventional with state of the art methods of caries diagnosis.*)

4 Management of pain and anxiety

4   Management of pain and anxiety
G. J. ROBERTS

4.1   INTRODUCTION

The need for good management of anxiety and pain in paediatric dentistry is paramount. A common cause of complaint from parents and their children is that a dentist hurt unnecessarily and that this has led to a variety of problems usually embraced by the term 'unco-operative'.

4.2   CHILDREN'S PERCEPTION OF PAIN

Without doubt, the effective and sympathetic management of pain and the associated anxiety is central to the practice of paediatric dentistry. A major difficulty for paediatric dentists are the varied responses of children of widely differing ages to painful stimuli. Infants up to about 2 years of age are unable to distinguish between pressure and pain. After the age of approximately 2 and up to the age of 10, children begin to have some understanding of 'hurt' and begin to distinguish it from pressure or 'a heavy push'. The problem is that it is not possible to identify which children are amenable to explanation and respond by being co-operative when challenged with local anaesthesia and dental treatment in the form of drillings or extractions.

   Children over the age of 10 are much more likely to be able to think abstractly and participate more actively in the decision to use local anaesthesia, sedation, or general anaesthesia. Indeed as children enter their teenage years they are rapidly becoming more and more like adults and are able to determine more directly, sometimes aggressively, whether or not a particular method of pain control will be used.

4.3   CONSENT

The issue of consent is superficially clear. Before you can do anything to a patient, even a simple examination, consent must be obtained. Consent may be implied, verbal, or written. The main purpose of written consent is to demonstrate *post hoc*, in the event of a dispute, that informed consent was obtained. It has the additional advantage of making clinicians and patients pause to consider the implications of what is planned and to weigh the advantages and disadvantages so that a reasoned and informed choice can be made. Many health trusts and other employing authorities are increasingly demanding that written consent is obtained for all procedures. This is especially difficult now as the lower age of consent is no longer specifically limited. The sole criterion is whether or not the patient is 'able to understand' the procedures and their implications. As a pragmatic rule the age of 16 years still acts as a guide. But if a procedure is proposed and a child under 16 years says 'no' then consent has been refused. Fortunately, in paediatric dentistry the prospect of a life-saving operation is rare so a refusal of consent can be managed by a change in the procedure or by establishing a temporal respite.

The current advice from the protection societies is that written consent must be obtained for a course of treatment. The plan of treatment proposed must indicate the nature and extent of the treatment and the approximate number of times that local anaesthesia and/or sedation is to be used. There is no need to obtain written consent for each separate time that sedation is used. If the plan of treatment changes and along with it the frequency or nature of sedation, then it is prudent to obtain written consent for the change. The greater risks associated with general anaesthesia require specific written consent for each and every occasion that treatment is carried out under general anaesthesia. Examples of suitably worded forms are available from the Medical Defence Societies.

4.4   SYSTEMIC PAIN CONTROL

Children may need pain control for 'toothache' for a day or two before the removal of carious teeth. Often, the teeth are also abscessed so that it is necessary to combine antibiotic therapy with analgesia to obtain optimum pain relief. Additionally, analgesia is required postoperatively usually after dento-alveolar surgery.

The most common method of administration is by mouth. Small children, and some recalcitrant adolescents, refuse to take tablets so liquid preparations are needed. If other methods of administration such as intramuscular or intravenous are required then these injections should be administered by clinical staff experienced with these special techniques. Rectal administration is increasingly common as absorption from the rectal mucosa is rapid. If such a route of administration is to be used, specific consent must be obtained. It should be remembered that the dose for children of different ages needs to be carefully estimated to avoid the risk of an overdose (dangerous) or of an underdose (ineffective). The parents must be advised that all drugs *must* be stored in a safe place. Bathroom cabinets or kitchen cabinets are the safest places as they are out of reach and out of sight of small children. Specific advice on prescribing for children can be obtained from a local pharmacist or the British National Formulary (BNF).

The dosages for children can be calculated on the basis of a percentage chart (Table 4.1). Often 'average' doses are used but the prescriber has the absolute responsibility to confirm that the dosages recommended are correct.

Table 4.1   Percentage method for calculating doses

Age (years)	Mean weight (kg)	Percentage of adult dose
1	10	25
3	14	33
5	18	40
7	23	50
12	37	75
14	50	80
16	58	90
Adult	68	100

Abstracted from *The British National Formulary*, No. 29, March 1995.

The common drugs used for pain control in children are paracetamol BNF, aspirin BNF and ibuprofen BNF. The potential side-effects and the dosages should be checked with the formulary before prescribing. Aspirin, which is a very effective analgesic in children should *not* be used on children under 12 years of age because of the risk of Reye's syndrome. If surgery is considered, the effects of aspirin on haemostasis should also be remembered and the operator be prepared to carry out more extensive use of local or systemic methods of controlling bleeding. The increase in asthma among children requires that this is considered before ibuprofen is prescribed. Narcotic analgesics such as codeine or morphine can be used on children but only after less powerful analgesics have been shown to be ineffective. As above, the dosage should be checked with the BNF.

4.5 METHODS OF PAIN CONTROL

The different methods of pain control vary from simple behaviour management to full intubation general anaesthesia in a hospital operating theatre (Fig. 4.1). There is a strong relationship between the perception of pain experienced and the degree of anxiety perceived by the patient. Painful procedures cause fear and anxiety; fear and anxiety intensify pain. This circle of cause and effect is central to the management of all patients. Good behaviour management reduces anxiety, which in turn reduces the perceived intensity of pain, which further reduces the experience of anxiety.

Behaviour management have been covered in detail in Chapter 2 and local anaesthetic techniques in Chapter 5. The majority of dental procedures on children can be carried out using a combination of these two techniques. This chapter will deal with the methods of sedation and general anaesthesia, applicable to dental treatment in children.

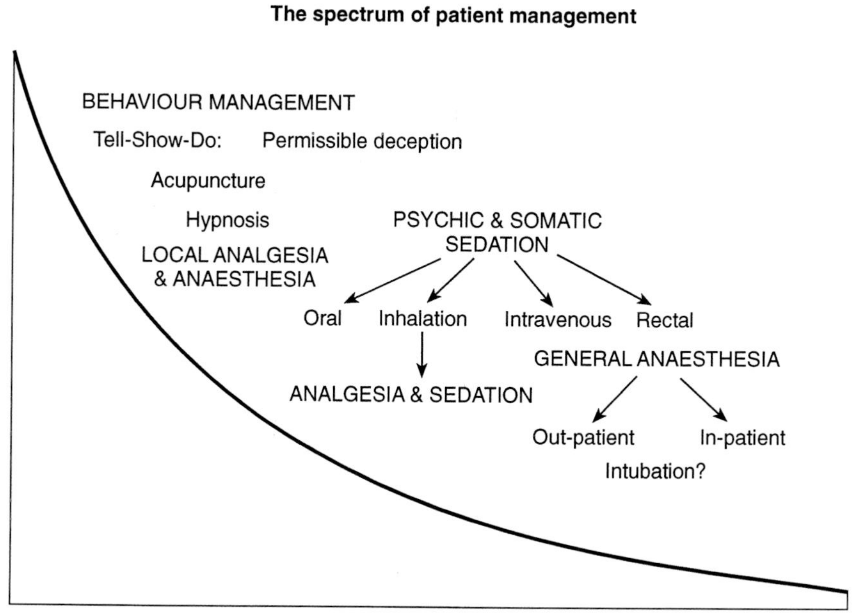

The spectrum of patient management

Fig. 4.1 This shows, on the left-hand scale, the approximate frequency with which a particular pain control technique is used, and on the bottom scale the increasing degree of physiological intrusion from local analgesia, through sedation and general anaesthesia.

4.6   MEDICAL STATUS

The wide variety of medical problems makes it difficult to be precise about the management strategy appropriate for each patient. Detailed descriptions of management of a variety of medical problems appear in a comprehensive book by Scully and Cawson (1993). As regards sedation, the American Society of Anesthesiologists' (ASA) classification provides an excellent guide to the type of sedation or anaesthesia appropriate to an individual patient's medical and behavioural problems (Table 4.2).

The decision as to whether a patient should be treated under general anaesthesia or local anaesthesia, or local anaesthesia with sedation depends on a combination of factors, the most important of which are:

(1)   the age of the child;

(2)   the degree of surgical trauma involved;

(3)   the perceived anxiety and how the patient may (or has) responded to similar levels of surgical trauma;

(4)   the complexity of the operative procedure;

(5)   the medical status of the child.

There are no hard and fast rules, and every procedure in every child must be assessed individually and the different elements considered in collaboration with the parents' and where appropriate with the child. For example, the younger the child the greater the likelihood of a need for general anaesthesia. At the other end of the age range it is unlikely that a 15 year old will need general anaesthesia for simple orthodontic extractions, although this might be required for moderately complex surgery, such as exposing and bonding an impacted canine. The degree of trauma involved is also another factor; a single extraction is most likely to be carried out under local anaesthesia, removal of the four first permanent molars is most likely to be carried out under general anaesthesia. Anxiety perceived as excessive, especially after after an attempt at treatment under local anaesthesia and sedation, would lead to simple treatment such as conservative dentistry being carried out under a general anaesthetic usually involving endotracheal intubation. Serious medical problems, e.g. cystic fibrosis with the associated respiratory problems would justify using sedation for more traumatic surgery such as removal of impacted canines, but it would be appropriate to carry out this treatment in a hospital environment. The degree of intellectual and/or physical impairment in handicapped children would also be a factor to be

Table 4.2   The American Society of Anesthesiologists' (ASA) physical status classification

Classification	Description
Class I	A healthy patient
Class II	A patient with mild systemic disease, e.g. diet controlled diabetes, asthma well controlled with drugs
Class III	A patient with severe systemic disease that is not incapacitating, e.g. insulin-dependent diabetes, congenital heart disease
Class IV	A patient with incapacitating systemic disease that is a constant threat to life, e.g. cystic fibrosis, congenital heart disease with cyanosis.
Class V	A moribund patient not expected to survive for 24 h with or without operation

considered. As indicated above, each child and their individual problems should be assessed on its merits and an appropriate method of pain control used.

Notwithstanding the above discussion, the vast majority of children are amenable to satisfactory treatment using behaviour management and local anaesthesia alone, largely because they fall into ASA class I with a few in ASA class II. General anaesthesia carries with it a finite risk of serious morbidity and even death. No child should be submitted to a general anaesthetic without consideration of this potentially devastating outcome. Intermediate between the minimally intrusive techniques of local anaesthesia and the major intrusion of general anaesthesia are the techniques of sedation (Fig. 4.1).

4.7 SEDATION TECHNIQUES

Sedation is defined as:

A state of depression of the central nervous system which reduces anxiety thus enabling treatment to be carried out satisfactorily. During sedation the patient will be able to independently maintain his airway, independently maintain an open mouth, and respond sensibly to verbal commands. In addition the patient will retain adequate function of protective reflexes such as the laryngeal reflex. The drugs used should carry a margin of safety sufficient to render unintended loss of consciousness extremely unlikely.

The routes of administration of sedative drugs of practical use in clinical paediatric dentistry are oral, inhalational, and intravenous. Other routes such as rectal or intranasal are little used and currently, intravenous sedation is unsuitable for the operator/sedationist when working on children. Current developments in intravenous techniques, especially the use of infusion pumps and patient-controlled analgesia (PCA) may prove to be sufficiently effective and safe for use by the operator/sedationist, but further research is required.

4.7.1 General facilities

The use of sedative drugs carries the risk of inadvertent loss of consciousness. Although the techniques are designed to reduce this risk to a minimum it should always be borne in mind that every time a sedative is given to a patient there is a risk of an idiosyncratic reaction to the drug which may result in unexpected loss of consciousness. The clinician must arrange the clinical session so that sedation without or *with* complications can proceed smoothly and safely. This includes the need for all patients who are having sedation to be accompanied. This can be anyone, relative or friend, sufficiently mature to understand the implications and potential problems of caring for a child during the later stages of recovery. In addition, the clinical facilities need to include suitable resuscitation equipment coupled with the knowledge and skills to use them.

4.7.2 Emergency equipment

Suitable emergency equipment must be available *easily* to hand. In any emergency time is of the utmost importance. For this reason emergency equipment and drugs should be within arms reach of the operator and ready for immediate use. Training of the dental surgeon and his or her staff is required before sedation techniques are used in surgery premises for the first time and further training should take place at regular intervals of not more than 1 year. It is essential that each member of the dental team knows exactly what is required of them in an emergency. The dental surgeon has the responsibility of ensuring the easy availability of drugs, particularly oxygen, and to see that the drugs in the emergency kit are not past their 'use by' date.

4.7.3   Emergency equipment for the dental surgeon

The following are items of equipment which a *dental surgeon* should be prepared to use in an emergency.

1. High volume suction for clearing the airways of saliva, debris, and blood. This must be capable of reaching the floor as a patient may be removed from the dental chair to lie on the floor to enable resuscitation.
2. An emergency supply of oxygen. A regularly working supply of oxygen from an inhalation sedation unit is an alternative.
3. Positive pressure ventilation apparatus with a self-inflating bag.
4. Face masks to fit children and adolescents.
5. Three sizes of oral airways.

    Note: These items should form part of an armamentarium of any dentist when treating patients using local anaesthesia alone.

4.7.4   Emergency drugs

Suitable emergency drugs must be available and because of the need for speed, the drugs must be stored with the emergency equipment. Training of the dental surgeon and their staff in the use of drugs has the same requirements as for equipment. It is the dental surgeon's duty to ensure the availability of drugs, particularly oxygen, and to see that they are not past their 'use by' date.

4.7.5   Emergency drugs for the dental surgeon

The following are drugs which the dentist should be prepared to use in an emergency.

1. Oxygen.
2. Adrenaline hydrochloride 1 mg/ml (1000 μg/ml), i.e. 1:1000 on a 1 ml ampoule for subcutaneous or intramuscular injection. The IMS Min-I-Jet system is particularly quick and easy to use.
3. Hydrocortisone sodium phosphate 100 mg per vial. To be made up to 1 ml with physiological saline immediately before use. For intravenous injection.
4. In addition to the above drugs suitable needles and syringes should be available to enable drugs to be drawn up and administered parenterally.
5. Flumazenil (benzodiazepine anatagonist) for reversing unexpected over-sedation from orally, intravenously, or rectally administered benzodiazepine.

4.7.6   Emergency equipment for medically qualified and staff trained in advanced life support

1. A laryngoscope, endotracheal tubes, and forceps to manipulate the endotracheal tubes during intubation.
2. A cricothyrotomy kit.
3. An electrocardiograph.
4. A defibrillator.

4.7.7 Emergency drugs for medically qualified and/or specially trained staff

1. Adrenaline 1:10 000 × 10 ml vials.
2. Atropine 1 mg/10 ml × 10 ml vials.
3. Calcium chloride 10 per cent × 10 ml vials.
4. Lignocaine 100 mg/10 ml (1 per cent) × 10 ml vials.
5. Isoprenaline 0.2 mg/ml × 10 ml vials.
6. Frusemide 80 mg/8 ml × 8 ml vials.
7. Sodium bicarbonate 8.4 per cent × 50 ml vials.
8. Glucose 50 per cent × 50 ml vials.
9. Naloxone 4 mg/ml x 1 ml vials.
10. Aminophylline 250 mg/10 ml × 10 ml vials.
11. Diazemuls 10 mg/2 ml × 2 ml vials.
12. Flumazenil 500 μg/5 ml × 5 ml vials.

Many of these drugs are available in prefilled syringes. It is the responsibility of the dentist to ensure the availability of the drugs required by the medical staff who may be called to deal with an emergency. Equally, it is the responsibility of the same medical staff to advise the dental surgeon of his or her precise requirements with regard to emergency drugs. This advice must be in writing.

Dental surgeons and their staff should at least be capable of providing basic life support; i.e. **A**irways, **B**reathing, **C**irculation (**ABC**). These can be reviewed by reading the following: European Resuscitation Council Guidelines for basic and advanced life support. *Resuscitation,* (1992). 24, 103–10.

4.8 GENERAL FACILITIES

There should be a suitable area where the child can sit quietly before the operation so that if appropriate, the sedative can be administered then the child monitored while it is taking effect. As a general rule it is not wise to let children have medication at home as quiet supervision of the child within the surgery premises is prudent. A journey to the surgery under the increasing influence of a mood-altering drug is not the most propitious way of preparing distressed children for treatment. These strictures do not apply to inhalation sedation or intravenous sedation. However, the general facilities suitable for providing care apply equally to oral, inhalational and intravenous sedation. During treatment there must be effective suction equipment and in the event of a power failure, a mechanically operated backup. Once treatment is complete the child should be able to sit (or lie) quietly until sufficiently recovered to be sent home accompanied by a responsible relative or friend. This will usually be a parent.

4.9 CLINICAL STATUS OF A SEDATED PATIENT

The sedative drugs, depending on the concentration used, cause a variety of effects from mild sedation, deep sedation, general anaesthesia and, in excessive concentrations, even death. It is important that dental surgeons working with children have a very clear idea of the clinical status of sedated patients. These are:

(1) the patient's eyes are open;
(2) the patient is able to respond verbally to questions;

(3) the patient is able to independently maintain an open mouth;

(4) the patient is able to independently maintain a patent airway;

(5) the ability to swallow.

All these criteria are evidence of 'light' sedation. The patients exhibiting these signs are sedated and quite clearly conscious. For this reason it is important not to let a child go to sleep in the dental chair while receiving treatment with sedation as closed eyes may be a sign of sleep, over-sedation, loss of consciousness, or cardiovascular collapse.

4.10 ORAL SEDATION

The only special equipment needed for this is a set of properly calibrated bathroom scales to enable the correct dose of sedative to be estimated for each patient. The drugs used for children vary from chloral hydrate to the benzodiazepines. One which is widely used is diazepam, a benzodiazepine which is usually administerd at a dosage of 250 μg/kg. For a 6 year old child this is approximately 5 g but could be as as low as 3.9 or high as 6.6 g. For a much older patient, for example a 15 year old, the average dose would be 13.6 g and vary from 9.7 to 18.9 g. These ranges are based on the 3rd, 50th, and 97th percentiles of the weights of children at 6 and 15 years respectively. It is clear that these dosages are likely to have a considerable depressive effect on the patient's physiological state, but lower dosages do not have any discernible effect on children's behaviour in the dental chair. For this reason the facilities outlined above are necessary in the unlikely event of loss of consciousness. The patient may require up to an hour of supervised postoperative recovery.

A further important strategy is to have a check-list so that the dental surgeon can be sure that all important elements of sedation have been properly considered and, for example, that the child has a responsible companion who will accompany the child and ensure safe delivery to the child's home.

4.10.1 Pre-operative instructions

These should be provided in writing and cover such points as ensuring that a suitable companion brings the child to and from the surgery, that a light meal only is eaten 2 or more hours before an appointment for sedation. In this context, a light meal is a cup of tea and a slice of toast. Postoperatively, suitable arrangements need to be made to ensure that the child plays quietly at home. In addition to these specific points 'local' rules are likely to apply.

4.10.2 Clinical technique

The following clinical regimen has been found to be practicable in clinical practice:

(1) on arrival of patient check that pre-operative instructions have been followed;

(2) weigh the patient and estimate the dose of diazepam;

(3) have the dosage checked by a second person;

(4) administer the diazepam approximately 1 h before treatment is due to start;

(5) allow the patient to sit in a 'quiet' room;

(6) once ready, to start and complete treatment with (or without) local anaesthesia;

(7) once treatment is complete, to allow the patient to recover in the quiet room until ready to return home;

(8) give companion postoperative instructions.

In this way the simple method of oral sedation will be relatively effective. This rather muted statement about the efficacy of oral sedation is made because the effects of oral sedation may be to improve patients' behaviour, make the behaviour worse, or have no effect, all in approximately equal proportions.

4.11 INHALATION SEDATION

This is synomous with inhalation of oxygen/nitrous oxide gas mixtures in relatively low concentrations, usually 20–50 per cent nitrous oxide. The technique is unique as the operator is able to titrate the gas against each individual patient. That is to say, the operator increases the concentration to the patient, observes the effect, and as appropriate, increases (or sometimes decreases) the concentration to obtain optimum sedation in each individual patient.

Inhalation sedation consists of three elements (Fig. 4.2):

1. The administration of low-to-moderate concentrations of nitrous oxide in oxygen to patients who remain conscious. The precise concentration of nitrous oxide is carefully titrated to the needs of each individual patient.

2. As the nitrous oxide begins to exert its pharmacological effects, the patient is subjected to a steady flow of reassuring and semi-hypnotic suggestion. This establishes and maintains rapport with the patient.

3. The use of equipment which exceeds the current BSI Standard for safety cutout devices installed within inhalation sedation equipment. This means that it is not possible to administer 100 per cent nitrous oxide either accidentally or deliberately. This is an important and critical clinical safety feature which is essential for the operator/sedationist.

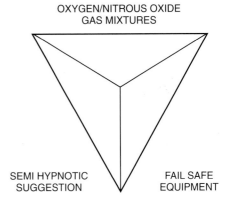

Fig. 4.2 The triad of elements of relative analgesia.

4.11.1 Equipment for inhalation sedation with oxygen/nitrous oxide gas mixtures

The most widely used equipment for inhalation sedation is the Quantiflex MDM (Fig. 4.3), which enables the operator to deliver carefully controlled volumes and concentrations of gases to the patient. In addition to the machine head that controls the delivery of gases, it is also necessary to have a suitable assembly for the gas cylinders, either a mobile stand (Fig. 4.4) or a pipeline system with cylinders stored remote from the machine head (Fig. 4.5).

4.11.2 Clinical technique

Of the inhalation sedation techniques available, the following is the easiest, the most flexible, and the least likely to cause surgery pollution. The control unit for the Quantiflex MDM (Fig. 4.3) has a single control for the total flow of gases, and a central, vertically placed, dial is turned to regulate simultaneously the percentage flow of both gases. Either of these controls can be changed without altering the other. The actual percentage of gases being delivered is monitored by looking at the flow meters for oxygen and nitrous oxide, respectively. There are 15 steps to the technique:

1. Check the machine.
2. Select the appropriate size of nasal mask and clean it with alcohol.

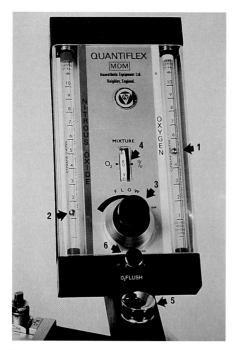

Fig. 4.3 The MDM inhalation sedation unit.

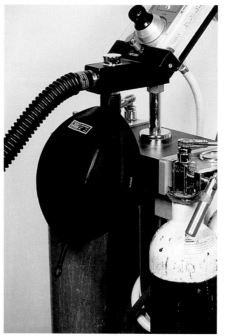

Fig. 4.4 The mobile cylinder stand showing the upper part of the oxygen and nitrous oxide cylinders and the reservoir bag.

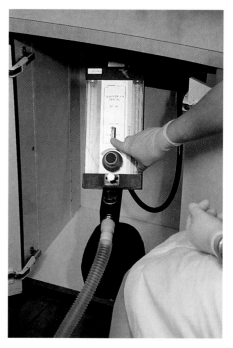

Fig. 4.5 The MDM unit mounted inobtrusively under a worktop.

3. Connect up the scavenging pipe.

4. Set the mixture dial to 100 per cent oxygen.

5. Settle the patient in the dental chair.

6. Turn the flow control to 3 l/min and allow the reservoir bag to fill with oxygen.

7. With the patient's help, position the nasal mask gently and comfortably to preclude any leaks. If necessary explain the way the mask is used.

8. Turn the flow control knob to the left until the flow rate of oxygen (litres/minute) matches the patient's tidal volume. This can be monitored by watching the reservoir bag, and should take 15–20 seconds. When the patient inspires the reservoir bag gets smaller. When the patient breathes out the reservoir bag gets larger as it fills with the mixture of gases emanating from the machine.

9. Simultaneously, reassure the patient about the sensations that will be felt. Encourage the patient to concentrate on breathing gently through the nose. If the reservoir bag appears to be getting too empty then the flow of oxygen should be increased until the flow rate in l/min matches the patient's minute volume.

10. Turn the mixture dial vertically to 90 per cent oxygen (10 per cent nitrous oxide). Wait 60 s.

11. Turn the mixture dial to 80 per cent oxygen (20 per cent nitrous oxide). Wait 60 s. Above this level the operator should exercise more caution and consider whether further increments should be only 5 per cent. With experience, operators will be able to judge whether further increments are needed.

12. At the appropriate level of sedation dental treatment can be started.

13. To bring about recovery turn the mixture dial to 100 per cent oxygen and oxygenate the patient for 2 min before removing the nasal mask.

14. Turn the flow control to zero and switch off the machine.
15. The patient should breathe ambient air for a further 5 min before leaving the dental chair. The patient should be allowed to recover for a total period of 15 min before leaving.

At all times the patient must remain conscious. This is judged by the five clinically discernible signs described previously.

The above method of administration is the basic technique that is required in the early stages of clinical experience for any operator. This method ensures that the changes experienced by the patient do not occur so quickly that the patient is unable to cope. Once the operator has sufficient skill and confidence the stages can be 'concertinaed', e.g. by starting at 20 per cent nitrous oxide and reducing the time intervals between increments.

The initial time intervals of 60 s are used because clinical experience shows that shorter intervals between increments can lead to too rapid an induction and overdosage.

4.11.3 The correct level of clinical sedation

One of the problems for the inexperienced clinician is to determine whether or not the patient is adequately sedated for treatment to start. By careful attention to signs and symptoms experienced by the patient the dentist will soon be able to decide whether the patient is ready for treatment.

The very rapid uptake and elimination of nitrous oxide requires the operator to be acutely vigilant so that the patient does not become sedated too rapidly.

4.11.4 Objective signs

The objective signs showing the patient is ready for treatment are (Fig. 4.6):

(1) the patient is awake;
(2) the patient is relaxed and comfortable;
(3) the patient responds coherently to verbal instructions;
(4) pulse rate is normal;
(5) blood pressure is normal;
(6) respiration is normal;
(7) skin colour is normal;
(8) pupils are normal and contract normally if a light is shone into them;
(9) the laryngeal reflex is normal;
(10) the gag reflex is reduced;
(11) reaction to painful stimuli is lessened;
(12) there is a general reduction in spontaneous movements;
(13) the mouth is maintained open on request (Fig. 4.7).

4.11.5 Subjective symptoms

Subjective symptoms experienced by the patient are (Fig 4.8):

(1) mental and physical relaxation;
(2) a tingling sensation (paraesthesia) singly or in any combination of lips, fingers, toes, or over the whole body;
(3) mild intoxication and euphoria;

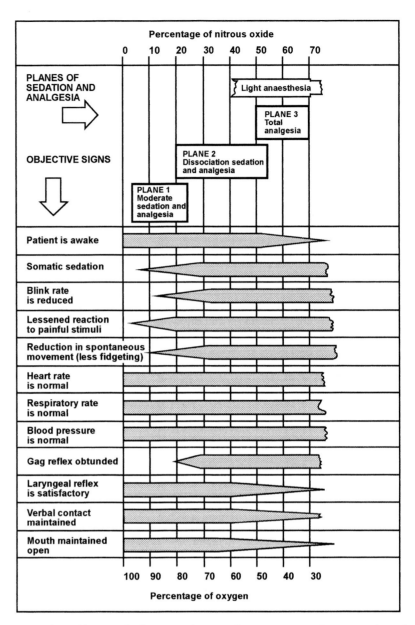

Fig. 4.6 Observable signs of sedation in relation to the concentration of nitrous oxide used.

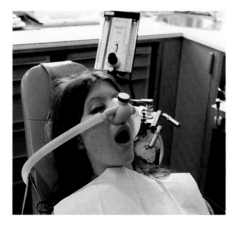

Fig. 4.7 The 'mouth open' sign.

(4) lethargy;

(5) a sense of detachment, sometimes interpreted as a floating or drifting sensation;

(6) a feeling of warmth;

(7) indifference to surroundings and the passage of time;

(8) dreaming;

(9) lessened awareness of pain.

If the patient tends to communicate less and less, and is allowing the mouth to close, then these are signs that the patient is becoming too deeply sedated. The concentration of nitrous oxide should be reduced by 10 or 15 per cent to prevent the patient moving into a state of total analgesia.

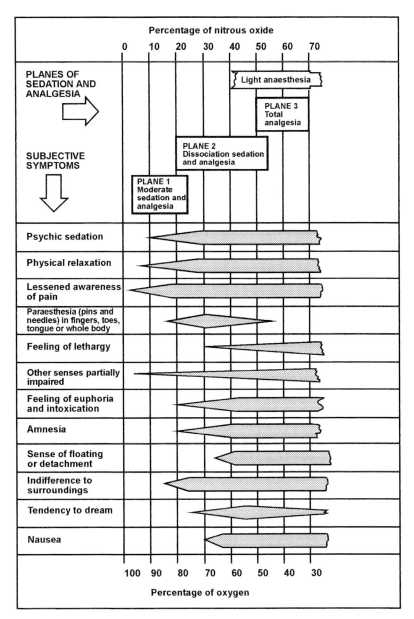

Fig. 4.8 Subjective symptoms experienced by the patient in relation to nitrous oxide concentration.

4.11.6 Monitoring

During sedation it is essential that the clinician monitors both the patient and the machinery. For healthy patients with ASA I or II, use of a radial pulse is sufficient. For patients with ASA III or IV, treatment within a hospital environment and pulse oximetry and/or electrocardiograph monitoring would be prudent. This applies to only a very small proportion of patients.

The patient

The clinician should pay careful attention to the patient's level of anxiety. This is achieved by assessing the patient's responses to an operative stimulus such as the dental drill. The level of sedation is assessed by the patient's demeanour compared with his or her pre-sedation behaviour. It is important to note that different patients exhibit similar levels of impairment at different concentrations of nitrous oxide. If the patient appears to be too heavily sedated then the concentration of nitrous oxide should be reduced.

Under hospital conditions a small number of patients with severe medical disorders may require continuous monitoring of pulse rate and blood pressure using an electronic pulse oximeter and blood pressure cuff. Such patients would be those with cystic fibrosis with marked lung scarring or children with severe congenital cardiac disease where there is high blood pressure or cyanosis.

The machinery

At all stages of inhalation sedation it is necessary to monitor intermittently the oxygen and nitrous oxide flow meters to verify that the machine is delivering the gases as required. In addition, it is essential to look at the reservoir bag to confirm that the patient is continuing to breathe through the nose the gases emanating from the machine. Little or no movement of the reservoir bag suggests that the patient is mouthbreathing, or that there is a gross leak, e.g. a poorly fitting nasal mask.

At present this is the only monitoring that is required for inhalation sedation for healthy patients. There is no need to use pulse oximetry (to measure blood oxygenation) or capnography (to measure exhaled carbon dioxide levels) as is currently recommended for patients being sedated with intravenously administered drugs.

4.11.7   The planes of inhalation sedation

The administration of oxygen/nitrous oxide gas mixtures for sedating child patients induces three levels or planes of analgesia and sedation.

Plane 1: moderate sedation and analgesia

This plane is usually obtained with concentrations of 5–25 per cent nitrous oxide (95–75 per cent oxygen). As the patient is being encouraged to inhale the mixture of gases through the nose, it is necessary to reassure him or her that the sensations described by the clinician may not always be experienced. The patient may feel tingling in the fingers, toes, cheeks, tongue, back, head, or chest. There is a marked sense of relaxation, the pain threshold is raised, and there is a diminution of fear and anxiety. The patient will be obviously relaxed and will respond clearly and sensibly to questions and commands.

Other senses such as hearing, vision, touch and proprioception are impaired in addition to the sensation of pain being reduced. The pupils are normal in appearance, and contract when a light is shone into them. The peri-oral musculature, so often tensed involuntarily by the patient during treatment, is more easily retracted when the dental surgeon attempts to obtain good access for operative work.

The absence of any side-effects makes this an extremely useful plane when working on moderately anxious patients.

Plane 2: dissociation sedation and analgesia

This plane is usually obtained with concentrations of 20–55 per cent nitrous oxide (80–45 per cent oxygen). As with plane 1, patients do not always experience all the symptoms. This should be remembered when reassuring and encouraging them.

As the patient enters this plane, psychological symptoms, described as dissociation or detachment from the environment, are experienced. Sometimes this dissociation is minimal, at other times it is profound. It may also take the form of a euphoria similar to alcoholic intoxication (witness the laughing gas parties of the mid-nineteenth century). The patient may feel suffused by a warm wave, and may experience a slight humming or buzzing in the ears, and a drowsiness or light-headedness sometimes described by the patient as a 'floaty' or 'woozy' feeling.

The overall demeanour of the patient will be relaxed and acquiescent. Apart from the overall appearance of relaxation, one of the few tangible physical signs is a reduction in the blink rate. At the deeper level of this plane of sedation the psychological effects become more pronounced. Occasionally, a patient will repeat words or phrases several times in succession. The words repeated may or may not make sense.

There is a noticeable tendency for the patient to dream, the dreams usually being of a pleasant nature. It is believed by many operators that the dreams experienced by the patient are to some extent conditioned by the ideas and thoughts introduced by the dental surgeon during the induction phase of sedation. The sedative effect is considerably pronounced, with both psychosedation and somatic sedation being present.

The psychosedation takes the form of a relaxed demeanour, and a willingness on the part of the previously unwilling patient to allow treatment regarded as frightening or especially traumatic. The somatic sedation takes the form of physical relaxation, unresisting peri-oral musculature, and occasionally an arm or leg sliding off the side of the dental chair indicating profound relaxation.

The analgesic effect is probably accentuated by the sedation and sense of detachment. The patient is still able to respond to questions and commands, although there may be a considerable mental effort involved in thinking out the answer. The response is usually delayed and sluggish. Paraesthesia may be more pronounced and cover a greater area of the body than in plane 1. The patient is nevertheless obviously conscious and can demonstrate this by keeping the mouth wide open to assist the dental surgeon during operative treatment. On recovery, the patient may exhibit total amnesia. Nausea is a rare side-effect and very occasionally (in less than 0.003 per cent of administrations) a patient may vomit.

Plane 3: total analgesia

This plane is usually obtained with concentrations of 50–70 per cent nitrous oxide (50–30 per cent oxygen). It has been claimed, that analgesia is so complete that extraction of teeth may be carried out in this plane. This has not been my experience. In this plane there is an increased tendency to dream. It is important to recognize that in a small number of patients as little as 50 per cent nitrous oxide may bring about *loss of consciousness*. It is for this reason that dentists must exercise considerable caution if the concentration of gas coming from the machine rises above 40 per cent nitrous oxide.

If the patient does become too deeply sedated and enters this third plane of total analgesia, he or she begins to lose the ability to maintain independently an open mouth and will be unable to co-operate by responding to the dentist's requests. If this 'open mouth' sign is lost, the operator can be sure that the patient is too deep in the plane of total analgesia and within a few minutes is likely to enter the plane of light anaesthesia. It is for this reason that a mouth prop must *never* be used, for if a prop is used the open mouth sign would not function.

If sedation is too deep and the patient shows signs of failing to co-operate, then the dentist should reduce the concentration of nitrous oxide by 10 or 15 per cent for a couple of minutes. If it is considered necessary to lighten the sedation even more rapidly, the nasal hood should be removed and the patient allowed to breathe ambient air. The patient will return to a lighter plane within 15–20 s.

This plane of total analgesia is regarded as a buffer zone between the clinically useful planes of moderate and dissociation sedation and analgesia, and the potentially hazardous plane of light anaesthesia.

4.11.8   Clinical application

The technique of nitrous oxide sedation can be used for a wide range of procedures involving the cutting of hard or soft tissue where local anaesthesia will usually be needed to supplement the general analgesia from the nitrous oxide. The major disadvantage (or minor if handled properly) is the inconvenience of the nasal hood restricting access to the upper incisor area if an apicectomy is required. This problem can be overcome by careful retraction of the upper lip and counterpressure from the thumb held on the bridge of the nose.

4.11.9   Scavenging

Effective scavenging equipment is extremely simple in design (Fig. 4.9). This design of scavenger can be used on a normal relative analgesia machine without any specific modifications to the machine itself. All that is required is a slight change in the design of the nasal hood and the tubing leading from the machine to the hood. First, the expiratory and/or air entrainment valve on the nasal hood itself is removed and replaced with a simple blank. This is possible as the sedation technique which uses air-entrainment is obsolete. Secondly, the tube leading from the machine is doubled in diameter, to lower airway resistance, and only a single tube leads from the machine to the nasal mask. The second tube, also doubled in diameter leads from the nasal mask to a specially devised exhaust pipe built into the wall or floor of the surgery. If considered essential, negative pressure can be applied to the exit pipe to increase the efficiency of the scavenging.

Surgery contamination is also affected by the *modus operandi* of the dental surgeon. Considerable care needs to be taken to discourage the patients from mouthbreathing, to use rubber dam whenever possible, and ensure that full recovery is carried out with the nasal hood in place. In this way the levels of surgery pollution can be kept to a minimum. Careful studies on the effects of nitrous oxide on dental personnel show that in scavenged surgeries there is no threshold of harmful effect. In unscavenged surgeries, beyond 5 h a week of exposure leads to detectable influences on the ability of female staff to become pregnant. Clearly, good practice requires that scavenging is used at all times so that the potentially harmful effects of operating room exposure are eliminated.

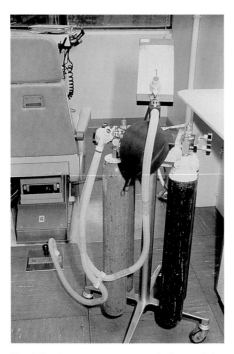

Fig. 4.9 Scavenging system applied to an RA machine with outlet in the floor.

4.12   INTRAVENOUS SEDATION

The circumstances when intravenous sedation can be used in paediatric dentistry are limited, although there is a slow but steady trend to extending its use especially in adolescents. The standard regimen is to use 0.07 mg/kg of midazolam infused slowly until the signs of satisfactory sedation are reached. This usually entails a loading dose of 2 mg followed by further increments as appropriate.

The technique requires the insertion of a small gauge needle which is allowed to remain *in situ* until the treatment for that visit is complete. This applies to manual infusion by the dental surgeon, diffusion pump infusion supervised by the dental surgeon, and patient controlled anaesthesia (PCA). For anxious children this is an almost insuperable problem as 'the needle' is the cause of their fear. Nevertheless, there appears to be a group of older children, usually adolescents requiring dento-alveolar surgery, who are willing to allow the placement of a needle in the dorsum of the hand or the antecubital fossa for infusion of benzodiazepine drugs.

4.12.1   Equipment for intravenous sedation

The general surgery set up is the same as for inhalation sedation. A disposable tray should be prepared with the following:

(1) a 5 ml syringe;
(2) a butterfly needle;
(3) adhesive tape;
(4) a green needle gauge 21;
(5) isopropyl alcohol swab;
(6) a single ampoule of the intravenous sedation drug;
(7) an ampoule of flumazenil (for urgent reversal of benzodiazepine sedation);
(8) a tourniquet.

The technique can be carried out as shown in the following sections.

4.12.2   Intravenous agents

There are many intravenous agents available in the BNF, but for dental purposes the practical choice is between midazolam, a benzodiazepine which is water soluble and well tolerated by tissues (important if some midazolam inadvertently becomes deposited outside rather than inside a vein) and propofol which leads to rapid sedation and rapid recovery. Unfortunately, the risk of unintended loss of consciousness is high with propofol because of the narrow therapeutic range of the drug which leads quickly to anaesthesia. Currently, the drug is used for sedation when there is a separate 'sedationist' present who is able to devote their attention entirely to the level of consciousness of the patient. Current research, especially with PCA may soon lead to a technique sufficiently well controlled for the operator/sedationist.

4.12.3   Intravenous access

The two most common sites of access are the antecubital fossa and the dorsum of the hand. In children especially, the antecubital fossa carries with it the danger of the needle causing damage to the vein and surrounding structures if the arm is bent during sedation. For this reason the dorsum of the hand is the preferred site.

4.12.4   Procedure

1. The patient's medical history is checked.
2. The arm is extended and a tourniquet applied.

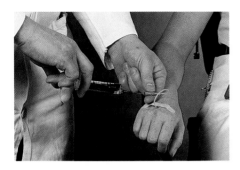

Fig. 4.10 Intravenous administration of midazolam through a vein in the dorsum of the hand.

3. The pulse oximeter and blood pressure cuff are applied to the contralateral arm. *Note*: a very anxious patient might be distressed by these procedures so they can be left until the patient is sedated.

4. The butterfly needle is inserted into the vein and taped into place.

5. The patient is asked to touch the tip of the nose to demonstrate good neuromotor control.

6. The first dose of drug is administered over 30 s (Fig. 4.10).

7. The patients' response is assessed after 2 minutes to determine whether further (smaller) increments of the sedative agent are required.

8. Dental treatment is carried out. If sedation becomes inadequate further increments of the sedative agent may given.

9. Once dental treatment is complete, the patient is allowed to recover sufficiently to be helped to the recovery area.

10. Recovery must be under the supervisory eye of specially trained personnel.

11. Once the patient is 'street fit', they are discharged into the care of an accompanying adult.

12. Postoperative instructions are given.

4.13   UNEXPECTED LOSS OF CONSCIOUSNESS

On the rare occasions when the patient becomes unconscious the dentist and their staff should follow the following routine.

1. Cease the operative procedure immediately.

2. Ensure that the mouth is cleared of all fluids by using high-volume suction.

3. Turn the patient on to his or her side in the 'recovery' position (Fig. 4.11).

4. Consider the administration of 100 per cent oxygen.

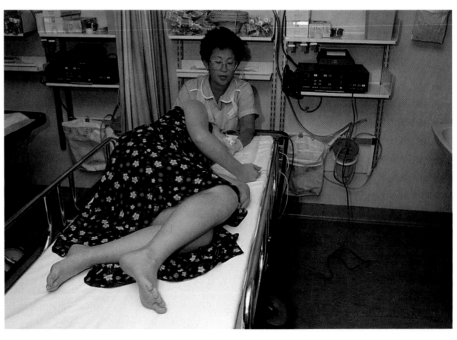

Fig. 4.11   Recovery position following general anaesthesia.

5. If intravenous sedation is being used, leave *in situ* the cannula or needle in the event that emergency drugs will be needed to hasten return of consciousness.

6. Consider monitoring pulse, blood pressure, and respiration. Be ready to start resuscitation.

7. Dentist to stay with the patient until full signs of being awake are present (eyes open, independent maintenance of the airways, and verbal contact).

8. Follow up of the patient by review within 3 days.

9. Full documentation of the incident.

10. Inform the patient's general medical practitioner of the incident.

4.14   GENERAL ANAESTHESIA

The use of general anaesthesia in dentistry has a wide application, usually for the extraction of teeth. Fortunately, the use of general anaesthesia in dentistry has reduced, due partly to the reduction in dental disease, but also to the increasing use of sedation. Nevertheless, there will always be a need for general anaesthesia in dentistry for children.

4.14.1   Type of anaesthesia

In dentistry, anaesthesia falls into three main groups:

(1) out-patient short case 'dental chair' anaesthesia;

(2) out-patient/day-stay 'intubation' anaesthesia;

(3) in-patient/hospital stay 'intubation' anaesthesia.

Within these three broad categories there are many variations used by different anaesthetists working under different circumstances. The introduction of these three types of anaesthesia is necessary as the preliminary assessment of patients for anaesthesia is carried out by the dental surgeon. In this way the general management for the patient can be organized, the correct information given to the parents and child, and the appropriate time allocated to the operative procedure.

Fortunately, the number of dentists carrying out general anaesthesia is reducing, hopefully to zero. Anaesthesia is a highly skilled clinical technique which requires a significant period of postgraduate training. The proper basis for this training is a first degree or diploma in medicine. This, by definition, precludes dentists from training in general anaesthesia. Nevertheless, the organization of dental general anaesthesia lists, at least in the preliminary stages, is performed by the dental surgeon. There is a need to understand the type of anaesthesia and the implications of the underlying medical condition as this is a factor in determining the circumstance under which anaesthesia is to be administered.

4.14.2   Facilities and staff for general anaesthesia

These need to be considered especially carefully as the potential for disastrous complications is greater than with any other technique of pain control. Apart from the obvious array of drugs (see above) and special equipment for endotracheal intubation, the additional monitoring such as an electrocardiograph, pulse oximeter, capnograph, and transcutaneous nerve stimulation are considered by many anaesthetists to be essential. In addition, for resuscitation, a defibrillator, cricothyroid needle, laryngoscopes, and special drugs for use by medically trained personnel (see above).

4.14.3   Definition of anaesthesia

The state of anaesthesia is defined as 'The absence of sensation artificially induced by the administration of gases or the injection of drugs or a combination of both'. The important feature of anaesthesia is that the patient is completely without the ability to independently maintain physiological function, such as breathing and protective reflexes, and is acutely vulnerable to the loss of any foreign bodies or fluids down the throat.

4.14.4   Out-patient 'short case' general anaesthesia

This is designed for patients who are ASA class I or class II where relatively short, 2–10 min, procedures such as simple dental extractions are intended. The induction is usually by the intravenous injection of sodium methohexitone (1.5 mg/kg) over 20–30 s in an unpremedicated patient in the supine position. An increasingly used alternative is propofol, also given intravenously (2.5 mg/kg) over 20–30 s. For children with extreme anxiety it is occasionally feasible to premedicate the child with diazepam (see above). It is usual to have a parent or 'carer' in the surgery with the child to help allay any anxiety expressed by the child at the time of induction. If venepuncture is difficult it is feasible to induce the child with 30 per cent oxygen and 70 per cent nitrous oxide, supplementing this with 2–3 per cent halothane or fluothane. Whichever method of induction is used it is common to maintain anaesthesia by a mixture of oxygen, nitrous oxide, and halothane.

Once anaesthesia is achieved it is necessary to pack the oropharynx with gauze to protect the airway. A recent and increasingly used technique is to place a pharyngeal cuff to protect the airway. (Fig. 4.12) This also needs some light packing. Monitoring for this type of anaesthesia usually consists of an electrocardiograph, oxygen saturation and a blood pressure cuff.

Treatment usually consisting of simple extractions is then carried out, the gauze removed and the patient turned into the recovery position. The huge advantage of methohexitone is its rapid induction and early recovery. Thus, patients are very quickly able to be placed in a quiet recovery room so that they can be monitored during the final phases of recovery.

This is usually judged to be complete when the child is able to drink a glass of water without being sick and able to stand without swaying or appearing dizzy. Although the child is deemed 'street fit', once he/she has arrived home the combined effects of anxiety, the general anaesthetic, and the dental surgery, make it necessary for the child to play 'quietly at home' for the rest of that day.

4.14.5   Out-patient 'day-stay' general anaesthesia

This is a natural extension of 'short case' dental anaesthesia and is reserved for ASA class I or class II usually on a day-stay basis. In general terms, the patients require dental treatment that lasts more than 10 min. The procedures commonly performed in this way are minor oral surgery such as removal of supernumeraries, complex and compound odontomes, exposing and bonding impacted teeth, or extensive conservative dentistry in children unable to accept such treatment when awake.

Anaesthetic induction is similar to that for 'short case' anaesthesia but with the addition of a neuromuscular paralysing agent such as atracurium 0.5 mg/kg

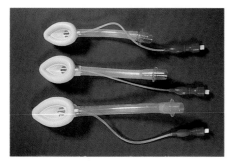

Fig. 4.12   Different sizes of pharyngeal cuff.

body weight to enable the anaesthetist to ventilate the patient artificially. It is immediately apparent that this form of anaesthesia is a much greater intrusion upon the patient's physiological state. Nevertheless, the same principles of protecting the airways apply.

It is usual to carry out such procedures with the airways maintained and protected by the placement of an endotracheal tube. From the point of view of the dental surgeon, the tube should be passed nasotracheally. If this is not possible or there is a positive indication against this an orotracheal tube will be used. In addition to the tube the throat will be packed with gauze. Once the patient is stabilized, treatment can progress at optimum speed and efficiency. If conservation is required it is prudent to use a rubber dam as good isolation is essential for a high standard of operative dentistry (Fig. 4.13). Surgical procedures can also proceed at optimum speed with local anaesthesia (2 per cent lignocaine with 1:1000 adrenaline) infliltrated into the area of surgery to reduce bleeding and to help visual assessment of bone and tooth tissues during surgery. This will also reduce the risk of cardiac dysrhythmias associated with procedures that stimulate pain receptors in the distribution of the trigeminal nerve. The monitoring is usually the same as 'short procedure' general anaesthesia with the addition of a capnograph and an inspired oxygen monitor. In addition, electrical stimulation of the calf muscle may be used to identify the return of paralysed muscles to normal neuromuscular excitability.

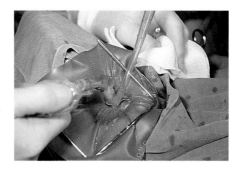

Fig. 4.13 Rubber dam applied during general anaesthesia.

Once treatment is complete the patient is placed in the recovery position and wheeled to a recovery suite where a nurse and duplicate resuscitation equipment are available. The recovery from such extensive anaesthesia is such that the patient may not be able to return home for several hours. Usually it is necessary to have access to a car as the children are never quite as 'street fit' as those who have had a short anaesthetic, so public transport is best avoided.

4.14.6 In-patient/hospital stay 'intubation' anaesthesia

Patients who are unfit for short or medium length general anaesthetics are usually in ASA class III. These patients have a medical problem that constitutes a significant increased risk so anaesthetists advise that they are treated in a hospital operating theatre, which is always close to the facilites of an intensive care unit. The dental surgery is no more complex than that carried out for 'short-' and 'day-stay' anaesthesia, but the underlying medical condition requires the increased level of care that *may* be needed in the operating theatre environment.

A typical approach to such anaesthesia is as follows.

1. Premedication: temazepam 0.5 mg/kg orally, 30–60 min before the anticipated time of anaesthetic induction. The maximum dose is 20 mg.
2. EMLA® cream on the dorsum of *both* hands, 60 min before anaesthetic induction.
3. Induction of anaesthesia using intravenous methohexitone or propofol.
4. Intravenous atracurium 0.5 mg/kg body weight.
5. Placement of a nasotracheal or an orotracheal tube.
6. Packing of the throat with gauze.
7. Completion of dental treatment.
8. Recovery of the patient.

4.15 SUMMARY

1. Most patients can be treated using local anaesthesia and good behaviour management.
2. A significant minority of patients will require some form of sedation to enable them to undergo dental treatment.
3. A small minority of patients require general anaesthesia.
4. All techniques require careful and systematic assessment before being used.
5. Dentists and their staff require careful training and regular updates in the techniques of anaesthesia and sedation for children.

4.16 FURTHER READING

Report of the the Working Party on Training in Dental Anaesthesia. (1993). Standing Dental Advisory Committee, Department of Health, United Kingdom. (*An excellent guide to sedation and anaesthesia in general dental practice and community dental practice.*)

Lindsay, S. J. E. and Yates, J. A. The effectiveness of oral diazepam in anxious child dental patients. (1985). *British Dental Journal*, **159**,149–53. (*The only objective study on the efficacy of oral premedication.*)

Coplans, M. P. and Green, R. A. (eds) (1983). Cardiovascular effects of dental anaesthesia. *Anaesthesia and and sedation in dentistry*. Elsevier, Amsterdam. (*An excellent review of the subject.*)

European Resuscitation Council Guidelines for basic and advanced life support. (1992). *Resuscitation* **24**, 103–10. (*Guidelines that all practitioners should read and put into effect.*)

Scully, C. and Cawson, R. A. (1993). *Medical problems in dentistry*. Wright, London. (*The most comprehensive account of how to cope with medical problems.*)

Roberts, G. J. and Rosenbaum, N. L. (1991). A colour atlas of dental analgesia and sedation. Wolfe Publishing, London. (*All you need to know about local analgesia and sedation.*)

5 Local anaesthesia for children

5 Local anaesthesia for children

J. G. MEECHAN

5.1 INTRODUCTION

This chapter considers the use of local anaesthesia in children and describes methods of injection which should produce minimal discomfort. The complications and contra-indications to the use of local anaesthesia in children are also discussed. The major use of local anaesthetics is in providing operative pain control; however, it should not be forgotten that these drugs can be used as diagnostic tools and also in the control of haemorrhage.

5.2 SURFACE ANAESTHESIA

Surface anaesthesia can be achieved by physical or pharmacological methods (topical anaesthetics). The physical method employed in dentistry involves the use of ethyl chloride and relies on the latent heat of evaporation of this volatile liquid to reduce the temperature of the surface tissue to produce anaesthesia. This method is rarely used in children as it is difficult to direct the stream of liquid accurately without involving associated sensitive structures such as teeth. In addition, the general anaesthetic action of ethyl chloride should not be forgotten.

5.2.1 Intra-oral topical agents

Topical anaesthetics work well in children and flavoured varieties can be especially popular. Topical anaesthetics will anaesthetize 2–3 mm depth of surface tissue when used properly. The following points are worth noting when using intra-oral topical anaesthetics:

(1) the area of application should be dried;
(2) the anaesthetic should be applied over a limited area;
(3) the anaesthetic should be applied for sufficient time.

A number of different preparations varying in the active agent and in concentration are available for intra-oral use. In the United Kingdom the agents most commonly employed are lignocaine and benzocaine. Topical anaesthetics are provided as sprays, solutions, creams, or ointments. Sprays are the least convenient as they are difficult to direct. Some sprays taste unpleasant and can lead to excess salivation if they inadvertantly reach the tongue. In addition, unless a metered dose is delivered, the quantity of anaesthetic used is poorly controlled. It is important to limit the amount of topical anaesthetic used because the active

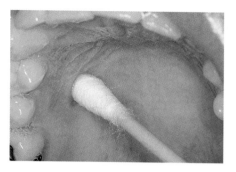

Fig. 5.1 Use of a cotton bud to apply topical anaesthetic over a limited area.

agent is present in greater concentration in topical preparations than local anaesthetic solutions and uptake from the mucosa is rapid. Systemic uptake will be even quicker in damaged tissue. An effective method of application is to spread some cream on the end of a cotton bud (Fig. 5.1). All of the conventional intra-oral topical anaesthetics are equally effective when used on reflected mucosa. The length of time of administration is crucial for the success of topical anaesthetics. Applications of about 15 s or so are useless. An application time of at least 2 min is required. It is important that topical anaesthetics are given sufficient time to work, because for many children this will be their initial experience of intra-oral pain control techniques, and if the first method encountered is unsuccessful then confidence in the operator and their armamentarium will not be established.

5.2.2 EMLA®

EMLA® cream (a 5 per cent eutectic mixture of prilocaine and lignocaine) is the first topical anaesthetic which has been shown to produce effective surface anaesthesia of intact skin and thus is a useful adjunct to the provision of general anaesthesia in children as it allows pain-free venepuncture. When used on skin it has to be applied for 1 h and is thus only appropriate for elective general anaesthetics. Clinical trials of the use of EMLA® intra-orally have shown it to be more effective than conventional local anaesthetics when used on attached gingiva such as the hard palate and interdental papillae; however, it is no more effective than conventional topical agents when applied to reflected mucosa. The 5 min application of EMLA® in the maxillary buccal sulcus has been shown to have no effect on the response of primary teeth to pulp testing. At present the intra-oral use of EMLA® is not recommended by its manufacturers.

5.2.3 Controlled release devices

The use of topically active agents incorporated into materials which will adhere to mucosa and allow slow-release of the agent is a potential growth area in the field of local anaesthetic delivery. Such techniques might prove of value in paediatric dentistry. Clinical studies investigating the release of lignocaine from intra-oral patches have shown some promise but as yet such devices are not in routine use.

5.2.4 Jet injectors

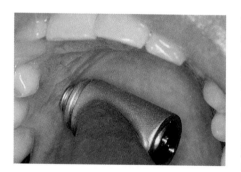

Fig. 5.2 The jet injector. (By kind permission of *Dental Update*.)

Jet injectors belong in a category somewhere between topical and local anaesthesia but will be discussed here for completeness. These devices allow anaesthesia of the surface and to a depth of over 1 cm without the use of a needle, by forcing a jet of solution through the tissue under high pressure (Fig. 5.2). Conventional local anaesthetic solutions are used in specialized syringes and have been successful in children with bleeding diatheses where deep injection is contra-indicated. Jet injection has been used both as the sole means of achieving local anaesthesia and prior to conventional techniques. Some practitioners have used jet injection alone or in combination with sedation to allow pain-free extraction of primary teeth. Nevertheless, the use of jet injection is not widespread for a number of reasons. Expensive equipment is required, soft tissue damage can be produced if a careless technique is employed, and the specialized syringes can be frightening to children both in appearance and in the sound produced during anaesthetic delivery. In addition, the unpleasant taste of anaesthetic solution which can accompany the use of this technique can be off-putting.

5.3   NON-PHARMACOLOGICAL METHODS OF PAIN CONTROL

A number of non-pharmacological methods of reducing the pain of operative dentistry are now available including the use of electrical stimulation and radio waves. Hypnosis also belongs in this category.

Electro-analgesia or TENS (transcutaneous electronic nerve stimulation) has been shown to be very effective in providing anaesthesia for restorative procedures in children aged 3–12 years. The technique has also been used to provide pain control during extraction of primary teeth. It can also be used as a 'deep topical' to reduce the pain of local anaesthetic injections. In younger children the level of stimulation is controlled by the operator; however, children over 10 years old can sufficiently understand the method to be able to control the level of stimulus themselves.

The basis of TENS blocking transmission of the acute pain of dental operative procedures is attributed to the fact that large myelinated nerve fibres (such as those responding to touch) have a lower threshold for electrical stimulation than do smaller unmyelinated pain fibres. Stimulation of these fibres by current from the TENS machine closes the 'gate' to central transmission of the signal from the pain fibres. This is quite different from the use of TENS in the treatment of chronic pain where the release of endogenous pain-killers such as β-endorphins is stimulated. In addition, older patients alter the level of stimulation received from the machine themselves, this feeling of control can allay anxiety and aid in pain management.

Non-pharmacological methods of pain control offer two advantages. First, systemic toxicity will not occur, and secondly the soft tissue anaesthesia resolves at the end of the procedure reducing the chances of self-inflicted trauma.

Hypnosis can be used as an adjunct to local anaesthesia in children by decreasing the pulse rate and the incidence of crying. It appears to be most effective in young children.

5.4   LOCAL ANAESTHETIC SOLUTIONS

A number of local anaesthetic solutions are now available that can provide anaesthesia from 10 min to over 6 h. There are few, if any, indications for the use of the so-called 'long-acting' agents in children. The gold standard is lignocaine with adrenaline. Unless there is a true allergy to lignocaine then 2 per cent lignocaine with 1:80 000 adrenaline is the solution of choice in the United Kingdom. 'Short-acting' agents such as plain lignocaine are seldom employed as the sole agent because, although pulpal anaesthesia may be short-lived, soft tissue effects can still last over an hour or so. More importantly, the efficacy of plain solutions is much less than those which contain a vasoconstrictor.

5.5   TECHNIQUES OF LOCAL ANAESTHESIA IN CHILDREN

There are no techniques of local anaesthetic administration that are unique to children; however, modifications to standard methods are sometimes required. As far as positioning the child is concerned the upper body should be about 30° to the vertical. Sitting upright can increase the chances of a faint while at the other extreme (fully supine) the child may feel ill at ease. When there is a choice of sites at which to administer the first local anaesthetic injection the primary maxillary molar area should be chosen as this is the region which is most easily anaesthetized with the least discomfort.

5.5.1   Infiltration anaesthesia

Infiltration anaesthesia is the method of choice in the maxilla. The infiltration of 0.5–1.0 ml of local anaesthetic is sufficient for pulpal anaesthesia of most teeth in children. The objective is to deposit local anaesthetic solution as close as possible to the apex of the tooth of interest; however, the presence of bone prevents direct apposition. As the apices of most teeth are closer to the buccal side a buccal approach is employed and the needle is directed towards the apex after insertion through reflected mucosa. Direct deposition under the periosteum can be painful therefore a compromise is made and the solution is delivered supraperiosteally. The one area where pulpal anaesthesia can prove troublesome in the child's maxilla is the upper first permanent molar region where the proximity of the zygomatic buttress can inhibit the spread of solution to the apical area (see below).

In the mandible the use of buccal infiltration anaesthesia will often produce pulpal anaesthesia of the primary teeth; however, it is usually unreliable when operating on the permanent dentition with the possible exception of the lower incisor teeth. The most reliable form of anaesthesia in the mandible is inferior dental block anaesthesia.

5.5.2   Regional block anaesthesia

Inferior dental and lingual nerve blocks

The administration of the inferior dental and lingual nerve block is easier to perform successfully in children compared with adults. A common fault in adults is placement of the needle too low on the ramus of the mandible with deposition of solution inferior to the mandibular foramen. In children, the mandibular foramen is low in relation to the occlusal plane (Fig. 5.3), and it is difficult to place the needle inferior to the mandibular foramen if it is introduced parallel to the occlusal plane. Thus in children it is easier to ensure that the solution is deposited around the nerve before it enters the mandibular canal.

The technique of administration is identical to that used in adults and is best performed with the child's mouth fully open. The direct approach introducing the needle from the primary molars of the opposite side is recommended as less needle movement is required once the tissues have been entered with this method compared with the indirect technique. The operator's non-dominant hand supports the mandible with the thumb intra-orally in the retromolar region of the mandible and the index or middle finger extra-orally at the posterior border of the ramus at the same height as the thumb. The needle is advanced from the primary molar region of the opposite side with the syringe held parallel to the mandibular occlusal plane. The needle is inserted through mucosa in the mandibular retromolar region medial to the pterygomandibular raphe midway between the raphe and the anterior border of the ascending ramus of the mandible aiming for a point half-way between the operator's thumb and index finger. The height of insertion is about 5 mm above the mandibular occlusal plane, although in young children entry at the height of the occlusal plane should also be successful. The needle should be advanced until the medial border of the mandible is reached. In young children bone will be reached after about 15 mm and thus a 25 mm needle can be used; however, in older children a long (35 mm) needle should be employed as penetration up to 25 mm may be required. Once bone has been touched the needle is withdrawn slightly until it is supraperiosteal, aspiration performed, and 1.5 ml of solution deposited. The lingual nerve is blocked by withdrawing the needle half-way, aspirating again

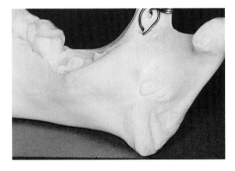

Fig. 5.3 The mandibular foramen is below the occlusal plane in children. (By kind permission of *Dental Update.*)

and depositing most of the remaining solution at this point, and the final contents of the cartridge are expelled as the needle is withdrawn through the tissues. A common fault is to contact bone only a few millimetres following insertion, and in most children this will lead to unsuccessful anaesthesia. This usually occurs due to entry at too obtuse an angle and if so the needle should not be completely withdrawn but pulled back a couple of millimetres, and then advanced parallel to the ramus for about 1 cm with the barrel of the syringe over the mandibular teeth of the same side. The body of the syringe is then repositioned across the primary molars or premolars of the opposite side and advanced towards the medial border of the ramus.

Long buccal, mental and incisive blocks

The long buccal injection usually equates to a buccal infiltration in children.

The mental (or incisive nerve block) is readily administered in children as the orientation of the mental foramen is such that it faces forward rather than posteriorly as in adults (Fig. 5.4). Thus it is easier for solution to diffuse through the foramen when approached from an anterior direction. The needle is advanced in the buccal sulcus and directed towards the region between the first and second primary molar apices. A mental nerve block provides excellent soft tissue anaesthesia; however, it is not as reliable as an inferior dental block as far as pulpal anaesthesia is concerned.

The pulps of lower incisor teeth may not be satisfactorily anaesthetized by inferior dental or mental block injections due to cross-over supply from the contralateral inferior dental nerve; often a buccal infiltration adjacent to the tooth of interest is sufficient to deal with this supply.

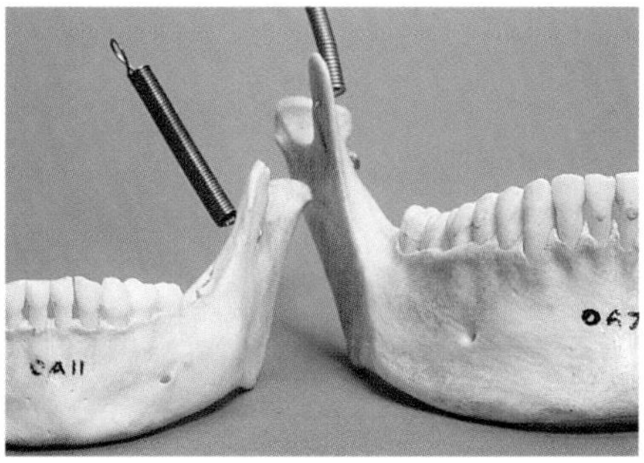

Fig. 5.4 The mental foramen faces anteriorly in children (left) compared with posteriorly in adults. (By kind permission of *Dental Update.*)

Maxillary block techniques

The use of regional block techniques is seldom if ever required in a child's maxilla. Greater palatine and nasopalatine nerve blocks are avoided by infiltrating local anaesthetic solution through already anaesthetized buccal papillae and 'chasing' the anaesthetic through to the palatal mucosa (see below). This technique is equally effective in anaesthetizing lingual gingivae in the lower jaw if infiltration or mental block techniques have been used (it is obviously not needed if a lingual block has been administered with an inferior dental block injection).

The effects of an infra-orbital block are often achieved by infiltation anaesthesia in the canine/maxillary first primary molar region in young children.

5.5.3   Intraligamentary anaesthesia

Intraligamentary or periodontal ligament (p.d.l.) anaesthesia is a very effective technique in children (Fig. 5.5) and is a method of intra-osseous injection with local anaesthetic reaching the cancellous space in the bone via the periodontal ligament. This method allows the use of small amounts of local anaesthetic solution, and the recommended dose per root is 0.2 ml. Although pulpal anaesthesia is not due to ischaemia the technique is significantly more successful when a vasoconstrictor-containing solution is employed. The anaesthetic of choice is 2 per cent lignocaine with 1:80 000 adrenaline. Sensible dose limitations must be used as entry into the circulation of intra-osseously administered drugs is as rapid as by the intravenous route.

The technique involves inserting a needle at an angle of approximately 30° to the long axis of the tooth into the gingival sulcus at the mesiobuccal aspect of each root and advancing the needle until firm resistance is met. Different authors

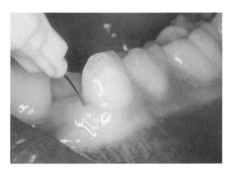

Fig. 5.5 Intraligamentary injection in a child.

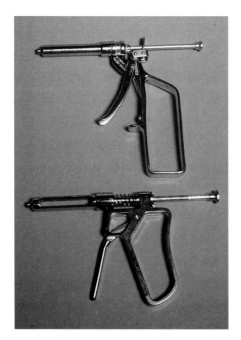

Fig. 5.6 Pistol grip intraligamentary syringes.

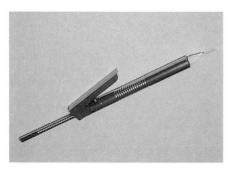

Fig. 5.7 A pen grip intraligamentary syringe. This is a less aggressive looking instrument than the pistol grip type and is preferred in children.

recommend different orientations for the bevel. It would seem sensible to have the bevel facing the bone when solution is being expelled; however, it has never been demonstrated that the direction to which the bevel faces affects the efficacy of the technique. The needle will not advance far down the ligament as even the finest needle is many times wider than a healthy periodontal ligament. The needle normally remains wedged at the alveolar crest. The solution is then injected under firm controlled pressure until 0.2 ml has been delivered. The application of the appropriate pressure is easier with specialized syringes (Figs 5.6 and 5.7) but the technique is equally effective with conventional dental syringes. Another advantage of the specialized syringes is that they deliver a set dose per depression of the trigger (0.06–0.2 ml depending on design). When using conventional syringes for intraligamentary injections the recommended dose of 0.2 ml for each root can be visualized as this is approximately the volume of the rubber bung in the cartridge. It is important not to inject too quickly; about 15 s per depression of the specialized syringe lever is needed, and it is also best to wait about 5 s after the injection before withdrawing the needle to allow the expressed solution to diffuse through the bone otherwise it escapes via the gingival sulcus into the mouth.

Intraligamentary anaesthesia reduces, but does not completely eliminate, the soft tissue anaesthesia which accompanies regional block anaesthesia in the mandible, and should therefore reduce the occurrence of self-mutilation of lip and tongue.

Intraligamentary anaesthesia is often mistakenly considered a 'one tooth' anaesthetic. This is not the case as adjacent teeth may exhibit anaesthesia and care must be used if this method is being used as a diagnostic tool in the location of a painful tooth.

There are few indications for the use of the p.d.l. technique in the maxilla because reliable pain-free anaesthesia should be possible in all regions of the maxilla using infiltration techniques. In the maxilla intraligamentary anaesthesia is best considered as a supplementary method of achieving pain control if conventional techniques have failed. However, this technique can be invaluable in the mandible and can eliminate the need for uncomfortable regional block injections.

5.6 PAIN-FREE LOCAL ANAESTHESIA

The administration of pain-free local anaesthesia depends upon a number of factors which are within the control of the operator. These factors relate to:

(1) equipment
(2) materials
(3) techniques.

5.6.1 Equipment

All components of the local anaesthetic delivery system can contribute to the discomfort of the injection. Needles should be sharp and the finest available gauge should be used. The narrowest needle used in dentistry is 30 gauge. A narrow gauge does not interfere with the ability to aspirate blood but it is worth noting that narrow needles are more likely to penetrate blood vessels than their wider counterparts.

The choice of syringe used for conventional local anaesthetic injections in children must allow aspiration both before and during the injection of the anaesthetic solution. There is evidence that inadvertent intravascular injection is more likely to occur in younger patients and positive aspirate incidences of 20 per cent of inferior dental block injections in the 7–12 year age group have been reported.

The construction of the anaesthetic cartridge can also contribute to the discomfort experienced during injection. The type of cartridge used should be one which allows depression of the rubber bung at a constant rate with a constant force. Cartridges which produce a juddering action should not be employed.

5.6.2 Materials

In the past heating the contents of local anaesthetic cartridges to body temperature prior to injection has been advised. There is no sound basis for this recommendation. There is ample evidence to suggest that patients cannot differentiate between local anaesthetics ranging in temperature from 21 to 37°C. Indeed storage of cartridges at higher temperatures can be detrimental to the solution as this can increase the chances of bacterial contamination, decrease the activity of adrenaline in the solution due to increased oxidation, and finally decrease the pH of the solution. However, cartridges stored in a refrigerator should be allowed to reach room temperature before use.

A reduction in the pH of the injected solution will increase the discomfort of the injection. Local anaesthetic solutions vary in their pH, those containing vasoconstrictors having lower values. Two per cent plain lignocaine has a pH of 6.8 compared with pH 3.2 for 2 per cent lignocaine with 1:80 000 adrenaline. Thus if minimal sensation is to be produced it may be worthwhile using a small dose of a plain lignocaine solution as an initial injection before using a vasoconstrictor-containing solution as the definitive local anaesthetic.

5.6.3 Techniques

Posterior maxillary buccal infiltrations

Assuming the proper materials and equipment have been chosen then the following technique can be used to reduce the discomfort of buccal infiltration injections in the maxilla posterior to the canine:

(1) dry the mucosa and apply a topical anaesthetic for 2 min;

(2) wipe off excess topical anaesthetic;

(3) stretch the mucosa;

(4) distract the patient (stretching the mucosa and gentle pressure on the lip between finger and thumb can achieve this);

(5) insert needle;

(6) aspirate, if positive then reposition needle without withdrawing from mucosa and when negative proceed;

(7) inject 0.5–1.0 ml supraperiosteally very slowly (15–30 s).

Anterior maxillary buccal infiltrations

Injection in the anterior aspect of the maxilla can be uncomfortable if some preparatory steps are not taken. Using the method described in steps (1)–(6) above about 0.2 ml of local anaesthetic is deposited painlessly in the first primary molar buccal sulcus on the side to be treated (Fig. 5.8). The next injection is placed anteriorly to this a minute later when soft tissue anaesthesia has spread radially from the initial injection site and further 0.2 ml increments are placed in the anterior aspect of the already anaesthetized area until the tooth of interest is

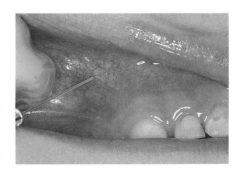

Fig. 5.8 Buccal infiltration injection in the upper primary molar region. (By kind permission of *Dental Update*.)

reached. The buccal infiltration of 0.5–1.0 ml can now be delivered painlessly through the already anaesthetized soft tissue.

Palatal anaesthesia

Injection directly into the palatal mucosa is painful. In some individuals the deposition of the solution close to a cotton wool bud coated with topical anaesthetic and applied with firm pressure for 2 min produces little discomfort especially when the pressure on the bud is increased simultaneously with needle insertion and the child is warned of this pressure increase (Fig. 5.9). However, as mentioned earlier, conventional topical anaesthetics are not very effective on the attached mucosa of the hard palate and this method is not successful with all individuals. A more reliable method of reducing the discomfort of palatal injections is to approach the palatal mucosa via already anaesthetized buccal interdental papillae. This is most readily achieved using ultra-short (12 mm) needles, which are inserted into the base of the interdental papilla at an angle of approximately 90° to the surface. The needle is advanced palatally while injecting local anaesthetic into the papilla. This is performed through both distal and mesial papillae and when a vasoconstrictor-containing solution is used blanching should be seen around the palatal gingival margin (Figs 5.10–5.12). With practice this technique can be used without the needle breaching the palatal mucosal surface which prevents the unpleasant-tasting solution inadvertently appearing in the mouth. This method usually provides sufficient anaesthesia for extractions; however, it may be supplemented by a painless gingival sulcus injection on the palatal side.

Other methods of reducing the discomfort of palatal injections which have been suggested are the use of jet injection (see above) or the use of local anaesthetic agents which exhibit excellent diffusion and allow sufficient infiltration to provide hard and soft tissue anaesthesia of the palate following buccal infiltration. Such a local anaesthetic is the amide articaine; however, this material is, at present, not widely used in the United Kingdom.

Mandibular anaesthesia

Inferior dental block injections can be uncomfortable but infiltration anaesthesia is not successful in the posterior permanent dentition. However, the use of very slow buccal infiltration anaesthesia following topical anaesthetic application in the mental foramen region can produce sufficient buccal and pulpal anaesthesia in the anterior mandibular teeth, and lingual anaesthesia can be obtained by chasing through the buccal papillae as described for palatal injections above. Alternatively, intraligamental (p.d.l.) injections may be employed to anaesthetize any of the mandibular teeth. Studies in adults have suggested that p.d.l. techniques are less unpleasant than conventional methods, but many children find delivery of anaesthetic solution via the periodontal ligament uncomfortable. The discomfort can be overcome by the following methods. The mesial buccal papilla can be treated with topical anaesthetic applied with pressure. While pressure is still being applied a papillary injection is administered followed by the intraligamental injection. However, as conventional topical local anaesthetics are not very effective on attached gingiva this method is not successful with all children. Alternatively, and this is usually more successful than the previous method in reducing pain, a small dose buccal infiltration is given apical to the tooth (this can be given as one depression of the p.d.l. syringe). This is followed by a papillary injection which should be painless, and finally by the intraligamental injection (Figs 5.13–5.15). Lingual gingival anaesthesia is obtained via the

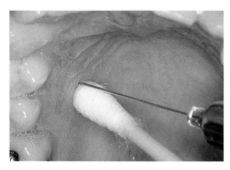

Fig. 5.9 Use of pressure and topical anaesthesia to lessen discomfort of a palatal injection. (By kind permission of *Dental Update*.)

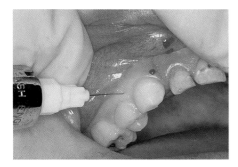

Fig. 5.10 Advancing local anaesthetic towards the palate via the buccal papilla. (By kind permission of *Dental Update.*)

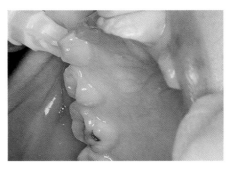

Fig. 5.11 Palatal view of Fig. 15.10 showing blanching of palate. (By kind permission of *Dental Update.*)

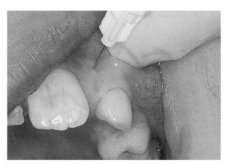

Fig. 5.12 It is simple to advance towards the palate when there is spacing of the teeth. (By kind permission of *Dental Update.*)

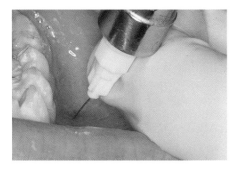

Fig. 5.13 Small dose buccal infiltration in lower premolar region for removal of lower second premolar.

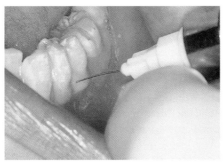

Fig. 5.14 Papillary injection after buccal infiltration.

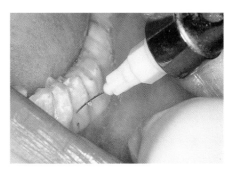

Fig. 5.15 Intraligamentary injection after papillary injection.

periodontal ligament by directing the needle through the interdental space (Fig. 5.16).

The techniques described produce minimal discomfort during local anaesthetic administration in children. When these methods are combined with relative analgesia the production of injection pain is even less likely to arise. When pain-free reliable local anaesthesia is achieved in children confidence is gained both by the child and the operator and a sound basis for a satisfactory professional relationship is established. This means that many of the treatments which were traditionally performed under general anaesthesia (such as multiple-quadrant extractions and minor oral surgery) can readily be performed in the conscious sedated child.

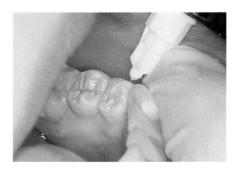

Fig. 5.16 Lingual view of Fig. 5.15 showing blanching of lingual gingiva.

5.7 COMPLICATIONS OF LOCAL ANAESTHESIA IN CHILDREN

Complications can be classified as localized and generalized and divided into early and late.

5.7.1 Generalized complications

Psychogenic

The most common psychogenic complication of local anaesthesia is fainting. The chances of this happening are reduced by sympathetic management and administration of the anaesthetic to children in the semi-supine position.

Allergy

Allergy to local anaesthetics is a very rare occurrence, especially to the amide group to which most of the commonly used dental local anaesthetics (such as lignocaine and prilocaine) belong. The only member of the ester group of local anaesthetics that is routinely used in the United Kingdom is benzocaine which is available as a topical anaesthetic preparation. Allergy can manifest in a variety of forms ranging from a minor localized reaction to the medical emergency of anaphylactic shock. If there is any suggestion that a child is allergic to a local anaesthetic they should be referred for allergy testing to the local dermatology or clinical pharmacology department. Such testing will confirm or refute the diagnosis and in addition should determine which alternative local anaesthetic can safely be used on the child. The majority of referrals prove to have no local anaesthetic allergy.

Toxicity

Overdosage of local anaesthetics leading to toxicity is rarely a problem in adults but can readily occur in children. Children over 6 months of age absorb local anaesthetics more rapidly than adults; however, this is balanced by the fact that children have a relatively larger volume of distribution and elimination is also rapid due to a relatively large liver. Nevertheless, doses which are well below toxic levels in adults can produce problems in children and fatalities attributable to dental local anaesthetic overdose have been reported. As with all drugs dosages should be related to body weight. The maximum dose of lignocaine for adults is 4.4 mg/kg. This is an easy dose to remember if one notes that the largest 2 per cent lignocaine anaesthetic cartridges available in the United Kingdom are 2.2 ml which means they contain 44 mg lignocaine. Thus a safe maximum dose is one-tenth of the largest cartridge available per kilogram. If the tenth of a cartridge per kilogram rule is adhered to then overdosage will not occur. Prilocaine, the other commonly used local anaesthetic drug in the United Kingdom has a maximum dose of 6.6 mg/ml and as it is presented normally as a 3 per cent solution the rule is one-eleventh of the cartridge per kilogram. When it is noted that a typical 5 year old weighs 20 kg it is easy to see that overdosage can easily occur unless care is exercised. The use of vasoconstrictor-containing local anaesthetics for definitive local anaesthesia is recommended in children as agents such as adrenaline might reduce the entry of local anaesthetic agents into the circulation. In addition, as vasoconstrictor-containing solutions are more effective, the need for multiple repeat injections is reduced.

Cardiovascular effects

Cardiovascular effects of the injection of a dental local anaesthetic solution will be due to the combined action of the anaesthetic agent and the vasoconstrictor.

Local anaesthetics affect the cardiovascular system by direct action on cardiac tissue and the peripheral vasculature, and also indirectly via inhibition of the autonomic nerves which regulate cardiac and peripheral vascular function. Most local anaesthetic agents will decrease cardiac excitability, and indeed lignocaine is used in the treatment of cardiac arrhythmias.

Both vasoconstrictors commonly used in the United Kingdom, namely adrenaline and felypressin can influence cardiovascular function. In addition to the beneficial effect of peripheral vasoconstriction for surgical procedures, adrenaline has both direct and indirect effects on the heart and the doses used in clinical dentistry will increase cardiac output, although this is unlikely to be hazardous in healthy children. Felypressin at high doses causes coronary artery vasocon-striction but the plasma levels which produce this are unlikely to be achieved during clinical dentistry.

Central nervous system effects

The fact that local anaesthetic agents influence activity in nerves other than peripheral sensory nerves is obvious to any practitioner who has inadvertently paralysed the peripheral branches of the motor facial nerve during a mandibular block injection. Similarly, the central nervous system is not immune to the effects of local anaesthetic agents. Indeed plasma concentrations of local anaesthetics which are incapable of influencing peripheral nerve function can profoundly affect the central nervous system. At low doses the effect is excitatory as central nervous system inhibitory fibres are blocked, at high doses the effect is depressant and can lead to unconsciousness and respiratory arrest. Fatalities due to local anaesthetic overdosage in children are generally due to central nervous tissue depression.

Methaemoglobinaemia

Some local anaesthetics cause specific adverse reactions when given in over-dosage and the main toxic effect of prilocaine is cyanosis due to methaemoglobin-aemia. In methaemoglobinaemia the ferrous iron of normal haemoglobin is converted to the ferric form, which cannot combine with oxygen.

Treatment of toxicity

The best treatment of toxicity is prevention. Prevention is aided by:

(1) aspiration;
(2) slow injection;
(3) dose limitation.

When a toxic reaction occurs then the procedure is:

(1) stop the dental treatment;
(2) call for medical assistance;
(3) protect the patient from injury;
(4) monitor vital signs;
(5) provide basic life support.

Drug interactions

Specialist advice from the appropriate physician should be requested in the treat-ment of children on significant long-term drug therapy. Apparently innocuous drug combinations can interact and cause significant problems in children, for example an episode of methaemoglobinaemia has been reported in a 3 month old child following the application of EMLA®. It was concluded from that case that prilocaine (in the EMLA®) had interacted with a sulphonamide (which can also produce methaemoglobinaemia) that the child was already receiving.

Infection

The introduction of agents which can produce generalized infection such as HIV and hepatitis is a complication which should not occur when appropriate cross-infection control measures are employed.

5.7.2 Early localized complications

Pain

Pain resulting from local anaesthetic injections can occur at the time of the injection due to: the needle penetrating mucosa; too rapid an injection; or injection into an inappropriate site. The sites at which injection may be painful include:

(1) intra-epithelial;
(2) subperiosteal;
(3) into the nerve trunk;
(4) intravascular.

Intra-epithelial injection is uncomfortable as a result of ballooning of the tissues at the commencement of the injection due to lack of dispersion of the solution.

Subperiosteal injection may produce pain both at the time of injection and post-operatively. The initial pain is due to injection into a confined space causing stripping of the periosteum from bone.

Direct contact of the nerve trunk by the needle produces an electric shock type of sensation and immediate anaesthesia. This is most likely to occur in the lingual and inferior dental nerves during inferior dental nerve blocks. Unfortunately, this complication is more common with experienced operators as it represents good location of the needle. When it occurs solution should not be injected at that point but delivered after the needle has been withdrawn slightly to avoid intraneural injection.

Intravascular injection

Accidental intravascular injections can easily occur in children if aspiration is not performed.

Intravascular injections can cause local pain if the vessel penetrated is an artery and spasm occurs. Intravenous injections can produce systemic effects which may be alarming, such as tachycardia and palpitations.

Intra-arterial injections are much rarer than intravenous injections; however, the effects of an intra-arterial injection can be alarming. Such effects range from local pain and cutaneous blanching (Fig. 5.17) to severe intracranial problems. The rare cases of hemiplegia following local anaesthetic injections which have been reported can be accounted for by rapid intra-arterial injection producing sufficient intracranial blood levels of the local anaesthetic to produce central nervous tissue depression.

Failure of local anaesthesia

Inability to complete the prescribed treatment due to failure of the local anaesthetic can be due to a number of causes including the following:

(1) anatomy
(2) pathology
(3) operator technique.

Anatomical causes of failed local anaesthesia can result from either bony anatomy or accessory innervation. Bony anatomy can inhibit the diffusion of

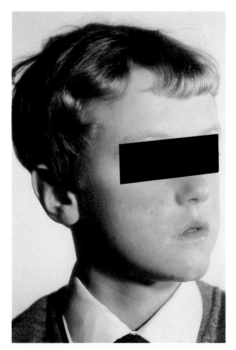

Fig. 5.17 Blanching of the cheek after intra-arterial injection in a child.

solution to the apical region when infiltration techniques are used and this can occur in children in the upper first permanent molar region due to a low zygomatic buttress. To overcome this problem the anaesthetic is infiltrated both mesially and distally to the upper first molar/zygomatic buttress region.

Accessory innervation may also produce failed local anaesthesia. In the upper molar region this may be due to pulpal supply from the greater palatine nerves, which can be blocked by supplementary palatal anaesthesia. In the mandible accessory supply from the cervical nerves will not be blocked by inferior dental, lingual, and long buccal blocks and may require supplementary injections in the lingual sulcus. The commonest area of accessory supply occurs near the mid-line where bilateral supply often necessitates supplemental injections when regional block techniques are employed.

The presence of acute infection interferes with the action of local anaesthetics. This is partly due to the reduction in tissue pH decreasing the number of union-ized local anaesthetic molecules, which in turn inhibits their diffusion through lipid to the site of action (the number of ionized versus unionized molecules is governed by pH and the pKa of the agent). In addition nerve endings stimulated by the presence of acute infection are hyperalgesic.

Regional block and intraligamental methods of local anaesthesia are technique dependent and often failure of these forms of local anaesthesia are due to the operator. This cause of failure becomes less common with experience. Infiltration anaesthesia is a very simple method which is readily mastered by novices and when this injection fails reasons other than operator technique should be sought.

Motor nerve paralysis

Paralysis of the facial nerve can occur following deposition of local anaesthetic solution within the substance of the parotid gland due to malpositioning of the needle during inferior dental block injections. The terminal branches of the facial nerve run through the parotid gland and will be paralysed by the anaesthetic agent. The most dramatic manifestation of this complication is loss of the ability to close the eyelids on the affected side and necessitates the provision of an eye patch until paralysis wears off.

This side-effect is probably more common in adults as the anatomy of the child's mandible is such that inability to palpate successfully the medial aspect of the mandible with the needle is uncommon.

Although paralysis of the eyelid is most often due to faulty technique during inferior dental block anaesthesia, the use of excessive amounts of solution in the maxillary buccal sulcus can also cause it.

Interference with special senses

Interference with vision and hearing after the intra-oral injection of local anaesthetics have been reported. Such occurrences most probably result from accidental intra-arterial injection.

Haematoma formation

Penetration of a blood vessel can occur during local anaesthetic administration; however, haematoma formation is rarely a problem unless it occurs in muscle following inferior dental block techniques when it may lead to trismus (see below).

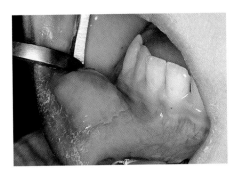

Fig. 5.18 Self-inflicted trauma following an inferior dental block injection. (By kind permission of *Dental Update.*)

5.7.3   Late localized complications

Self-inflicted trauma

Self-inflicted trauma is common following local anaesthetic injections in children and may follow regional techniques in the mandible and infiltration anaesthesia in the maxilla. The commonest site is the lower lip (Fig. 5.18); however, the tongue and upper lip can also be affected.

It can be prevented by adequate explanation to the patient and parent by the clinician.

The use of periodontal ligament techniques may reduce the frequency of this complication; however, it must be stressed that soft-tissue anaesthesia is not completely avoided with this method in all cases.

Oral ulceration

Occasionally, children will develop oral ulceration a few days following local anaesthetic injections. This is usually due to trauma initiating an aphthous ulcer; however, rarely needle trauma may activate a latent form of herpes simplex.

Long-lasting anaesthesia

Long-lasting anaesthesia can result from direct trauma to a nerve trunk from the needle or from injection of solution into the nerve. This may occur after regional block techniques but is a rare complication.

Trismus

Trismus may follow inferior dental block injections and is usually the result of bleeding within muscle due to penetration of a blood vessel by the needle. However, injection of solution directly into muscle tissue may also result in trismus. The condition is self-resolving; however, it may take a few weeks before normal opening is restored.

Infection

Localized infection due to the introduction of bacteria at the injection site is a complication which is rarely encountered

Developmental defects

Local anaesthetic agents are cytotoxic to the cells of the enamel organ and it is possible that the incorporation of these agents into the developing tooth germ could cause developmental defects. There is experimental evidence that such defects can arise following intraligamental injections in primary teeth in animal models; however, such occurrences in humans have not been reported. In addition to cytotoxic effects of the anaesthetic agent it is possible that physical damage to permanent successors from the needle could result from overenthusiastic use of intraligamentary anaesthesia in the primary dentition.

5.8   CONTRA-INDICATIONS TO LOCAL ANAESTHESIA IN CHILDREN

In certain children some local anaesthetic materials will be contra-indicated, in others specific techniques are not advised.

5.8.1 General

Immaturity

Very young children are not suited to treatment under local anaesthesia as they will not provide the degree of co-operation required for the completion of treatment. A child who cannot differentiate between painful and non-painful stimuli (such as pressure) is not suitable for treatment under local anaesthesia.

Mental or physical handicap

Where the degree of handicap precludes co-operation local anaesthesia is contraindicated.

Treatment factors

Certain factors related to the proposed treatment may preclude the use of local anaesthesia. These factors include time and access.

Prolonged treatment sessions, especially if some discomfort may be produced such as during surgical procedures, cannot satisfactorily be completed under local anaesthesia. It is unreasonable to expect a child to co-operate for more than 30–40 min under such circumstances even when sedated.

Similarly, where access proves difficult or uncomfortable, for example during biopsies of the posterior part of the tongue or soft palate, satisfactory co-operation may not be possible under local anaesthesia.

Acute infection

As mentioned above acute infection reduces the efficacy of local anaesthesia.

5.8.2 Specific agents

Allergy

Allergy to a specific agent or group of agents is an absolute contra-indication to the use of that local anaesthetic.

Medical conditions

Some medical conditions present relative contra-indications to the use of some agents. For example in liver disease the dose of amide local anaesthetics should be reduced. Ester local anaesthetics should be avoided in children who have a deficiency of the enzyme pseudocholinesterase.

Poor blood supply

The use of vasoconstrictor-containing local anaesthetic solutions should be avoided in areas where the blood supply has been compromised, for example after therapeutic irradiation.

5.8.3 Specific techniques

Bleeding diatheses

Injection into deep tissues should be avoided in patients with bleeding diatheses such as haemophilia. Inferior dental block techniques should be avoided. This can be overcome by the use of intraligamental injections in the mandible in such patients for restorative dentistry.

Susceptibility to endocarditis

Intraligamentary anaesthesia will produce a bacteraemia. In patients susceptible to endocarditis this method should not be used for procedures in which gingival manipulation would not normally be involved as it is unreasonable to provide antibiotic prophylaxis for the anaesthetic when other methods of local anaesthesia can be employed; if antibiotic prophylaxis has been provided to cover the operative procedure then of course intraligamental injections can be employed.

Incomplete root formation

The use of intraligamental techniques for restorative procedures on permanent teeth with poorly formed roots could lead to avulsion of the tooth if inappropriate force is applied during the injection.

Trismus

Trismus can preclude the intra-oral approach to the inferior dental nerve block. The external approach to this nerve is not recommended in children.

Epilepsy

As seizure disorders can be triggered by pulsing stimuli (such as pulses of light) it is perhaps unwise to use electro-analgesia in epileptic children.

5.9   SUMMARY

1. Surface anaesthesia is best achieved with a topical agent on a cotton bud applied to dry mucosa for 2 min.
2. Buccal infiltration anaesthesia is successful in the maxilla.
3. Regional block anaesthesia is successful in the mandible.
4. Intraligamentary anaesthesia is successful in children. This method may be first choice in the mandible and as a supplementary technique in the maxilla.
5. Pain-free local anaesthesia in the maxilla is possible with buccal infiltration and by anaesthetizing the palate via the buccal papillae.
6. In the mandible intraligamental techniques may be used to avoid the discomfort of regional block injections.
7. Complications of local anaesthesia are reduced by careful technique and sensible dose limitations.
8. Contra-indications to local anaesthesia may be related to certain agents or to specific techniques.

5.10   FURTHER READING

Malamed, S. F. (1990). *Handbook of local anesthesia*. Mosby, St Louis. (*An excellent reference book.*)

Meechan, J. G. (1992). Intraligmentary anaesthesia: a review of literature. *Journal of Dentistry*, **20**, 325. (*A critical assessment of periodontal ligament anaesthesia.*)

Moore, P. A. (1992). Preventing local anesthetic toxicity. *Journal of the American Dental Association*, **123**, 60. (*A salutary case report of a paediatric local anaesthetic fatality.*)

6 Dental caries

6 Dental caries

A. J. RUGG-GUNN

6.1 DEVELOPMENT OF DENTAL CARIES

Almost all research on the process of dental caries supports the chemoparasitic theory proposed by W. D. Miller in 1890. This is now more commonly known as the acidogenic theory of caries aetiology. The main features of the caries process are: (a) fermentation of dietary sugars by micro-organisms in plaque on the tooth surface to organic acids; (b) rapid acid formation which lowers the pH at the enamel surface below the level (the critical pH) at which enamel will dissolve; (c) when sugar is no longer available to the plaque micro-organisms, the pH within plaque will rise due to the outward diffusion of acids, and their metabolism and neutralization in plaque so that remineralization of enamel can occur, and (d) dental caries progresses only when demineralization is greater than remineralization.

One of the interesting features of an early carious lesion of the enamel is that the lesion is subsurface; that is, most of the mineral loss occurs beneath a relatively intact enamel surface. This contrasts strongly with the histological appearance of enamel after a clean tooth surface has been exposed to acid, where the surface is etched and there is no subsurface lesion. This dissolution of the surface of enamel, or etching, is a feature of erosion of enamel caused, among other things, by dietary acids. The explanation for the intact surface layer in enamel caries seems to lie in diffusion dynamics: the layer of dental plaque on the tooth surface acting as a partial barrier to diffusion.

Dental plaque forms on tooth surfaces which are not cleaned and is readily apparent if toothbrushing is stopped for 2–3 days. Contrary to popular opinion, plaque does not consist of food debris, but is 70 per cent micro-organisms — about 100 million organisms per mg of plaque. When plaque is young, cocci predominate but as plaque ages the proportions of filamentous organisms and veillonellae increase. Diet influences the composition of the plaque flora considerably, with mutans streptococci much more numerous when the diet is rich in sugar, and these organisms are particularly good at metabolizing sugars to acids.

Knowledge of the dental caries process increased considerably with the development of pH electrodes, particularly micro-electrodes which could be inserted into plaque before, during, and after the ingestion of various foods. The pioneer of this area of research was Robert Stephan, and the plot of plaque pH against time (Fig. 6.1) has become known as the Stephan curve.

Within 2–3 min of eating sugar or rinsing with a solution of sugar, plaque pH falls from an average of about 6.8 to near pH 5, taking about 40 min to return to its original value.

The clinical appearance of these early lesions is now well recognized (Figs 6.2–6.5). They appear as a white area which coincides with the distribution of plaque. This might be around the gingival margin, as in Fig. 6.2, or between

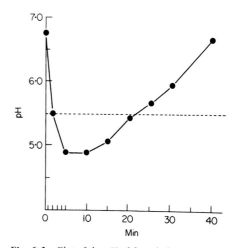

Fig. 6.1 Plot of the pH of dental plaque against time: this is commonly known as a Stephan curve. The curve was produced by rinsing with a 10 per cent glucose solution. The dotted line represents a typical value of pH below which enamel will dissolve (the critical pH). (Reproduced from Jenkins (1978) with permission.)

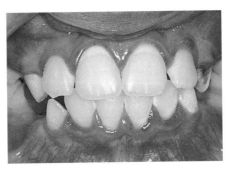

Fig. 6.2 Clinical appearance of pre-cavitation carious lesions on the buccal surfaces of maxillary incisor teeth.

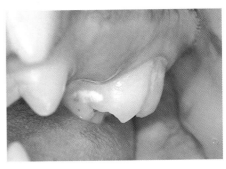

Fig. 6.3 Clinical appearance of a pre-cavitation carious lesion on the mesial surface of a maxillary first molar tooth.

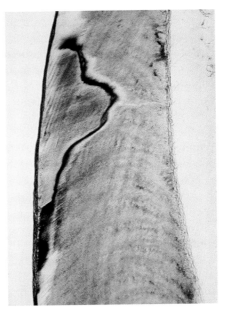

Fig. 6.4 Longitudinal ground section through a carious lesion of the type shown in Fig. 6.3, examined in water by polarized light × 50. (Reproduced from Soames and Southam with permission.)

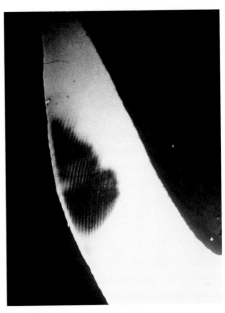

Fig. 6.5 Micro-radiograph of a longitudinal ground section through a lesion of the type shown in Figs. 6.3 and 6.4. The body of the lesion shows marked radiolucency (loss of mineral) in contrast to sound enamel and the surface layer: × 70. (Reproduced from Soames and Southam with permission.)

the teeth, as in Fig. 6.3. A histological section through a lesion such as that shown in Fig. 6.3 would look like Fig. 6.4 and a micro-radiograph like Fig. 6.5 — in both, the subsurface body of the lesion and surface zone can be seen clearly. If the process of dental caries continues, support for the surface layer will become so weak that it will crumble like an eggshell, creating a cavity. Once a cavity is formed, the process of dental caries continues in a more sheltered environment and the protein matrix of enamel and then dentine is removed by proteolytic enzymes produced by plaque organisms.

The ability of early carious lesions ('pre-cavitation carious lesions') to remineralize is now well understood; periods of demineralization are interspersed with periods of remineralization, and the outcome — health or disease — is the result of a push in one direction or the other on this dynamic see-saw. The shorter the time during which plaque-covered teeth are exposed to acid attack and the longer the time during which plaque pH is high and remineralization can occur, the greater is the opportunity for a carious lesion to heal. Satisfactory healing of the carious lesion can only occur if the surface layer is unbroken, and this is why the 'pre-cavitation' stage in the process of dental caries is so relevant to preventive dentistry. Once the surface has been broken and a cavity has formed, it is usually necessary to restore the tooth surface with a filling. The first stages of dental caries — to the visible 'white spot' pre-cavitation lesion stage — can occur within a few weeks if conditions are very favourable to its development. In the general population, though, it commonly takes 2–4 years for caries to progress through enamel into dentine.

The most important of the natural defences against dental caries is saliva. If salivary flow is impaired, dental caries can progress very rapidly. Saliva has many functions, which are listed in Table 6.1. The presence of food in the mouth is a powerful stimulus to salivation, with strong-tasting acid foods being the best stimulants. Saliva not only physically removes sugars and acids produced by plaque from the mouth, but it has a most important role in buffering the pH in saliva and within plaque. Fast-flowing saliva is alkaline — reaching pH values of 7.5–8.0 — and is vitally important in raising the pH of dental plaque previously lowered by exposure to sugar. Because teeth consist largely of calcium and phosphate, the concentration of calcium and phosphate, in saliva and plaque is thought to be important in determining the progression or regression of caries. Also, it is well-known that fluoride aids the remineralization process. Although it may seem sensible to try to maximize the availability of calcium, phosphate and fluoride in the environs of the tooth, in practice, fluoride is much the most important.

Key Points

Dental Caries:
- occurs in plaque-covered areas frequently exposed to dietary sugars
- the initial lesion is subsurface before the thin surface layer collapses
- the initial or pre-cavitation lesion is reversible
- saliva plays an essential part in caries prevention

Table 6.1   The general functions of saliva

Digestive functions
    Assisting the mastication of food
    Forming a bolus
    Assisting in swallowing of bolus
    Taste perception
    Metabolism of starch

Protective functions
    Ensuring comfort through lubrication
    Preventing dessication of oral mucosa, gingivae, and lips
    Antimicrobial
        lavage
        bacteriostatic, bacteriocidal
        inhibiting adhesion of bacteria
        aggregation of bacteria
    Buffering
        within saliva
        within dental plaque
    Removal of toxins (including carcinogens)
    Aids speech

6.2   THE EPIDEMIOLOGY OF DENTAL CARIES

Dental caries is one of our most prevalent diseases and yet there is considerable variation in its occurrence between countries, regions within countries, areas within regions, social and ethnic groups. One of the tasks of epidemiology is to record the level of disease and the variation between groups. A second task is to record changes in dental caries levels in populations over time, while a third task is to try to explain these variations.

The United Kingdom has one of the best series of national statistics on dental caries. The dental health of adults and children has been recorded every 10 years, beginning with the Adult Dental Health Survey of 1968 (Table 6.2). The advantages of this series of surveys are: (a) that they are national, using sound sampling methods to obtain representative samples of the populations; (b) they include both clinical and sociological data, giving the interaction between knowledge, attitude, behaviour, and disease; and (c) methods are well-described and carefully standardized, resulting in meaningful longitudinal information.

Ravages of dental caries were so severe in the past that the extent of disease in a population was measured by the proportion of the population with no natural teeth — or edentulousness. A marked decrease in the per cent edentulous between 1968 and 1988 was recorded, especially in adults aged 35–44 years.

For younger people, it is common to record the prevalence (the proportion of people affected) and the severity (number of teeth affected per person) of dental

Table 6.2   National surveys of children's and adults' dental health in the United Kingdom

Children	
England and Wales	1973
United Kingdom*	1983
United Kingdom*	1993
Adults	
England and Wales	1968
Scotland	1972
United Kingdom*	1978
United Kingdom*	1988

* England, Wales, Scotland, and Northern Ireland.

Table 6.3   Decay experience of 5 year old children (primary teeth), 12 and 14 year old children (permanent teeth) in England and Wales, as recorded in national surveys

	1973	**1983**	**1993**
5 years			
Per cent affected	72	49	45
Mean dmft	4.0	1.8	1.8
12 years			
Per cent affected	93	79	50
Mean DMFT	4.8	2.9	1.2
14 years			
Per cent affected	96	88	59
Mean DMFT	7.4	4.7	1.9

dmft, DMFT: decayed, missing, and filled teeth.

caries. The drastic improvement in both of these parameters in England and Wales between 1973 and 1993 is shown in Table 6.3. About half of all children are now 'caries-free'. What is of concern is opinion that in the youngest age groups the improvement is not continuing and indeed there are signs that caries experience is increasing in some areas.

A world decline in caries, first noticed during the 1970s, has been recorded in a large number of industrialized countries. The dental health of older children continued to improve in the 1980s but caries experience in primary teeth, measured at ages 5 or 6 years, had stayed fairly constant. The Nordic countries used to have very high caries experience and the drastic improvement in all five Nordic countries can be seen in Fig. 6.6, although it occurred somewhat later in Iceland. One of the most dramatic improvements has been recorded in Switzerland where the mean DMFT (decayed, missing, filled teeth) in 12 year olds fell from 8.0 in 1964, to 5.1 in 1972, 3.0 in 1980, to 1.1 in 1992. In 15 year olds it fell from 13.9 DMFT in 1964 to 2.2 DMFT in 1992. Caries experience in Australian children has been well recorded indicating a dramatic improvement in dental health (Fig. 6.7). Reports from North America indicate that caries prevalence and severity in the permanent dentition have continued to decline since 1982 in Canada and the United States but that caries experience in the primary dentition may have stabilized since about 1986–87.

While dental surveys of school children have been quite common, there is much less information on the dental health of pre-school children mainly because access to them is more difficult. The prevalence and severity of dental caries in British pre-school children was reviewed by Holt, and in pre-school children around the world by Holm. In most European countries, North America, and Australia, caries experience has declined in parallel with the increasing use of fluoride toothpastes, although this decline appears to have stopped in the United Kingdom. Caries experience of pre-school children in South-East Asia, Central America, and parts of Africa is high and there are discernable trends of increasing prevalence in parallel with the rise in availability of sugar-containing snacks.

While the state of the permanent dentition in children has improved dramatically in many countries, caries in primary teeth is still a considerable problem in

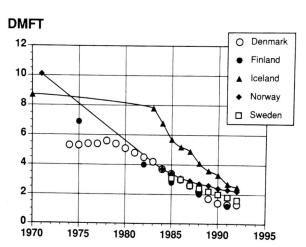

Fig. 6.6 Caries experience (DMFT) for 12 year old children in Nordic countries. (Reproduced from von der Fehr with kind permission of the *International Dental Journal*.)

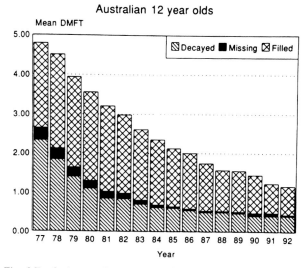

Fig. 6.7 Caries experience in Australian 12 year olds. (Reproduced from Spencer with kind permission of the *International Dental Journal*.)

pre-school and school children. In industrialized countries caries experience is highest in the more deprived groups of society and often in ethnic minority groups. In developing countries, the reverse social trend is observed, with the better off, urban children having the most caries experience. Most of these variations in children's dental health can be explained in terms of the preventive role of fluoride and the caries-inducing role of sugary snacks. In adults, provision of dental services and patient preference for treatments can have a major effect on the state of the dentition in addition to the aetiological and preventive roles of sugar and fluoride.

Key Points

Dental caries:

- epidemiology indicates the size of the problem of caries and changes over time
- since 1968 there have been surveys every 10 years of adult's and children's dental health in the United Kingdom
- prevalence and extent have fallen markedly since the late 1970s in many countries
- remains a problem in pre-school children in many countries

6.3 CARIES DIAGNOSIS AND CLINICAL CHARACTERISTICS

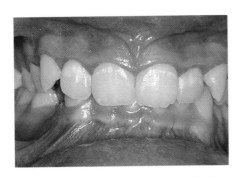

Fig. 6.8 Clinical appearance of pre-cavitation carious lesions on the labial and approximal surfaces of maxillary incisor teeth.

Caries diagnosis is frequently difficult because of the continuum of dental caries. The initial demineralization is invisible to the eye and the first visible sign is faint whiteness of the intact enamel surface especially when the tooth surface is dried well. As demineralization progresses, the whiteness of the lesion increases and the surface shine changes to a matt finish. During this time the surface is still intact and examples of these lesions are given in Figs 6.2, 6.3, and 6.8. The greatest mineral loss occurs beneath the surface layer which eventually gets so undermined that it collapses and a cavity is formed. The maxillary canine tooth shown in Fig. 6.9 has extensive carious lesions including a newly formed cavity in the white lesion near the gingival margin and an older cavity, which has taken up some stain. If demineralization and removal of the protein matrix of dentine progress, total destruction of the tooth will follow.

There are very good reasons for dividing carious lesions into pre-cavitation lesions, where the surface outline is still intact, and cavities, where the surface integrity has been lost. Only in exceptional circumstances (e.g. over-riding aesthetic considerations) should pre-cavitation lesions be restored. It is usual to restore cavities — to restore the function and aesthetics of the tooth and prevent further caries progression — although in rare situations (especially on exposed surfaces) caries progression can arrest and the tooth need not be restored. Recognizing pre-cavitation lesions is important as they are a warning sign and prevention must be vigorously persued. Under favourable conditions these pre-cavitation lesions can regress (remineralize) to the appearance of a sound surface or, at least, remain as a pre-cavitation lesion without progressing to a cavity.

Dental caries can be confused with developmental defects of tooth formation. There are numerous causes of interruption of tooth development with defects varying from very minor whiteness of enamel to gross abnormalities of tooth structure (Chapter 12). A number of signs help the clinician to distinguish between developmental defects and dental caries. First, dental caries tends to occur at predilection sites — it rarely occurs on cusps or incisal edges while developmental defects are not uncommon there. Second, and most important, developmental defects tend to follow incremental lines of enamel while pre-cavitation carious lesions, especially on labial/buccal tooth surfaces, tend to follow the present or previous line of the gingival margin. This is because dental caries occurs beneath plaque and plaque is often found adjacent to the gingival margin. This is illustrated in Figs 6.2 and 6.8; while in Fig. 6.2 pre-cavitation carious lesions are observed adjacent to the gingival margin, indicating present caries attack, the pre-cavitation lesions shown in Fig. 6.8 are some distance from the present gingival margin, indicating past caries attack when the gingival margin was more coronal. From the preventive viewpoint, the situation shown in Fig. 6.2 calls for immediate action, while the person illustrated in Fig. 6.8 should be congratulated as the previous caries attack (which might have recurred about 2 years previously) has been overcome and the enamel newly exposed by the naturally receding gingivae is sound. This situation is often called 'tide-mark caries' — whether these white areas will disappear completely is difficult to say but some improvement can be expected through further remineralization and natural abrasion.

Cavitation may be easy to record on accessible buccal or lingual (free smooth) surfaces but is definitely more difficult in pits and fissures and approximal surfaces. There has been much work assessing the accuracy of various methods in detecting carious cavities on fissure and approximal surfaces. These methods have included the eye alone (visual), the eye plus probe (visual tactile), radiography (usually bitewing radiographs), and electrical resistance methods (ERM). (see section 3.9, Further reading) The accuracy or validity of a diagnostic method can be quantified by calculating 'sensitivity' and 'specificity'.

Sensitivity is the proportion of carious surfaces that are detected by the method under test, i.e. a measure of the true positive diagnoses; for example, if a method detected 80 per cent of carious cavities, the sensitivity will be 0.80 or 80 per cent. Specificity is the proportion of surfaces that are not carious which are recorded by the method under test as non-carious, i.e. a measure of true negatives; for example, if a method recorded as non-carious 70 per cent of all the non-carious surfaces, the specificity of the method would be 0.70 or 70 per cent.

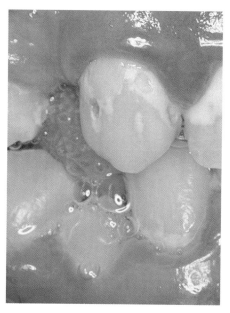

Fig. 6.9 Maxillary permanent canine tooth showing a variety of carious lesions. Plaque has been removed. Much of the enamel has pre-cavitation carious lesions but cavitation has occurred in three places.

Caries Treatment:	**Key Points**
● pre-cavitation lesion — prevention	
● cavitation lesion — restoration and prevention	

As far as diagnoses of carious cavitation or caries into dentine in occlusal surfaces are concerned, the general conclusions are that visual examination has high specificity (near 0.9 or 90 per cent) but low or moderate sensitivity (0.6–0.7): thus cavities are missed but there is little over filling. Using ERM as a means of detecting fissure caries is of growing interest, with several research workers reporting both high sensitivity and specificity.

Diagnosis of caries on approximal surfaces is difficult and bitewing radiographs have been used as an adjunct for many years. Using 'caries into dentine' assessed on histological examination as the validating criterion, Downer reported that radiolucency at or beyond the amelodentinal junction had a sensitivity of 0.73 and a specificity of 0.97, i.e. if these surfaces with radiolucencies to the amelodentinal junction had been restored, there would be little over-filling, but some lesions into dentine would not have been restored.

Fibre-optic transillumination (FOTI) has been suggested as an adjunct to clinical examination and an alternative to radiological examination of approximal surfaces. A very fine light source is placed in the interproximal area (Fig. 6.10). Mitropoulos reported that FOTI recorded slightly fewer lesions into dentine than bitewing radiographs in a study of 12–13 year old children. Sensitivity was reported to be 0.73 and specificity 0.99. Thus, very few surfaces recorded as sound (no lesion in dentine) on bitewing radiographs were recorded carious using FOTI.

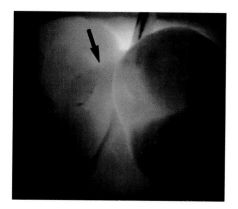

Fig. 6.10 Fibre-optic transillumination (FOTI) of approximal surfaces of posterior permanent teeth. The arrow points to a shadow caused by an approximal carious lesion. (Illustration from Mitropoulos with kind permission of *Caries Research*.)

Key Points   Caries diagnosis:

- visual–tactile supported by bitewing radiographs remains the most satisfactory method
- electrical resistance measurement is the most promising newer method
- systematic and random errors in diagnosis are great

6.4   PREVENTION OF DENTAL CARIES

The dramatic improvement in dental health, especially in children, in many developed countries during the past 15 years is proof that prevention works. Dental caries is not inevitable; the causes are well known and discouraging caries development and encouraging caries healing are realities to be grasped. Failure to do so is, at least, to provide second class dental care.

There are four practical pillars to the prevention of dental caries: diet, fluoride, plaque control, and fissure sealing. Each of these will be considered in turn before being brought together in treatment planning.

Prevention of caries is so easy in theory but in practice involves many skills. The main reason for this is that control of the aetiological agents — plaque and sugar — involve a change in behaviour. There is no 'magic bullet' that can be applied to teeth which will render them totally resistant to caries. Fissure sealants come close to this but they are expensive to apply, some fall off, and they only prevent caries of pits and fissures. The value of fluoride is that it can be delivered in a variety of ways, some of which require minimal action by the patient. Of the four practical methods listed, diet and fluoride remain the most important.

6.4.1   Nutrition and diet in caries control

There is very extensive information on the effect of nutrition and diet on dental caries. Although it has been recognized for many years that sugar is the main dietary cause of dental caries, there remain a number of areas where some clarification is desirable. These are:

1. Does nutrition while teeth are forming influence future susceptibility to dental caries?
2. Are all sugars and sugar-containing foods equally cariogenic?
3. Is frequency of eating the only variable of any importance?
4. What are the main sources of sugars in the diet?
5. Is there any benefit in using non-sugar sweeteners?

Each of these issues will be considered in turn.

The pre-eruptive influence of diet

The Health Education Authority, London, has said quite clearly, in its influential publication *The Scientific Basis for Dental Health Education*, that fluoride was the only nutrient that had any pre-eruptive influence on a tooth's future caries susceptibility. This seems a reasonable conclusion for well-nourished populations but whether this is also true for less well-nourished populations is unclear as caries development in those populations seems more rapid than in their well-nourished counterparts for any given level of sugar intake. Malnourished children may have less well developed salivary glands resulting in less, and poorer quality, salivary flow. They may have a higher prevalence of hypoplastic dental enamel which has been associated with higher caries experience, although the relationship between hypoplasia and caries is not necessary causal. There is no doubt that fluoride is protective against dental caries but its effect is mainly post-eruptive. Some other trace elements may influence caries development — e.g. molybdenum, strontium — but their effect is minor compared with that of fluoride.

Cariogenicity of sugars and sugar-containing foods

There is some evidence that sucrose is the most cariogenic sugar but the other common dietary sugars, glucose, fructose, and maltose are not far behind; there is little advantage in substituting these sugars, or glucose or fructose syrups, for sucrose in order to reduce cariogenicity. Lactose is less cariogenic. Adolescent children in developed countries ingest about 100 g of sugars per day. About two-thirds of this total daily sugars intake comes from so-called 'added sugars' or 'free sugars'. These have also been called non-milk extrinsic (NME) sugars to distinguish them from milk sugar (lactose in milk) and intrinsic sugars (in fruit and vegetables). This distinction is important in dietary advice as neither lactose in milk nor intrinsic sugars are seen as a threat to dental health; it is the NME sugars, or free sugars as WHO calls them, which are responsible for the epidemic of dental caries during the twentieth century. Staple starchy foods — potatoes, bread, rice, pasta — are not a cause of dental caries but mixtures of finely ground heat-treated starch and sugars — such as occurs in biscuits — are likely to be as cariogenic as sugars themselves.

Frequency of eating

There is much evidence that frequency of eating sugars is important in caries development and educators are right to advise reducing frequency of sugar intake. But it is wrong to suggest that quantity of sugar is unimportant as there is also much evidence that the amount of sugar eaten per day is positively related to caries development. This is not surprising as in free-living people there is a strong correlation between amount eaten per day and frequency of eating sugary foods. Advice should be to reduce both amount and frequency.

Sources of sugars in the diet

Two-thirds for NME sugars in English school children are in confectionery, soft drinks and table sugar, and it is not surprising that these are the targets in dental health education (Table 6.4). In young children, sugar-containing fruit-flavoured drinks are a major threat to dental health and a frequent cause of 'rampant' caries (Fig. 6.11). Numerous reports have highlighted the damage caused by these drinks especially if given in dinky or reservoir feeders or lightweight bottles which can be easily left with the young child. Unnecessary addition of extra sugar to milk feeds is also a cause of caries in young children.

Non-sugar sweeteners

Those allowed for use in foods and drinks in the United Kingdom are given in Table 6.5; the list is very similar for most countries. There is much evidence that they are non-cariogenic or virtually so. The intense sweeteners and xylitol are non-cariogenic while the other bulk sweeteners can be metabolized by plaque bacteria but the rate is so slow that these sweeteners can be considered safe

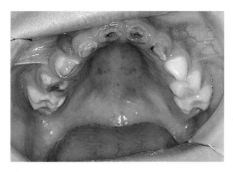

Fig. 6.11 'Rampant caries' in 3 year old child caused by frequent and prolonged use of a bottle containing fruit-flavoured sugar-containing drink.

Table 6.4 Mean daily intake of non-milk extrinsic sugars from various dietary sources (as grams and as per cent of sugars intake) in two surveys of about 400 12 year old English children in 1980 and 1990

		1980		1990		
		%	g	g	%	
Confectionery		29	24	30	33	
Soft drinks	71%	19	15	24	27	60% 72%
Table sugar		23	19	11	12	
Biscuits and cakes		11	10	10	11	
Sweet puddings		9	7	5	6	
Breakfast cereals		2	2	5	5	
Syrups and preserves		3	3	2	2	
Other sources		3	3	3	4	
All sources		100	83	90	100	

Table 6.5 Permitted sweeteners in foods (United Kingdom)

Bulk sweeteners
    Sorbitol
    Mannitol
    Hydrogenated glucose syrup*
    Isomalt*
    Xylitol*
    Lactitol[†]
Intense sweeteners
    Saccharin
    Acesulfame K*
    Aspartame*
    Thaumatin*

* permitted 1982.
[†] permitted 1988.

for teeth. The use of non-sugar sweeteners is growing rapidly particularly in confectionery and soft drinks. Confectionery products which have passed a well-established acidogenicity test can be labelled with the Mr Happy-Tooth logo (Fig. 6.12) which is a protected trademark, which informs the purchaser and consumer that these products are dentally safe. Toothfriendly sweets are available (in 1994) in about 26 countries; in Switzerland about 20 per cent of confectionery sold carries the Toothfriendly (or Mr Happy-Tooth) logo. There is good evidence that sugarless chewing gums are not only non-cariogenic but also positively prevent dental caries, by stimulating salivary flow.

The bulk sweeteners can have a laxative effect and should not be given to children below 3 years of age. People vary in their sensitivity to these polyols as some adults in the Turku sugar studies were consuming up to 100 g of xylitol per day without effect.

Dietary advice for the prevention of dental caries

The basic advice is straightforward — reduce the frequency and amount of intake of NME sugars. It is important that advice for dental health is compatible with advice for general health. For many years there has been a consensus in the United Kingdom and in many other countries on dietary goals. These are: reduce consumption of fats, especially saturated fatty acids, NME sugars and alcohol, and increase consumption of staple starchy foods, fresh fruit, and vegetables. The most common targets set by Governments are that fats should provide no more than 35 per cent and NME sugars between 0 and 10 per cent of food energy intake; present consumption levels for adolescents are about 40 per cent for fat and 17 per cent for NME sugars. Dietary advice for the under 5 year olds should be cautious, guarding against over-restriction of fat intake but intake of NME sugars is acknowledged to be too high in this group. Some sick children require special diets which have to be high in sugars intake in order to be calorie-sufficient — particularly those with disorders of protein and fat metabolism — and dentists should be prepared to liaise with dietitians in order to ensure that these children's diets are best for general and dental health.

Dietary advice should be at two levels. First, every patient should receive basic advice. This especially applies to parents of young children who need to be given the correct advice at the appropriate age of the child. They need constant encouragement to resist the pressures of commercial food and drink companies to buy products generally high in NME sugars, and often fats. Confectionery is not only the most important source of sugars in the diet of adolescents, but is now the second most important source of dietary fats.

Dietary advice is often too negative; energy which has been provided by confectionery has to be replaced and it is very important to emphasize positive eating habits. The variety of foods available has increased enormously in most countries in recent years; we must use this increased choice to assist our patients to make better food choices — in broad terms this means increasing consumption of starchy foods, fresh fruit, and vegetables.

The second level of advice is a more thorough analysis of the diet of children with a caries problem. A well accepted method is the 3 day diary record. One practical drawback of this method is that it requires at least three visits — an introductory visit where the patient is motivated and informed about the procedure and the diet diary given out, the diary collection visit, and a separate visit for advice and to agree targets. Each of these stages is important. At the first visit it is vital that the patient and parent appreciate that there is a dental problem and that you are offering your expert advice to help them overcome this problem. Once motivated they must understand how the diary is to be completed. Any requests by parents for advice at the first visit should be parried and delayed until the third visit. At the third visit, advice must be *personal, practical,* and *positive* — all three of these are important. Food preference of children, cooking skills, food availability, and financial considerations vary enormously — advice must be personally tailored and practical for that patient. Positive advice has a much greater chance of acceptance than negative advice such as 'avoid this', 'don't eat that' — nagging is a de-motivator. Dietary changes are difficult, targets often have to be limited and constant reinforcement of advice and encouragement is essential. However, health gains can be considerable, to general as well as dental health and often to other members of the family, so that dietary advice is an essential part of care of children.

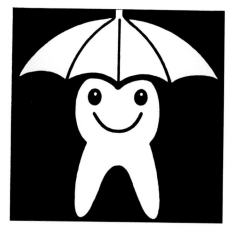

Fig. 6.12 Pictogram of Mr Happy-Tooth. This is the protected logo of the International Toothfriendly Association to be seen on products which have passed the internationally accepted toothfriendly test. (Reproduced by kind permission of the Association.)

6.4.2 Fluoride and caries control

Fluoride is effective at preventing caries because of a combination of properties all of which work in the same direction. The major property of fluoride seems to be its ability to increase remineralization of dental enamel but it also increases enamel's resistance to demineralization and decreases acid production in plaque. In the early days of fluoride research, fluoride's role in strengthening enamel against acid attack was considered paramount and ingestion of fluoride while teeth are forming was thought to be all-important. This pre-eruptive effect is important but now seems to be less important than the post-eruptive local intra-oral effect of fluoride. This division of action into pre-eruptive and post-eruptive has led to the development of systemic fluoride agents — those made to be swallowed — and topical fluoride agents — those made to be applied to teeth in the mouth and not to be swallowed. It is still useful to classify the several ways of delivering fluoride in this way, not least because only one systemic method of giving fluoride should be offered but any number of topical methods. However, it should be appreciated that there is much cross-over in action between topical and systemic methods with systemic methods giving substantial topical benefit while they are in the mouth, and some fluoride given topically will be swallowed and incorporated into any teeth forming. Each of the methods will be considered in turn.

Water, salt, and milk

Fifty years ago, the fluoride concentration in the water supply to Grand Rapids, USA, was adjusted upwards to 1.0 p.p.m. (1.0 mg fluoride/L). Now, 56 per cent of the population (145 million people) in the United States received optionally fluoridated water; 43 of the 50 largest cities are fluoridated. Water fluoridation schemes have been introduced into 20 countries reaching about 230 million people. In Europe, water fluoridation is not widespread; Ireland is the exception with 60 per cent of its population receiving fluoridated water, and in the United Kingdom about 10 per cent (5.5 million) of the population live in fluoridated areas. Those who care for dental health of children should know the concentration of fluoride in the water supplies in their area. There is much evidence that water fluoridation cuts caries by half. It has the tremendous advantage of reaching the whole of the population and brings great benefit to those in greatest need who are frequently in the more deprived groups and least able to take advantage of other caries preventive measures.

The main alternative to water as a vehicle for fluoride, is salt. Schemes operate in Switzerland, France, Germany, and some countries in Central and South America. The concentration of fluoride in salt is usually 250 mg fluoride/kg salt. Although there is little doubt that salt fluoridation is effective, there are much less data on its effectiveness compared with water fluoridation. Milk is another vehicle for fluoride; fluoridized milk has been shown to be effective in caries prevention and trial schemes are currently operating in communities in several different countries. The usual concentration is 5 mg fluoride/L milk.

Fluoride dietary supplements

Soon after the effectiveness of water fluoridation became apparent, dentists looked for other ways of providing fluoride, especially to young children who received fluoride-deficient water. Providing fluoride in tablet form was an obvious choice. On the assumption that children consumed 1 litre of tap-water per day, tablets were made containing 1 mg fluoride; younger children would have half this dose. Since the first trial in 1960, the effectiveness in caries prevention of daily administration of fluoride tablets has been established clearly in a large number of trials. Drops are more practical for young children.

Although fluoride drops and tablets — often known as fluoride dietary supplements — have been used widely throughout the world as an alternative to water fluoridation, their use has changed and they are seldom now recommended universally for all children. Over the last 10 years there has been a reduction in the daily dosage of fluoride from tablets. This is also due to two main reasons: (a) the realization that the original dose was probably too high as children drink much less than 1 litre of water per day, and (b) fluoride is ingested from other sources by young children, particularly toothpastes but also drinks made in fluoridated areas.

Despite the above cautious commentary, fluoride tablets have an important place in preventive dentistry. Dentists wishing to recommend their use or prescribe them to patients should check the fluoride level of the child's drinking water, choose the current recommended dosage in that country, explain fully the use of fluoride dietary supplements to the parent, motivate the patient and parent and continually encourage them in their endeavours.

Fluoride toothpastes

World-wide, fluoride toothpastes are by far the most important vehicle for fluoride. For very many industrialized countries, the addition of fluoride to toothpaste became almost unwittingly the turning-point in caries prevention. In the United Kingdom, caries prevalence and experience reached a peak in the late 1950s and 1960s; by the mid-1970s, the caries decline had begun. While in 1970 virtually no toothpaste contained fluoride, by 1978, 97 per cent contained fluoride. Initially, the most popular fluoride concentration in toothpastes was 1000 p.p.m. (1 mg fluoride/g toothpaste). By 1980, it was clear that caries prevention increased if the fluoride concentration was raised from 1000 to 1500 p.p.m. and many toothpastes now contain this higher concentration. Paedodontists and manufacturers were then concerned that young children might ingest sufficient fluoride from toothpaste to cause visible developmental defects of enamel. This concern led to the development and marketing of toothpastes containing about 500 p.p.m. fluoride (0.5 mg/g toothpaste) as children's toothpastes. Trials showed that caries prevention was slightly less when the concentration was about 500 p.p.m. fluoride compared with 1000 or 1500 p.p.m. fluoride. Thus a compromise had to be reached between a high fluoride concentration for maximum caries prevention and a low fluoride concentration in children's toothpastes to lessen the possibility of discoloration of forming teeth. Opinions differ quite sharply as to whether it is necessary and sensible for young children to use a toothpaste containing 500 p.p.m. fluoride rather than 1000 p.p.m. fluoride and the age when a person should begin to use a 1500 p.p.m. fluoride toothpaste. On present evidence, a reasonable suggestion is: from 1 to 5 years, a 500 p.p.m. fluoride toothpaste; 6–11 years, a 1000 p.p.m. fluoride toothpaste; and over 11 years, a 1500 p.p.m. fluoride toothpaste.

The Health Education Authority has for many years recommended that children put a pea-size amount on their brush and, although there is some disagreement between experts, this seems sensible advice. Parents should supervise the brushing of their children's teeth. In older children, excessive rinsing after brushing is unnecessary and may be counterproductive in washing fluoride away from the tooth's environment.

Fluoride mouthrinses

A large number of trials have demonstrated the ability of fluoride mouthrinses to prevent caries. Frequency of rinsing is important with daily rinsing more effective than weekly or fortnightly rinsing. For daily rinses, the concentration is usually 0.05 per cent sodium fluoride (about 225 p.p.m. fluoride) and for weekly rinses 0.2 per cent sodim fluoride (about 900 p.p.m. fluoride). In Scandinavia, the United States and Ireland, fluoride mouthrinsing has been the method of choice for school-based caries-preventive programmes. They were considered the major factor in reducing the very high caries experience in Sweden in the 1960s. It is fair to say that with the general decline in caries in children in these and other countries, health authorities have stopped many of these school-based programmes, relying on the home-based use of fluoride toothpaste instead.

Fluoride mouthrinses are extremely useful in the care of patients with specific caries-preventive problems. These might include: (a) patients with a number of pre-cavitation carious lesions, and (b) patients undergoing fixed or removable orthodontic therapy. As with all home therapy, patient selection, motivation, and encouragement are very important. Young children are likely to swallow rinses and it is usual only to recommend the use of fluoride rinses after 6 years of age.

Clinical application of fluoride solutions, gels and varnishes

These are concentrated solutions containing about 1 per cent fluoride; they are for use in the dental surgery and are not suitable for home use. Two per cent neutral sodium fluoride (9000 p.p.m. fluoride) was the first concentrated fluoride solution to become established, but the use of stannous fluoride solutions and acidulated phosphate fluoride (APF) gels applied in trays followed soon after. Their effectiveness has been established in many trials and there is little to choose between them. A common frequency of application is 6 monthly but increasing the frequency increases effectiveness.

More recently, fluoride varnishes have been developed, and have the advantage that application is quick, in that the varnish can get wet straight after application, while the application time for solutions and gels is 4 min. Varnishes are especially useful for young children and the taste of the varnish is acceptable too.

There has been concern over the amount of fluoride swallowed from gels and varnishes. There is a greater potential problem with gels as trays can be overloaded and the high salivary flow induced by the highly flavoured acid gel encourages swallowing. Guidelines for gel and tray application urge: (a) that the patient be upright; (b) the trays should be well-filling and should not be more than half full; (c) use of a saliva ejector; (d) wipe the mouth after the tray is removed and ask the patient to spit out (but not rinse); and (e) this technique should not be used in children under 5 years of age.

Combining fluoride therapies in a treatment plan for a patient

Although each individual method of giving fluoride is effective, a combination of two or more methods results in greater benefit. The golden rule is that there should only be *one* systemic method of delivering fluoride (water *or* salt *or* milk *or* drops/tablets) but any number of topical methods, subject to restrictions for young children mentioned above. Table 6.6 gives a guide as to which therapies might be appropriate depending upon water fluoride level, age and perceived caries risk. (see section 16.2.4.)

Table 6.6 Guidelines for planning fluoride therapy for patients

Risk groups	Under 6 years	6–15 years	Adults
Fluoridated community			
Low caries risk	Toothpaste	Toothpaste	Toothpaste
Average caries risk	Toothpaste	Toothpaste	Toothpaste
High caries risk	Toothpaste	Toothpaste	Toothpaste
	Topical varnish	Topical gel/ varnish	Topical gel/ varnish
		Mouthrinse	Mouthrinse
Low fluoride community — less than 0.3 p.p.m.			
Low caries risk	Toothpaste	Toothpaste	Toothpaste
Average caries risk	Toothpaste	Toothpaste	Toothpaste
	Drops/tablets	Tablets	Mouthrinse
High caries risk	Toothpaste	Toothpaste	Toothpaste
	Drops/tablets	Tablets	Topical gel/ varnish
	Topical varnish	Topical gel/ varnish	Mouthrinse
		Mouthrinse	

6.4.3 Fissure sealing

The idea of sealing pits and fissures in teeth from the oral environment is at least a century old, but it was not until the development of the 'acid etch' technique in the 1950s that fissure sealing was considered seriously. This discovery coincided with the results of early fluoride studies which showed that fissure surfaces were least protected and approximal and free-smooth surfaces the most protected by fluoride. Owing to the widespread use of fluoride, the majority of carious cavities now occur in pits and fissures. Thus, the combination of fluoride therapy and fissure sealing is very attractive.

The technique of fissure sealing is simple but very sensitive to water contamination.

Several materials have been used but the most successful and popular is bis GMA resin. Polyurethane materials were very poorly retained, while cyano-acrylate resins and glass ionomer cements were more retentive but not as good as bis GMA. Glass ionomer sealants contain substantial concentrations of fluoride and give some caries preventive effect despite short retention times. They may be used in the child with a high caries rate and are placed as soon as the fissure system of a newly erupted tooth is visible (without this intervention the tooth would probably be carious by the time it had gained occlusion and was accessible for conventional resin sealant). Glass ionomer cement is run into the fissures after the tooth has been washed and dried. A square of green occlusal adjustment wax is then burnished over the occlusal surface and will keep the sealant dry until it sets. Newer light cured glass ionomer cements may not be as beneficial in this situation as the fluoride may be 'locked in' and not as available for release.

Both filled and unfilled resins have been used successfully as sealants, and while some operators prefer clear sealants because of better flow and aesthetic characteristics and the assurance of being able to see underlying enamel through the sealant, others prefer a white or tinted sealant because it can be more easily checked (Chapter 7).

Key Points

Fissure sealing:
- prophylaxis before etching does not enhance retention but may be advisable when there is much plaque present
- etching with 30–40 per cent phosphoric acid for 20–30 s is now fairly standard
- washing, re-isolation, and drying are critical steps and contamination with saliva must be avoided — the use of rubber dam can assist this
- etched enamel not covered with sealant will remineralize within 24 h

While the first photo-initiated sealants were activated intra-orally by ultra-violet lights, most are now set by 'blue' lights which are less hazardous. Nevertheless, the use of a light shield is advisable to protect the operator's eyes.

There have been a large number of clinical trials on resin sealants; the longest so far lasting 15 years. A common result is for 50 per cent of sealants to be retained for at least 5 years. The younger the child and the further back in the mouth the tooth being sealed, the poorer the retention rate. Re-sealing teeth which had lost their sealant was not practised in the majority of trials for experimental purposes, but re-sealing would now be advocated. Stained fissures should always be investigated prior to sealing and any lesions into dentine restored with preventive resin restorations (Chapter 7).

Although the effectiveness of fissure sealant is beyond doubt, their cost-effectiveness is hotly debated. Sensible guidelines for patient selection and tooth

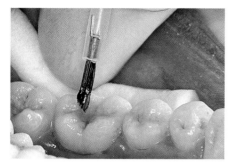

(a)

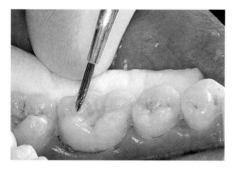

(b)

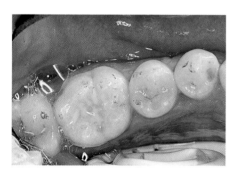

(c)

Fig. 6.13 Fissure sealant placement on a first permanent molar tooth: (a) etching gel applied with brush; (b) fissure sealant application after washing and drying; (c) occlusal analysis.

selection have been published by the British Society for Paediatric Dentistry, and these are given below.

Patient selection

1. Children with special needs. Fissure sealing of all occlusal surfaces of permanent teeth should be considered for those who are medically compromised, physically or mentally disabled, or having learning difficulties, or for those from a disadvantaged social background.
2. Children with extensive caries in their primary teeth should have all permanent molars sealed as soon as possible after their eruption.
3. Children with caries-free primary dentitions do not need to have first permanent molars sealed routinely; rather these teeth should be reviewed at regular intervals.

Tooth selection

1. Fissure sealants have the greatest benefit on the occlusal surfaces of permanent molar teeth. Other surfaces should not be neglected, in particular the cingulum pits of upper incisors. The sealing of primary molars is not normally advised.
2. Sealants should normally be applied as soon as the selected tooth has erupted sufficiently to permit moisture control.
3. Any child with occlusal caries in one first permanent molar should have the fissures of the sound first permanent molars sealed.
4. Occlusal caries affecting one or more first permanent molars indicates a need to seal the second permanent molars as soon as they have erupted sufficiently.

Technique

Clean and dry the tooth surface and ensure that there are no stained fissures. Isolate the tooth with saliva ejector, cotton wool rolls and dry tips, or with rubber dam. Etch the fissures with 30–40 per cent phosphoric acid for 20–30 s, wash for 30 s, and dry for 30 s. Deposit some resin (chemical or light cured) into the fissures and encourage the resin to flow into and along all the fissures. Do not to touch the etched areas with an instrument as this will destroy the etch pattern. Either light-cure (30 s) or wait for self-cure (3 min). After curing check the sealant to ensure no contamination has occurred and then check the occlusion (Fig. 6.13a–c). Excess material can be removed with a round diamond bur.

6.4.4 Toothbrushing and other methods of plaque removal

As dental caries is caused by bacteria in plaque fermenting dietary sugar to acids which dissolve enamel, it is logical to prevent caries by removing plaque from teeth, usually with a toothbrush. Unfortunately, many investigations indicate that caries reduction is not brought about by improved toothbrushing alone. However, it must be said straight away that, first, toothbrushing is a very important way of controlling gingivitis and periodontal disease and, second, that toothbrushing with toothpaste is a very important way of conveying fluoride to the tooth surface. The vital role of fluoride toothpastes in controlling dental caries over the past 20 years was emphasized previously.

The results of the few studies to investigate the effect of flossing on dental caries are mixed. Daily flossing of the teeth of young children reduced caries in one study but no preventive effect was observed in older children who flossed their own teeth.

Twenty years ago, in Kalstaad, Sweden, caries increments were virtually eliminated in children who had fortnightly prophylaxes and intensive preventive advice by dental hygienists. Other workers have tried to reproduce those sensational results (96 per cent caries reduction compared with a control group) but have failed to do so, illustrating the difficulty of extrapolating findings of trials from one country to another.

Plaque growth can be prevented by twice-daily rinsing with chlorhexidine but because of the intra-oral side-effects of chlorhexidine (changed taste sensation, poor taste, and tooth staining), it is usually recommended for short-term use only to aid periodontal care.

6.4.5 Treatment planning for caries prevention

The above summaries of the various methods of preventing dental caries have highlighted the advantages and disadvantages of the four practical methods of caries prevention: diet, fluoride, fissure sealing, and plaque control. Each is capable of preventing caries, but achieving changes in diet and toothbrushing, undertaking fissure sealing, and applying fluoride in the dental chair are all time-consuming. It is unrealistic to attempt to use each method to its maximum potential and it is necessary to agree an overall philosophy. Everyone should receive some advice in caries prevention and those perceived to be at greater risk of and from dental caries should receive a more thorough investigation and preventive treatment plan.

Four clear preventive messages are promoted by the Health Education Authority (HEA) in England (Table 6.7). This is the minimum advice. Parents of infants and young children should be advised on sensible eating habits; the abuse of sugar-containing fruit-flavoured drinks and the need for meals which will reduce the demand for sugar-laden snacks. Toothbrushing should be observed in the surgery giving an opportunity to discuss the type of toothbrush and toothpaste.

Some patients are more likely to develop dental caries than others, and these patients need more aggressive preventive advice and therapy. Effective toothbrushing with an appropriate fluoride toothpaste is an essential first goal. Other forms of fluoride therapy should be considered, as outlined above (Table 6.7): drops/tablets (if the drinking water is fluoride deficient), mouth rinses, and topical applications of solutions, gel or varnish. Dietary habits should be investigated using a 3 day diet diary and appropriate advice given that is personal, practical and positive. As toothbrushing, rinsing, and sugar control all require

Table 6.7 The scientific basis of dental health education

Summary

1. Reduce the consumption and especially the frequency of intake of sugar-containing food and drink and very acid drinks.
2. Clean the teeth thoroughly every day with a fluoride toothpaste.
3. Request your local water company to supply water with the optimum fluoride level.
4. Have an oral examination every year.

Health Education Authority (1996).

changes in life-style especially at home, continuous encouragement is essential. Fissure sealing is likely to be sensible, in line with the guidelines set out above.

The order in which the various caries preventive measures are scheduled in the treatment plan is of some importance. It is sensible to investigate toothbrushing early, as it is a good bridge between the home and the dental surgery and it gives proper emphasis to this vital preventive measure. If done first, it allows you to work on clean teeth. As investigation of diet and dietary advice requires at least three visits, it is sensible to introduce this by the second appointment. Fissure sealing can be commenced early in the treatment plan as a relatively easy procedure giving emphasis to prevention rather than restoration, while topical fluoride therapy could be carried out after fissure sealing. If fluoride dietary supplements and/or mouth rinses are going to be recommended, it is sensible to introduce them on the first or second appointment so that continuous encouragement in their use might be given at later appointments.

The above intensive preventive therapy is for patients 'at risk' of developing caries. This begs the question on how to predict future caries development. There has been much work on this topic with many risk factors or markers of caries risk proposed. Overall, the findings are not encouraging. The most successful are: past caries experience, saliva properties (flow rate, buffering power, and microbiological content), and social status. These can be used in combination to increase discriminatory power. Despite much work, one large American investigation showed that the best predictor of future caries increment in children was 'intuition of the dentist'.

Key Points

Prevention:

- the four practical methods of caries prevention are: sugar control, fluoride, fissure sealing, and plaque control
- the effects of these methods are additive
- treatment planning takes into account age, caries risk, water fluoride level, and co-operation
- diet advice in particular has to be personal, practical, and positive

6.5 SUMMARY

1. Dental caries is caused by dietary sugars being fermented by plaque bacteria to acid.
2. The pre-cavitation lesion is a danger sign indicating the need for prevention.
3. The four practical pillars to caries prevention are: diet, fluoride, fissure sealing and toothbrushing.
4. Preventive advice must be to parent and child and should be appropriate to the age and circumstances of the child.
5. Motivation and continuous encouragement is essential if prevention is to be successful.

6.6 FURTHER READING

British Society of Paediatric Dentistry (1992). A policy document on sugars and the dental health of children. *International Journal of Paediatric Dentistry*, **2**, 177–80. (*A short concensus view of the BSPD.*)

British Society of Paediatric Dentistry (1993). A policy document on fissure sealants. *International Journal of Paediatric Dentistry*, **3**, 99–100. (*A very short document giving the BSPD concesus view on patient and tooth selection.*)

Gordon, P. H. and Nunn, J. H. (1996). Fissure sealants. In *The prevention of oral disease* (ed. J. J. Murray), (3rd edn) pp. 78–94. Oxford University Press, Oxford. (*Like the above reviews, the emphasis is on the results of research rather than a 'cookbook'.*)

Health Education Authority (1996). *The scientific basis of dental health education* (4th edn). Health Education Authority, London. (*Often considered the 'bible' in DHE in the UK A consensus view of 'experts' in England.*)

Holm, A. K. (1990). Caries in the preschool child; international trends. *Journal of Dentistry*, **18**, 291–5. (*The only review of this subject worldwide — comprehensive.*)

Murray, J. J., Rugg-Gunn, A. J., and Jenkins, G. N. (1991). *Fluorides in caries prevention* (3rd edn). Butterworth-Heinemann, Oxford. (*Nineteen chapters, nearly 400 pages: the most comprehensive review of this subject.*)

Naylor, M. N. (1994). Second international conference on declining caries. *International Dental Journal*, **44** (Suppl. 1), 363–458. (*A special supplement containing 13 papers on changes in caries prevalence worldwide.*)

Rugg-Gunn, A. J. (1993). *Nutrition and dental health*. Oxford University Press, Oxford. (*Eighteen chapters, nearly 500 pages: the only comprehensive review of this subject.*)

Sutcliffe, P. (1996). Oral cleanliness and dental caries. In *The prevention of oral disease* (ed. J. J. Murray), (3rd edn) pp. 68–77. Oxford University Press, Oxford. (*A short, but comprehensive review of the evidence relating oral cleanliness and plaque to caries.*)

7 Operative treatment of dental caries

7   Operative treatment of dental caries

J. PAGE and R. R. WELBURY

7.1   INTRODUCTION

While there is no doubt that the best way to tackle the problem of dental caries is through an effective programme of prevention as outlined in the previous chapter, it is unfortunate that many children still suffer from the disease and its consequences. Hence there is a need for operative treatment to prevent the breakdown of the dentition.

Over the years the treatment of dental caries in children has been discussed and many attempts made to rationalize the management of the disease. Writing 150 years ago Harris was one of the first to address the problem of restoring the primary dentition. Even in those days he was emphasizing the importance of prevention by good toothbrushing. Caries could be arrested by 'plugging', but from his description he obviously found treatment for the young patient difficult and not as successful as in adults. However, he did emphasize the importance of looking after the teeth of children: 'If parents and guardians would pay more attention to the teeth of their children, the services of the dentist would much less frequently be required', and, 'Many persons suppose that the teeth, in the early periods of childhood, require no attention, and thus are guilty of the most culpable neglect of the future well-being of those entrusted to their care'. Unfortunately this statement still applies today.

The huge number of different techniques and materials that have been advocated over the years since Harris wrote those words testify to the fact that no ideal solutions have so far been found. Unfortunately, most treatments are advocated on the basis of dentists' clinical impressions and there have been very few objective studies that have attempted to discover which treatments succeed and which are a waste of time and effort.

It is not possible to cover the whole field of operative treatment for children in one chapter and the reader is directed to other texts for a fuller account of available techniques. However, it is possible to outline the rationale for providing operative treatment, to give advice on the selection of appropriate ways of providing care, and to describe a few of the more useful treatment methods.

7.2   REMOVE, RESTORE, OR LEAVE

When faced with a tooth that has caries the first decision has to be whether it requires treatment or not. It may be felt that the caries is so minor and prevention so effective that further progress of the lesion is unlikely. Less rationally it may be felt that a carious tooth with a non-vital pulp and near to exfoliation is unlikely to cause great problems and may be left to its own devices. Although this decision is not one of which the authors would approve there are significant reasons why it may be inadvisable to treat a particular tooth.

7.2.1   Reasons not to treat

These can be divided into several distinct categories.

1. *The damage done by treatment to:*

   (a) *The affected tooth.* However conservative the technique it is inevitable that some sound tooth tissue has to be removed when operative treatment is undertaken. This weakens the tooth and makes it more likely that problems such as cracking of the tooth or loss of vitality of the pulp may occur in the future.

Key Point

- Every time that a restoration is replaced more sound tissue has to be removed putting the tooth at further risk.

   (b) *The adjacent tooth.* It is almost inevitable when treating an approximal lesion that the adjacent tooth will be damaged. The outer surface has a far higher fluoride content than the rest of the enamel so that even a slight nick of the intact surface will remove this reservoir of fluoride. Additionally, it has been shown that early lesions that remineralize are less susceptible to caries than intact surfaces and these areas of the tooth are all too easily removed when preparing an adjacent tooth.

Key Point

- Early lesions that remineralize are less susceptible to caries.

   (c) *The periodontal tissues.* Dental treatment can cause both acute and long-term damage to the periodontium. It is virtually impossible to avoid damaging the interdental papillae when treating approximal caries. The papillae can be protected by using rubber dam and/or wedges and if well fitting restorations are placed the tissues will heal fairly rapidly but long-term damage can be more critical. Many adults can be seen to be suffering from over-enthusiastic treatment of approximal caries in their youth and while the relative importance of poor margins compared to bacterial plaque can be debated, the potential damage from approximal restorations is sufficient reason to avoid treatment unless a definite indication is present.

   (d) *The occlusion.* Poor restoration of the teeth can, over time, lead to considerable alteration of the occlusion. It is tempting when restoring occlusal surfaces to leave the material well clear of the opposing teeth to avoid difficulties or to be unconcerned if the filling is slightly 'high'. However, this can allow the teeth to erupt into contact again or the interocclusal position to change and alter the occlusion. Often this is felt to be of little concern but there are a large number of adults where the cumulative effect of many poorly restored teeth has severely disturbed the occlusion making further treatment difficult, time consuming, and expensive.

2. *The difficulty of diagnosis.* It is well known that it is difficult to diagnose dental caries accurately. Even when coarse criteria such as those developed for the United Kingdom Child Dental Health Surveys are used, there is wide variation between examiners. It is not just variations between examiners that need to be considered as there is also a marked difference between the same examiner on different occasions. The implications need to be considered in relation to the decision to treat or not.

3. *The slow rate of caries attack.* Caries usually progresses relatively slowly, although some individuals will show more rapid development than others. The majority of children and adolescents will have a low level of caries and progress of carious lesions will be slow. In general the older the child at the time that the caries is first diagnosed the slower the progression of the lesion.

However, a substantial group of children will have caries that develops rapidly.

4. *The fact that remineralization can arrest and repair enamel caries*. It has long been known that early smooth surface lesions are reversible and it is now accepted that the chief mechanism whereby fluoride reduces caries is by encouraging remineralization and that the remineralized early lesion is more resistant to caries than intact enamel. Although it is difficult to show reversal of lesions on radiographs many studies have demonstrated that a substantial proportion of early enamel lesions do not progress over many years.

5. *The short life of dental restorations*. Surveys of dental treatment have often shown a rather disappointing level of success. In general 50 per cent of amalgam restorations in permanent teeth can be expected to fail during the 10 years following placement. Some studies have shown an even poorer success rate when looking at primary teeth and this has been put forward as a reason for not treating these teeth.

7.2.2 Reasons to treat

1. *Adverse effects of neglect*. The fact that the treatment of approximal caries can cause damage to the affected tooth, the adjacent tooth, the periodontium, and the occlusion is a valid reason to think twice before putting bur to tooth. But, of course, a case could equally well be made that the neglect of treatment will cause as much or more damage. Lack of treatment can, and all too often does, lead to loss of contact with adjacent and opposing teeth, exposure of the pulp resulting in the development of periapical infection, and/or loss of the tooth.

2. *Unpredictability of the speed of attack*. While it is true that the rate of attack is usually slow it is quite possible for the rate in any one individual to be rapid so that any delay in treatment would not then be in the best interests of the child.

3. *Difficulty in assessing if a lesion is arrested or not*. Because of the normally slow rate of attack it is difficult to be sure if a lesion is arrested or merely developing very slowly. It is true that remineralization will arrest and repair early enamel lesions but there is, in fact, little evidence that remineralization of the dentine or the late enamel lesion is common.

4. *Success when careful treatment is provided*. The majority of published studies show that class II amalgam restorations in primary teeth have a poor life expectancy but this is not the experience of the careful dentist and some of these have published their results showing that the great majority of their restorations in primary teeth survive without further attention until they exfoliate. The treatment procedures used are not particularly difficult in comparison to others that dentists attempt on adults and it is difficult to avoid the conclusion that the reasons for poor results in some studies are due to poor patient management and lack of attention to detail. It should be the aim of the profession to develop better and more effective ways of treating the disease rather than throwing our hands up in surrender.

5. *Early treatment is more successful than late*. Small restorations are more successful than large and therefore if a carious lesion is going to need treatment it is better treated early rather than late. This was the rationale behind the early suggestions of Hyatt of a 'prophylactic filling' for pits and fissures and for the modern versions in the form of fissure sealants and preventive resin restorations. The fact that small restorations are often more successful makes for difficult decisions

when the management of caries involves preventive procedures which need both time to work and time to assess whether they have been effective.

7.2.3 Remove or restore

Once a decision has been made to treat a carious tooth a further decision has to be made as to whether to remove or restore it. This decision should take into account the following.

1. *The child.* Each child is an individual and treatment should be planned to provide the best that is possible for that individual. Too often treatment is given which is the most convenient for the parent or more likely the dentist. Is it really in the best interest of the child to remove a tooth which could be saved? In the United Kingdom general anaesthesia is still widely used for removing the teeth of young children despite the risks of death, it's unpleasantness, and the cost involved. It would seem that this procedure is often prescribed because of the preference of the dentist rather than that of the parent or child.

Key Point

- Treat the child — not the convenience of parents or dentist.

2. *The tooth.* It is not usually in a child's interest for a permanent tooth to be removed. However, if the pulp of a carious permanent tooth is exposed a considerable amount of treatment may be required to retain it, and the prognosis for the tooth would still be poor. It may therefore be in the child's long-term interest to lose it and to allow another tooth to take its place either by natural drift or with orthodontic assistance.

Primary teeth are often considered by parents and some dentists as being disposable items because there comes a time when they will be exfoliated naturally. However, it is an unusual child who thinks the same way! Loss of a tooth before its time has a considerable significance in a child's life. Losing a tooth early gives a message to the child that teeth are not valuable and not worth looking after. It can then be difficult to persuade a child to care for their teeth. A well restored primary dentition can be a source of pride to young children and an encouragement for them to look after the succeeding teeth.

It is usually more important and fortunately rather easier to save and restore a second primary molar than a first. While anterior teeth might be less important for the maintenance of space their premature loss can cause low esteem in both child and parent.

3. *The stage of the disease.* It is easier for both child and dentist to restore teeth at an early stage of decay. Later the pulp may become involved and subsequent restoration difficult making loss of the tooth more likely.

4. *The extent of the disease.* A large number of teeth requiring treatment may put a strain on a young child and less importantly on the parent and dentist.

Caries in children is significantly less than it was 20 years ago and it would be good to think that the dental profession would be able to restore the reduced number of decayed teeth that now present.

7.2.4 Diagnosis and treatment planning

This was discussed in Chapter 3 and will be only briefly outlined here. As stated above the treatment of carious teeth should be based on the needs of the child. The long-term objective should be to help the child reach adulthood with an intact permanent dentition, with no active caries, as few restored teeth as possible, and a positive attitude to their future dental health. If restoration is required it should be carried out to the highest standard possible in order to maximize longevity of the restoration and avoid retreatment.

Diagnosis

Careful diagnosis of the extent of the disease is required before treatment is undertaken. Each tooth needs to be looked at carefully and assessed as to the possible need for endodontic treatment and whether a simple or extensive restoration is required. Radiographs should be available if anything other than a very minimal restoration is to be placed. It can usually be assumed that if the marginal ridge of a primary molar is broken, due to undermining by caries, treatment of the pulp will be required. It would then be wise to consider the use of a preformed metal crown to restore the tooth.

- Destruction by caries of the marginal ridge of a primary molar indicates likely pulpal involvement.

Key Point

Treatment planning

Following diagnosis of the extent of caries in each tooth and the probable state of the pulp, a logical treatment plan should be made which would usually involve treating a quadrant of the mouth at a time. It used to be felt that multiple short visits placed least stress on a child particularly if they were under 6 years of age. However, the most important aspect of child management is to gain the confidence of the child and make sure that there is as little discomfort as possible. Once the tissues have been anaesthetized and the child is confident that there will be no pain it is usually best to complete treatment on a whole quadrant. The number of visits can then be kept to a minimum and a reservoir of co-operation maintained.

If a child is in pain then it matters little if an appointment is 5 min or 45. It is more important to make sure that there is no pain. It is critical that any dentist who is treating children is confident in using all available methods of local analgesia including infiltration, mandibular block, interpapillary, intraligamentous, and intraosseous techniques (Chapter 5).

7.3 DURABILITY OF RESTORATIONS

In contrast to the amount of useful research which has been carried out with regard to the diagnosis and prevention of dental caries, methods of treatment are still empirical. Treatment decisions ought to be based on sound scientific evidence but unfortunately despite the great effort that has been spent providing treatment over many years, little in the way of resources has been spent on clinical research into the success or otherwise of dental treatment methods. This is especially true with regard to the primary dentition.

There are few reports in the literature on the relative success in the primary dentition of different treatment methods or materials. The majority of those reports are retrospective and therefore need to be treated with caution.

7.3.1 Conventional restorative materials

Many different materials have been advocated over the years but as indicated above very little research has been carried out to find out which ones might be the most useful. Therefore the popularity of any particular material has depended

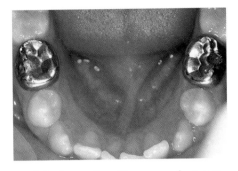

Fig. 7.1 Restoration of lower second primary molars with preformed crowns 7 years after placement.

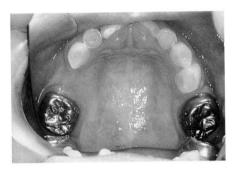

Fig. 7.2 Temporary restoration of carious upper first permanent molars with preformed crowns in an 8 year old child with a high caries rate.

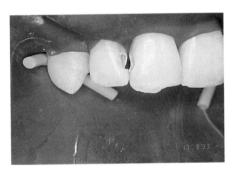

Fig. 7.3 Rubber dam placement prior to restoration of approximal lesions with composite resin. Dam stabilised with 'wedjets'. Wooden wedges removed showing retraction of gingivae.

on clinical impression and fashion. This section provides a brief overview of the materials which are both currently widely available and have been subject to some clinical research.

Silver amalgam

Silver amalgam has been used for restoring teeth for over 150 years and despite the fact that it is not tooth coloured and that there have been repeated concerns about its safety (largely unfounded) it is still widely used. This is probably because it is relatively easy to use, is tolerant of operator error and has yet to be bettered as a material for economically restoring posterior teeth. Modern non-gamma 2 alloy restorations have been shown to have extended lifetimes in permanent teeth when placed under good conditions and have also been shown to be much less sensitive to poor handling than tooth-coloured materials.

In clinical trials and retrospective studies no intracoronal material has so far performed more successfully than amalgam.

Preformed metal crown

These were introduced in 1950 and have gained wide acceptance in North America. In Europe they have been less popular, being seen by most dentists as too difficult to use, although in reality they are often easier to place than some intracoronal restorations (Fig. 7.1).

All published studies have shown preformed metal crowns to have a higher success rate in primary teeth than all other restorative materials. They are certainly the preferred treatment option for first primary molars with anything other than minimal caries.

Preformed crowns are also advocated for hypoplastic or carious first permanent molars where the approximal surfaces are involved. They act as provisional restorations prior either to strategic removal at age 9–12 years or later restoration with a cast crown (Fig. 7.2). Etched retained castings may now be used in hypoplastic teeth without involvement of the approximal surface.

Composite resin

Composite resins came on the market in the early 1970s and have been modified since then in an attempt to improve their properties. Current materials are still best applied to anterior teeth and small restorations in posterior teeth. The development of acid etching at the time that these materials were introduced has ensured that they have performed reasonably well in terms of marginal seal. They are sensitive to variations in technique and take longer to place than equivalent amalgam restorations. They must be placed in a dry field (Fig. 7.3).

The long-term success of composite resins is jeopardized by their instability in water. The best materials have maximum inorganic filler levels and low water absorption, but will deteriorate over time.

Key Point	• All composite resin and glass ionomer restorations must be placed in a dry field.

Glass ionomer

Glass ionomer cements came on to the market in the late 1970s and have also been modified since then in order to enhance their properties. Current materials are much improved and have some advantages over composite resins. Being made from glasses with a high fluoride content they provide a sustained release over an extended period, acting as a reservoir of fluoride and so protecting adjacent surfaces from caries progression.

They adhere to enamel and dentine without the need for acid etching, do not suffer from polymerization shrinkage, and, once set, are dimensionally stable in conditions of high humidity such as exist in the mouth (Fig. 7.4).

Similarly to composite resins it is imperative that they are placed in a dry field.

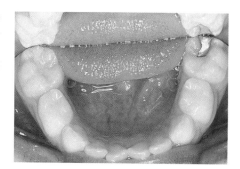

Fig. 7.4 Distal–occlusal restorations on both lower second primary molars after 3 years. One restored with conventional amalgam, the other with glass ionomer cement.

7.3.2 New restorative materials

Recently, a number of new materials have come to the market which aim to maximize the best qualities of both composite resins and glass ionomers. Some of these show promise and should be considered for the restoration of teeth in children. None of them have had more than short-term clinical trials so their widespread use is not yet justified.

They can be classified according to whether they retain the essential acid–base reaction of the glass ionomers or not.

Resin modified glass ionomer

These consist of a glass ionomer cement to which has been added a resin system which will allow the material to set quickly using light or chemical catalysts (or both) while allowing the acid–base reaction of the glass ionomer to take place. Thus, the materials will set albeit rather slowly without the need for the resin system and the essential qualities of a glass ionomer cement should be retained (Fig. 7.5).

Polyacid-modified composite resin

In contrast these materials have a much higher content of resin and the acid–base reaction of the glass ionomers does not take place. Therefore although they are easier to use (being pre-mixed in capsules), there is some doubt as to the longer-term benefits over conventional composite resins (Fig. 7.6).

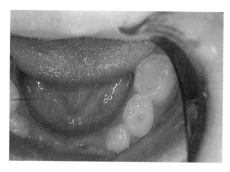

Fig. 7.5 Resin modified glass ionomer restoration after 2 years in a lower second primary molar.

7.4 RUBBER DAM

Most texts that discuss operative treatment for children advocate the use of rubber dam but it is used very little in practice despite many sound reasons for its adoption. In the United Kingdom less than 2 per cent of dentists use it routinely. It is perceived as a difficult technique that is expensive in time and arduous for the patient.

In fact, once mastered, the technique makes dental care for children easier and a higher standard of care can be achieved in less time than would otherwise be required. In addition it isolates the child from the operative field making treatment less invasive of their personal space.

The benefits can be divided into three main categories.

7.4.1 Safety

Damage of soft tissues

The risks of operative treatment include damage to the soft tissues of the mouth from rotary and hand instruments and the medicaments used in the provision of endodontic and other care. Rubber dam will go a long way to preventing damage of this type.

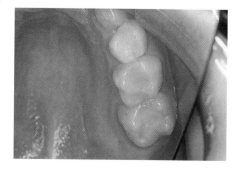

Fig. 7.6 Mesial–occlusal restoration after 1 year in an upper second primary molar with polyacid modified composite resin.

Risk of swallowing or inhalation

There is also the risk that these items may be lost in the patient's mouth and swallowed or even inhaled and there are reports in the literature to substantiate this risk.

Risk of cross-infection

In addition there is considerable risk that the use of high-speed rotary instruments distribute an aerosol of the patients saliva around the operating room putting dentist and staff at risk of infection. Again a risk that has been substantiated in the literature.

Nitrous oxide sedation

If this is used it is quite likely that mouth breathing by the child will increase the level of the gas in the environment again putting dentist and staff at risk. The use of rubber dam in this situation will make sure that exhaled gas is routed via the scavenging system attached to the nose piece. Usually less nitrous oxide will be required for a sedative effect, increasing the safety and effectiveness of the procedure.

7.4.2 Benefits to the child

Isolation

One of the reasons that dental treatment causes anxiety in patients is that the operative area is very close to and involved with all the most vital functions of the body such as sight, hearing, breathing, and eating. When operative treatment is being performed all these vital functions are put at risk and any sensible child would be concerned. It is useful to discuss these fears with child patients and explain how the risks can be reduced or eliminated.

Glasses should be used to protect the eyes and rubber dam to protect the airways and the oesophagus. By doing this and provided that good local analgesia has been obtained the child can feel themselves distanced from the operation. Sometimes it is even helpful to show the child their isolated teeth in a mirror. The view is so different from what they normally see in the mirror that they can divorce themselves from the reality of the situation.

Relaxation

The isolation of the operative area from the child will very often cause the child to become considerably relaxed — always provided that there is good pain control. It is common for both adult and child patients to fall asleep while undergoing treatment involving the use of rubber dam — a situation which rarely occurs without. This is a function of the safety perceived by the patient and the relaxed way in which the dental team can work with its assistance.

7.4.3 Benefits to the operator

Reduced stress

As noted above, once rubber dam has been placed the child will be at less risk from the procedures that will be used to restore their teeth. This reduces the effort required by the operator to protect the soft tissues of the mouth and the airways. Treatment can be carried out in a more relaxed and controlled manner lessening the stress of the procedure on the dental team.

Retraction of tongue and cheeks

Correctly placed rubber dam will gently pull the cheeks and tongue away from the operative area allowing the operator a better view of the area to be treated.

Retraction of gingival tissue

Rubber dam will gently pull the gingival tissues away from the cervical margin of the tooth, making it much easier to see the extent of any caries close to the margin and often bringing the cervical margin of a prepared cavity above the level of the gingival margin thus making restoration considerably easier. Interdentally, this retraction should be assisted by placing a wedge firmly between the adjacent teeth as soon as the dam has been placed. This wedge is placed horizontally below the contact area and above the dam thus compressing the interdental gingivae against the underlying bone. Approximal cavities can then be prepared, any damage from rotary instruments being inflicted on the wedge rather than the child's gingival tissue.

Quite often it can be difficult and time consuming to take the rubber dam between the contacts because of dental caries or broken restorations. It is possible to make life easier by using a 'trough technique', which involves snipping the rubber dam between the punched holes. All the benefits of rubber dam are retained except for the retraction and protection of the gingival tissues (Fig. 7.7).

Moisture control

As mentioned previously silver amalgam is probably the only restorative material that has any tolerance to being placed in a damp environment and there is no doubt that it and all other materials will perform much more satisfactorily if placed in a dry field. Rubber dam is the only technique that readily ensures a dry field.

7.4.4   Technique

Most texts on operative dentistry demonstrate techniques for the use of rubber dam. It is not intended to duplicate this effort but it would seem useful to point out features of the technique which have made life easier for the authors when using rubber dam with children.

Analgesia

Placement of rubber dam can be uncomfortable especially if a clamp is needed to retain it. Even if a clamp is not required the sharp cut edge of the dam can cause mild pain. Soft tissue analgesia can be obtained using infiltration in the buccal sulcus followed by an interpapillary injection. This will usually give sufficient analgesia to remove any discomfort from the dam. However, more profound analgesia may be required for the particular operative procedure that has to be performed.

Method of application

There are at least four different methods of placing the dam but most authorities recommend a method whereby the clamp is first placed on the tooth, the dam stretched over the clamp and then over the remaining teeth that are to be isolated. Because of the risk of the patient swallowing or inhaling a dropped or broken clamp before the dam is applied it is imperative that the clamp be restrained with a piece of floss tied or wrapped around the bow. This adds considerable inconvenience to the technique and the authors favour a simpler method whereby the clamp, dam, and frame are assembled together before application and taken to the tooth in one movement. Because the clamp is always on the outside of the dam relative to the patient there is no need to use floss to secure the clamp.

A 5 inch square of medium dam is stretched over an Ivory frame and a single hole punched in the middle of the square. This hole is for the tooth on which the clamp is going to be placed and further holes should be punched for any other teeth that need to be isolated. A winged clamp is placed in the first hole and the whole assembly carried to the tooth by the clamp forceps. The tooth that is going to be clamped can be seen through the hole and the clamp applied to it. The dam is then teased off the wings using either the fingers or a hand instrument. It can then be carried forward over the other teeth with the interdental dam being 'knifed' through the contact areas. It may need to be stabilized at the front using either floss, a small piece of rubber dam, a 'Wedjet' (Figs 7.3 and 7.7) or a wooden wedge.

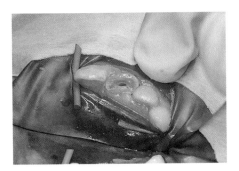

Fig. 7.7 'Trough technique' of rubber dam placement for an endodontic procedure on a broken down upper permanent central incisor. Dam stabilized with a 'wedjet'.

7.5   OPERATIVE TREATMENT OF PRIMARY TEETH

7.5.1   Pit and fissure caries

Pit and fissure caries is less of a problem in primary teeth than in permanent. The fissures are usually much shallower and less susceptible to decay so the presence of a cavity in the occlusal surface of a primary molar is a sign of high caries activity. Because of this it is quite likely that the children who require treatment of these surfaces will be young. However, treatment is not difficult and can usually be accomplished without problem. Infiltration analgesia should be given together with supplemental intrapapillary injection. Caries is removed using a 330 bur in a high speed handpiece. For restoration, although as indicated above silver amalgam has not so far been bettered in clinical trial, because occlusal caries in the primary dentition indicates high caries activity the material of choice may be a resin modified glass ionomer cement taking advantage of the caries preventive properties of the material (Fig. 7.5).

7.5.2   Approximal caries

Silver amalgam

Failure of amalgam itself as well as faults in the cavity design have been the most commonly reported causes of failure of approximal restorations in primary teeth. Attempts to overcome these deficiencies and to improve durability have come through alteration in cavity design and the choice of material used. A reduction in the size of the occlusal lock, rounded line angles and minimum extension for prevention all result in less destruction of sound tooth tissue. In addition, the 'minimal' approximal cavity with no occlusal 'dovetail' has been described for both amalgam and adhesive restorations, and incorporates some

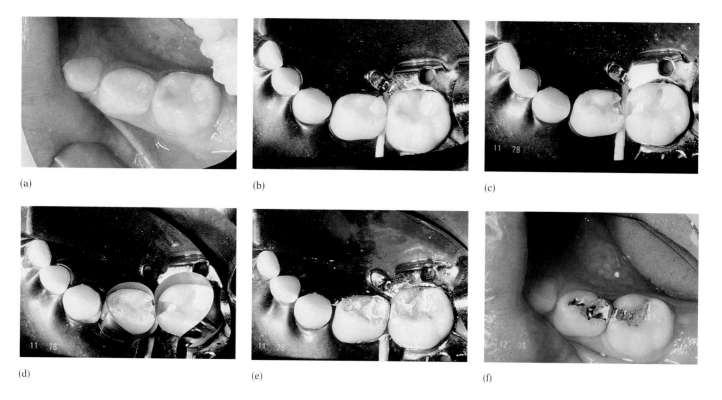

(a)   (b)   (c)

(d)   (e)   (f)

mechanical retention in the form of small internal resistance grooves placed with a very small round bur just inside the enamel–dentine junction. Figure 7.8a–f demonstrates the clinical stages in the placement of two-surface amalgam restorations in the primary dentition.

It is unlikely that the 'perfect cavity design' exists for an amalgam restoration in primary molars due to certain anatomical features:

(1) widened contact areas make a narrow box difficult to achieve;
(2) thin enamel means that cracking and fracture of parts of the crown are more common;
(3) primary teeth may undergo considerable wear under occlusal stress themselves and this in turn will affect the restorations.

It is therefore necessary to investigate other materials for use in restoring the primary dentition.

Fig. 7.8 (a)–(f) Technique sequence for the placement of two-surface amalgam restorations in lower primary molars. The first molar could have been restored with a preformed crown.

Composite resin

Composite resin has been used quite widely to restore primary teeth and results are generally acceptable. Cavity design is usually a modified approximal design with bevelling of margins to increase the amount of enamel available for etching and bonding.

The use of rubber dam is essential if a dry field is to be achieved. This fact together with the materials relative expense probably reflects the lack of widespread use of composite resin in many countries.

Glass ionomer cement

More studies exist using glass ionomer cements as opposed to composite resins. However, the cavity designs used in the different studies vary considerably and it is difficult to draw firm conclusions. Certainly, glass ionomer cement will undergo significantly more loss of anatomical form than amalgam in the approximal area and as such conventional glass ionomers have not been shown to be as durable as amalgam. However, the operator will need to balance this fact with the obvious mechanical and chemical advantages of the cement, namely its ability to bond to enamel and dentine thus requiring a more conservative preparation, and its ability to release fluoride.

Preformed metal crowns

Preformed metal crowns should be considered whenever posterior primary teeth (especially first molars) require restoration. They were originally developed to provide a 'restoration of last resort' for those teeth that were not salvageable by any other means. At the time that they were introduced in the early 1950s the only alternatives were silver or copper amalgam or a selection of cements, materials completely unsuited to the restoration of grossly carious teeth or those that had been weakened by pulp treatment. Over the years it has become apparent the life expectancy of these crowns is far better than any other restoration for primary posterior teeth and that they come close to the ideal of never having to be replaced prior to exfoliation. In addition, they are less demanding technically than intracoronal restorations in primary teeth.

They should therefore now be considered for any tooth where the dentist cannot be sure that an alternative would survive until the tooth is lost. It is unfair to put a child through more treatment situations than necessary because a less successful material was chosen which needs frequent replacement.

Prior to preparation, all caries is removed and any pulp treatment that may be required carried out. A recent pre-operative radiograph must be available to make sure that the periapical and inter-radicular tissues are healthy and that the tooth is unlikely to be exfoliated in the near future.

Preparation and fitting is easier if rubber dam is in place but even if this is not the case it is advisable to place wedges mesially and distally, gingival to the contact area (Fig. 7.9a). These wedges should be placed firmly using the applicator supplied with them or a pair of flat beaked pliers. It is essential that good soft tissue anaesthesia be obtained so that this procedure is not painful, although the wedges should compress the gingivae away from the contact area and not be driven into the tissue. The use of wedges in this manner protects the tissues and reduces the contamination of the operating field as well as making the margins of the preparation easier to see.

The mesial and distal surfaces of the tooth are removed using a 330 bur or a fine tapered fissure bur or diamond (Fig. 7.9b). It is important to cut through the tooth away from the contact area to avoid damage to the adjacent tooth. The bur should be angled away from the vertical so that a shoulder is not created at the gingival margin.

The same bur may be used for the whole preparation, although it can be quicker to use a larger diamond for the next stage which is to reduce the occlusal surface to allow 1.5–2 mm of space between the prepared tooth and its opposite number.

Many authorities advocate doing no more preparation than this but it takes little further time to reduce the buccal and lingual surfaces sufficiently to remove any undercuts above the gingival margin. Any sharp line angles are rounded off to avoid interferences which might prevent the crown seating.

The mesial and distal preparation might seem rather radical in comparison to that required when a cast crown is constructed for a permanent tooth, but the principles of retention and resistance of the two types of crown are different. A

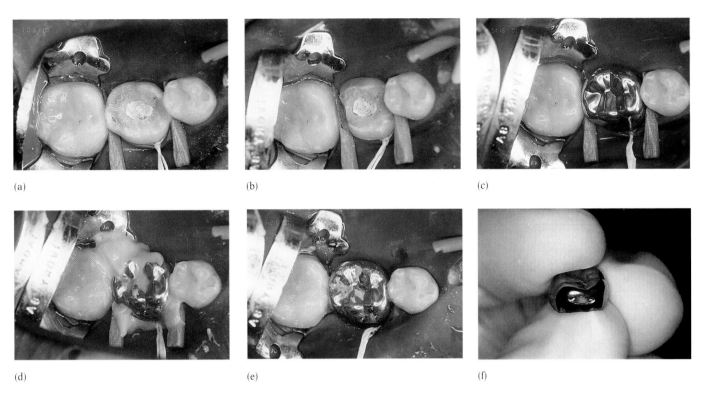

(a)   (b)   (c)

(d)   (e)   (f)

Fig. 7.9 (a) Rubber dam and wedges in place, pulpotomy and coronal reduction completed. (b) Mesial and distal surfaces reduced. (c) Crown 'try-in'. (d) Cementation of crown. (e) Excess cement removed prior to rubber dam removal and occlusal analysis. (f) Approximal hole in preformed crown prior to placement.

cast crown is retained by friction between the walls of the prepared tooth and the internal surface of the crown. It is therefore important to have near parallel walls of adequate height. A preformed metal crown is retained by contact between the margins of the crown and the undercut portion of the tooth below the gingiva. The shape of the preparation above the gingiva is relatively unimportant and difficulty in fitting these crowns is most often because of under-preparation. However, it is most important that a shoulder is not formed at the gingival margin as this would make the seating of a well adapted crown impossible.

Try the crown on, checking to feel that it is within the gingival crevice (Fig. 7.9c) by probing. If it rests *on* the gingival crevice then crimp in with some pliers. Again seat the crown. If it is over-extended cut down in that area with a stone or scissors and smooth off before retrying. Check contacts with adjacent teeth and finally polish the margins with a stone or rubber wheel. Wash and dry the tooth before cementation with a glass ionomer cement. Seat the crown from lingual to buccal pressing down firmly (Fig. 7.9d). Remove excess cement when set with a probe and dental floss (Fig. 7.9e), before removing rubber dam and checking the occlusion.

Although not proven statistically beneficial the authors favour making small holes in the approximal surfaces of the preformed crown, to confer the benefits to the adjacent teeth of fluoride release from the glass ionomer cement (Fig. 7.9f).

Figure 7.10a–d shows how the restoration of heavily carious primary molars with preformed crowns has maintained arch space and allowed permanent pre-molars to erupt into ideal occlusion.

7.5.3   Anterior teeth

The treatment of decayed primary incisors depends on the stage of decay and the age and co-operation of the patient. In the pre-school child caries of the upper primary incisors is usually as a result of 'nursing caries syndrome' due to the

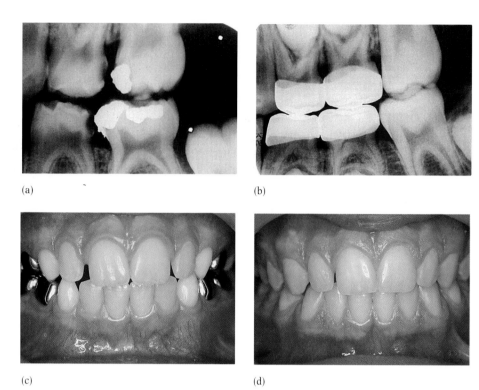

(a)   (b)

(c)   (d)

Fig. 7.10 (a) Carious upper and lower primary molars. (b) After placement of preformed crowns. (c) Occlusion in the mixed dentition. (d) 'Ideal' final occlusion in the permanent dentition.

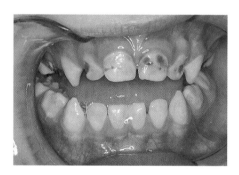

Fig. 7.11 Labial and approximal caries in upper anterior primary teeth.

frequent or prolonged consumption of fluids containing fermentable carbohydrate from a bottle or feeder cup (Fig. 6.11). The lower incisors are rarely affected as they are protected during suckling by the tongue and directly bathed in secretions from the submandibular and sublingual glands. In 'nursing caries' the progression of decay is rapid, commencing on the labial surfaces and quickly encircling the teeth. It is impossible to prepare satisfactory cavities for restoration and after a comprehensive preventive programme the most suitable form of restoration is the 'strip crown technique'. This utilizes celluloid crown forms and a light cured composite resin to restore crown morphology. Either calcium hydroxide or glass ionomer cement can be used as a lining and the high polishability of modern hybrid composites make them aesthetically as well as physically, suitable for this task.

In older children over 3 or 4 years of age new lesions of primary incisors, although not usually associated with the use of pacifiers do indicate high caries activity (Fig. 7.11). Such lesions do not progress so rapidly and usually appear on the mesial and distal surfaces and glass ionomer cement or composite resin can be used for restoration. Glass ionomer lacks the translucency of composite but has the useful advantages of being adhesive and releasing fluoride.

Fractures of the incisal edges in primary teeth, as in permanent teeth, should be restored with composite resin.

7.6   OPERATIVE TREATMENT OF PERMANENT TEETH

7.6.1   Pit and fissure caries

The pits and fissures are the major sites of caries activity in the child and adolescent. It is therefore most likely that the dentist be required to treat these surfaces rather than the approximal surfaces. Fortunately, they are easier to treat and it is

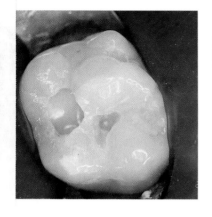
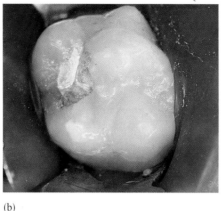

(a)   (b)

Fig. 7.12 (a) and (b) Upper first permanent molar after cavity preparation and final restoration. The occlusal contacts are not retained on enamel in the distal fissure and silver amalgam is the material of choice. The mesial fissure has been restored with a preventive resin restoration.

les ʿely that iatrogenic damage be caused. The two essentials to bear in mind are remove only the minimal amount of sound enamel that will allow clearing the ʿnelodentinal junction of caries and to make sure that occlusal contacts are noʿ st. If the occlusal contacts are retained on enamel, a resin or glass ionomer resʿation is a possibility. However, should it be necessary to remove more sound enamel so as to gain access to the dentinal caries it will be necessary to use a material that will not wear significantly nor cause wear to the opposing tooth. Silver amalgam is therefore the only practical choice and it should be explained to the patient and parent that the minor disadvantages of an amalgam restoration in a posterior tooth need to be balanced against the long-term success of the material (Fig. 7.12a and b).

Difficulty of diagnosis

The main problem with regard to occlusal caries is that it is impossible to diagnose consistently by clinical means and is seen on radiographs only when fairly advanced. All practising dentists will have had the experience of cleaning out a fissure which appeared to be reasonably sound only to find a huge cavity in the dentine below (Fig. 7.13a and b). However, it is unusual to experience the opposite and the risk of overtreatment of occlusal surfaces is low.

Oral hygiene and fluorides

It is possible to prevent occlusal caries by the assiduous use of good oral hygiene and fluoride therapy and some authorities advocate this approach rather than the use of fissure sealants. Fluoride has been shown to be effective in preventing occlusal caries. Although the percentage reduction of caries is always greater for smooth surfaces, the actual number of cavities saved is usually greater compared with approximal surfaces. However, at present most authorities would advocate the judicious use of fissure sealants and preventive resin restorations to control the disease.

Early intervention

Methods for the prevention of occlusal caries that rely on the dentist intervening date back to the days of Hyatt and Bödecker. Bödecker suggested that polishing and opening up the fissures would enable them to be kept clean and thus avoid breakdown, whereas Hyatt advocated cleaning out and cutting into the fissure so as to remove early caries prior to sealing with amalgam. The

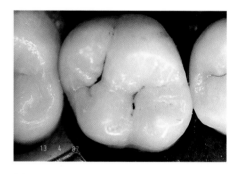

(a)

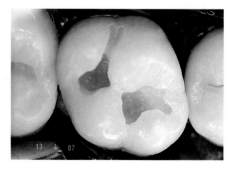

(b)

Fig. 7.13 (a) and (b) Extensive caries revealed after exploration of stained fissures.

advantage of producing a small and manageable restoration by anyone who has seen the destruction of an otherwise sound tooth by neglected occlusal caries is obvious.

Fissure sealants

There are now several materials that could be considered for fissure sealing. The early studies tended to support the use of composite resin and currently most fissure sealants on the market are either unfilled or lightly filled resins and these have been shown to be effective for most children. Resin sealants are not satisfactory in children who are highly caries active because there is poor resistance to secondary caries at the margins of the restoration. In this instance it is likely that a glass ionomer would give better protection (Chapter 6). The poor retention and resistance to wear of conventional glass ionomers is balanced by their high-fluoride release and it is likely that the problem of wear may be reduced with the newer resin modified glass ionomer cements and these merit a clinical trial against conventional resin sealants.

There has been continuing interest in the question as to whether caries sealed into teeth will progress or not. There is no doubt that if the possibility of leakage is eliminated, caries sealed under a restoration will become arrested and the bacterial count diminished. This has been shown to happen under amalgam restorations and under well placed fissure sealants. However, it only needs the failure of *one* part of the restoration for leakage to be re-established and the carious process to continue. Resins are not impervious to water and although the acid etch technique reduces marginal leakage considerably it is unwise to leave caries under a resin material because of the difficulty of monitoring.

Consideration needs to be given as to whether to use a clear, coloured, or opaque sealant or whether to use a filled resin. Early sealants were clear because it was felt to be important to be able to see through the material to make sure that caries was not developing under the material. Because of the difficulty of seeing whether sealant was still present, coloured materials were introduced and more recently some have been made opaque.

Sealants fail when the margins break down and this is often difficult to see if a clear sealant has been used. Additionally, if stained fissures have been sealed it can take some time to examine a surface to see the difference between the original staining and marginal leakage. When seeing children at subsequent recall appointments it can take a considerable time to examine all occlusal surfaces and determine whether further treatment is indicated. Therefore most authorities now advocate the use of an opaque (white) sealant. This is easily seen on recall and any degree of marginal staining is an indication for further investigation and resealing.

A number of studies have shown that the greatest success with sealants has been achieved when a filled resin (composite) has been used. In comparison with unfilled resins a composite is stronger, more rigid, and less likely to wear. The disadvantages of these materials is that they take longer to apply and more care needs to be taken of the occlusion so as to make sure that no excessive wear of the opposing tooth follows their placement. However, they would be the authors' choice as once placed they need less maintenance or supervision.

It is the authors' belief that stained fissures should not be sealed without being cleaned and investigated (Fig. 7.14a and b). Etching does remove a good deal of organic material but there is always a considerable amount of debris at the base of a fissure and this prevents adhesion of the sealant at that point. In addition, as pointed out above, it is impossible to be confident of the state of the tooth under a stained fissure.

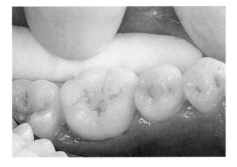

(a)

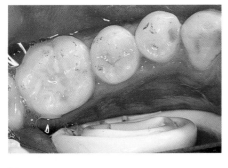

(b)

Fig. 7.14 (a) and (b) Stained fissures in first permanent molar before investigation and after sealing with an opaque sealant.

A procedure similar to that described by Bödecker as 'fissure eradication' should be carried out using a 330 bur or small stone to clean and round out the stained fissures. This will improve the retention of the sealant by removing the bulk of organic debris from the fissure and allowing a greater volume of sealant in the fissure, giving more strength and rigidity to the restoration. The procedure also makes it easier to see if there is a significant amount of caries in the dentine. If only a small amount of carious dentine needs to be removed it will be possible to use a composite resin to restore the cavity followed by sealing of the rest of the fissure system. This type of restoration is commonly called a preventive resin restoration (PRR).

Preventive resin restoration (PRR)

Local anaesthesia is necessary to achieve painless rubber dam application and cavity preparation. Initial exploration of the pit should be with a small round bur to the depth of the pit and then withdrawal in a circumferential motion around the periphery of the pit. This removes demineralized enamel from the walls of the fissure and aids removal of caries from the ADJ. If caries along the ADJ cannot be reached with hand instruments or bur it will be necessary to widen the access. Begin dentinal caries removal at the margin and extend to the depth of lesion until it is free of caries. Check there is no grossly undermined enamel and ensure the walls of the cavity are slightly undercut to give a cavo-surface angle of about 90°.

Dentine should be lined either with calcium hydroxide or glass ionomer cement before restoring the cavity and the remaining fissure system with a compatible filled composite and fissure sealant:

(1) etch cavity margins and fissure system — wash and dry;
(2) apply thin layer of unfilled resin to cavity and enamel margins — blow gently to distribute evenly and light cure;
(3) pack cavity with filled composite (do not overfill) — light cure;
(4) apply compatible fissure sealant over restoration and the rest of the fissure system — light cure.

It is possible to combine (3) and (4) and light cure once only after placement of the fissure sealant (Fig. 7.15a–h).

These minimal cavities are more conservative of sound tooth tissue than amalgam cavities and longevity trials of up to 7 years have shown PRR to be as durable as amalgam (Fig. 7.16a and b).

7.6.2 Approximal caries

The benefits of improved dental health among children has been most marked by a reduction in the prevalence of approximal caries. This is fortunate because it is much more difficult to avoid iatrogenic damage in this situation. In comparison with the management of occlusal caries where fissure sealing or the placement of preventive resin restorations should be considered at the first signs of caries, great thought should be given before interfering with approximal surfaces and early intervention is to be avoided.

Conventional cavity preparation embodies some severe disadvantages. Class II amalgam restorations sacrifice a large amount of sound tooth tissue if the dentist adheres to Black's principles of cavity preparation. However, more conservative designs are now advocated which are equally retentive (Fig. 7.17a and b).

The absolute physical and mechanical properties of composite resins are relatively good. However, clinical trials in approximal cavities have shown significant

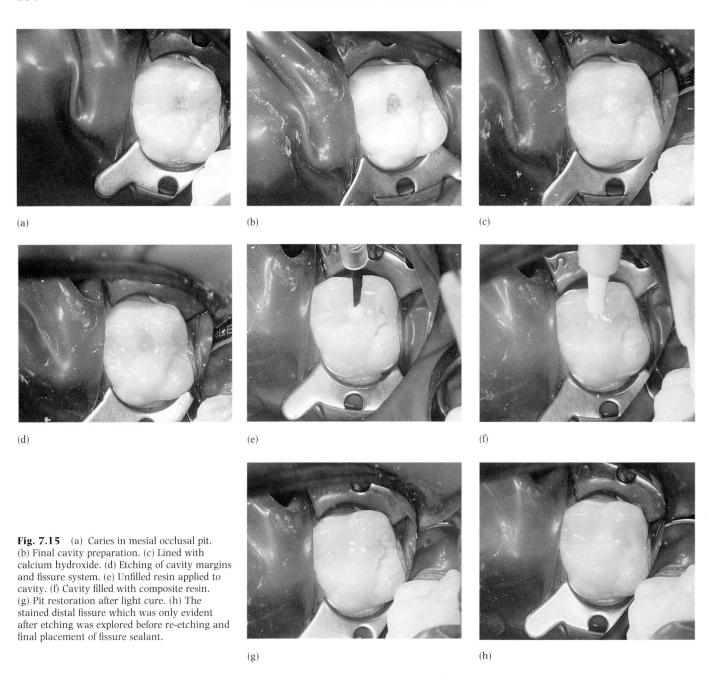

Fig. 7.15 (a) Caries in mesial occlusal pit. (b) Final cavity preparation. (c) Lined with calcium hydroxide. (d) Etching of cavity margins and fissure system. (e) Unfilled resin applied to cavity. (f) Cavity filled with composite resin. (g) Pit restoration after light cure. (h) The stained distal fissure which was only evident after etching was explored before re-etching and final placement of fissure sealant.

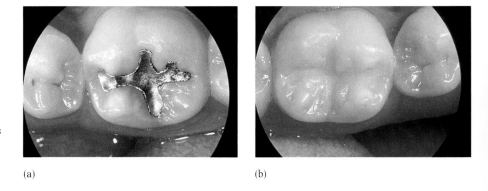

Fig. 7.16 (a) and (b) First permanent molars 7 years after placement of amalgam and composite restorations.

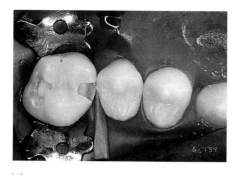

(a)

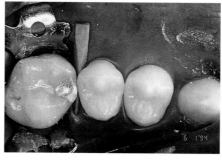

(b)

Fig. 7.17 (a) Cavities prepared in an upper first permanent molar. (b) Restoration of the distal–occlusal pit with a PRR and the mesial–occlusal cavity with silver amalgam.

wear after 4 or 5 years which may be a manifestation of fatigue within the resin matrix, or even as a result of bacterial degradation of the resin.

In summary, the loss of occlusal and approximal contact when using non-metallic restorative materials has not yet been solved and it would seem that material with a much lower coefficient of friction will have to be produced before tooth-coloured restoratives can be advocated for any situation where contact with opposing or adjacent posterior teeth is involved.

7.6.3 Anterior teeth

Approximal and gingival caries should be restored with composite resin to achieve satisfactory aesthetics, although glass ionomer cement with its adhesive properties and fluoride release should be considered in the patient with a high caries rate. If composite resin is used then the dentine should be lined either with a dentine bonding agent in a shallow cavity or with calcium hydroxide or glass ionomer cement in a deeper cavity. If too much calcium hydroxide is used it can 'shine through' a composite restoration, and therefore glass ionomer cement is a better cosmetic option as a liner in addition to its other properties.

Incisal edge lesions require composite resin restorations. Correct design of cavities together with the adhesive properties of glass ionomer cement and bonding properties of composite resin to both glass ionomer cement and enamel mean that dentine pins should only be used as a last resort (Fig. 7.18a and b).

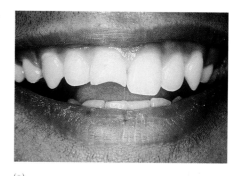

(a)

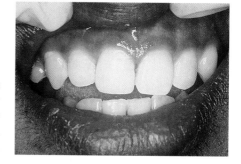

(b)

Fig. 7.18 (a) and (b) Incisal edge fracture restored with a hybrid composite resin.

7.7 TREATMENT OF THE CHILD WITH A HIGH CARIES RATE

The type of treatment instituted for patients with rampant caries depends on the patients' and parents' motivation towards dental treatment, the extent of decay and the age and co-operation of the child. Initial treatment, including temporary restorations, diet assessment, oral hygiene instruction, and home and professional fluoride treatments should be performed before any comprehensive restorative programme commences. However, in patients presenting with acute and severe signs and symptoms of gross caries, pain, abscess, sinus, or facial swelling, then immediate treatment is indicated. This may involve extractions and even a general anaesthetic in a young child. It is wiser to extract all teeth with a dubious prognosis under one general anaesthetic rather than have an acclimatization programme interrupted by a painful episode in the future.

Table 7.1 summarizes the preventive regimens that should be employed for rampant caries in different age groups.

Table 7.1 Prevention of rampant caries in children and adolescents

Primary dentition:	*0–5 years*
Dietary advice:	Dietary counselling with parents on good nursing techniques
Fluoride therapy:	Toothpaste
	Drops/Tablets if in area without water fluoridation
	Topical varnish application every 6 months
Plaque control:	Oral hygiene instructions to parents
	Toothbrushing with parental supervision
Early visit to dentist at about 12 months of age with 3–6 month recall	
Mixed dentition:	*5–12 years*
Dietary advice:	Dietary counselling with parents and patients
Fluoride therapy:	Toothpaste
	Tablets if in area without water fluoridation
	Mouthrinse
	Topical gel/varnish application every 6 months
Plaque control:	Oral hygiene instructions to patient
	Toothbrushing without parental supervision
	Disclosing tablets
Fissure sealants	
3–6 month recalls	
Permanent dentition:	*12 years+*
Dietary advice:	Dietary counselling with parents and patients
Fluoride therapy:	Toothpaste
	Mouthrinse
	Topical gel/varnish application every 6 months
Plaque control:	Oral hygiene instructions to patient
	Toothbrushing
	Disclosing tablets
	Interdental cleaning with floss or wood sticks
Fissure sealants	
3–6 month recalls	

Once rampant caries is under control, then comprehensive restorative treatment can be undertaken. This should aim to retain the primary dentition with the methods described in this and Chapter 8 and deliver the child pain-free into adolescence and adulthood.

7.8 SUMMARY

1. A full preventive programme must be instituted before any definitive restorations in a child with a high caries rate.
2. The preformed metal crown is the most durable restoration in the primary dentition for large cavities and endodontically treated teeth.
3. Composite resin restorations in permanent premolar and molar teeth should not be placed in areas of occlusal or approximal contact.
4. Resin modified glass ionomers and polyacid modified composite resins may have an increased role in the future in both the restoration of primary and permanent teeth.
5. Rubber dam should be placed, if at all possible, prior to the restoration of all teeth.
6. Stained fissures should be investigated early in order to conserve tooth tissue.

7.9 FURTHER READING

Curzon, M. E. J. and Roberts, J. S. (1996) *Kennedy's Paediatric Operative Dentistry* (4th edn) Wright London. *(A comprehensive text on the technical aspects of operative dentistry for children)*

Duggal, M. S., Curzon, M. E. J., Fayle, S. A., Pollard, M. A., and Robinson, A. J. (1995). *Restorative techniques in paediatric dentistry*. Martin Dunitz, London. *(A superb colour atlas and pictorial guide.)*

Harris, C. A. (1839). *The dental art*. Armstrong and Berry, Baltimore. *(An interesting historical guide.)*

Kidd, E. A. M. and Smith, B. G. N. (1990). *Pickard's manual of operative dentistry* (6th edn). Oxford University Press, Oxford. *(An ideal reference manual for restoration of permanent teeth.)*

Paterson, R. C., Watts, A., Saunders, W. P., and Pitts, N. B. (1991). *Modern concepts in the diagnosis and treatment of fissure caries*. Quintessence, London. *(A very practical and clear approach to the problem.)*

Reid, J. S., Challis, P. D., and Patterson, C. J. W. (1990). *Rubber dam in clinical practice*. Quintessence, London. *(This guide will prove to you that you can easily use rubber dam.)*

8 Paediatric endodontics

8 Paediatric endodontics

J. M. WHITWORTH and J. H. NUNN

8.1 INTRODUCTION

Contemporary advances in primary prevention have brought falling levels of dental disease in many of the world's developed countries. Nevertheless, there can be little room for complacency. Dental caries and traumatic dental injuries are still very prevalent and treatment of the widespread damage they inflict is still a major component of paediatric dental practice.

The principal goal of paediatric operative dentistry is to prevent the extension of dental disease and to restore damaged teeth to healthy function. In pursuit of this goal, a range of conservative endodontic procedures have developed which are able to provide predictable alternatives to extraction for many pulpally compromised primary and young permanent teeth. They are within the grasp of all practitioners and are central to the practice of paediatric dentistry.

While many of the general principles and operative procedures in paediatric endodontics are shared with adult endodontics, a number of important differences exist which justify the special coverage given in this chapter.

Disadvantages of unplanned extractions in the primary and mixed dentitions:

- loss of space, promoting malocclusion
- reduced masticatory function (especially posterior teeth)
- impaired speech development (especially anterior teeth)
- psychological disturbance (especially anterior teeth)
- anaesthetic and surgical traumas

Key Points

8.2 THE DENTAL PULP

Dental pulp is the living, soft tissue structure which resides in the coronal pulp chamber and root canals of primary and permanent teeth.

Histologically, it is composed of loose connective tissue which is surrounded on its periphery by a continuous layer of specialized secretory cells, the odontoblasts. Odontoblasts are unique to the dental pulp and are responsible for dentine deposition.

Blood vessels and nerves enter the pulp through the apical foramen and occasionally through lateral or accessory root canals. The pulps of primary and young permanent teeth, especially those with incomplete apices have a very rich blood supply. For this reason, immature permanent pulps have great healing capacity and generally respond well to treatment aimed at pulp preservation.

Sensory fibres of the trigeminal nerve also enter the pulp in large numbers. In mature teeth, two types of sensory neurons predominate. Myelinated, fast

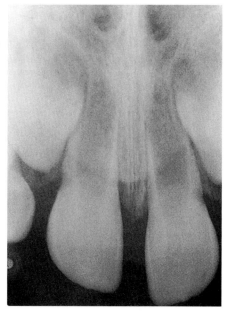

(a)

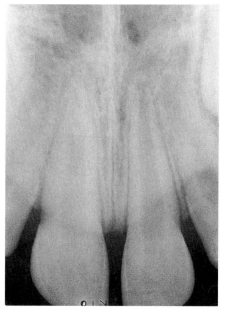

(b)

Fig. 8.1 Maturation of permanent incisors.
(a) Immature incisors showing short roots with incomplete, wide-open apices. The lateral walls of the roots are thin and structurally weak.
(b) The same teeth 2 years later, roots now almost complete following continued dentine deposition by healthy pulps.

reacting A (delta) fibres are the most numerous. Their threshold of stimulation is low, and they communicate the characteristic sharp, stabbing pain associated with dentine sensitivity and reversible pulpal inflammation. The other major group is the unmyelinated C fibres. They have a higher threshold of stimulation and convey the dull, intense pain characteristic of advanced, irreversible pulpal inflammation.

From a clinical standpoint, it is interesting to note that A (delta) fibres do not enter the pulp to any significant extent before tooth eruption. This may in part explain the occasional insensitivity of immature primary and permanent teeth to pulp sensitivity tests and to cavity preparation.

The most important function of the pulp is to lay down dentine which forms the basic structure of teeth, defines their general morphology, and provides them with mechanical strength and toughness.

Dentine deposition commences many months (primary teeth) or years (permanent teeth) before tooth eruption and while the crown of a newly erupted tooth has a mature external form, the pulp within still has considerable work to do in completing tooth development. Newly erupted teeth have short roots, and their apices are wide and often diverging, the so-called 'blunderbuss' apex (Fig. 8.1a). In addition, the dentine walls of the entire tooth are thin and relatively weak.

Provided the pulp remains healthy, dentine deposition will continue during the post-eruptive year for primary teeth, and the next 2–3 years for permanent teeth, transforming the tooth to its mature form (Fig. 8.1b). One of the key goals of paediatric dentistry is therefore to protect and preserve the pulps of teeth in a healthy state *at least* until this critical phase of tooth development is complete.

Loss of pulp vitality before a tooth has reached maturity may not only create unwanted pain and suffering, but may also leave the tooth vulnerable to fracture, and with an unfavourable crown–root ratio. Endodontic treatment of non-vital, immature teeth can also present special technical difficulties which may compromise the long-term prognosis of the tooth.

8.3   PULP PATHOSIS

The coronal dentine and pulp of a sound, newly erupted tooth is protected from injury by a hard, impervious layer of enamel. Breakdown of this barrier occurs most commonly in children due to caries (especially in posterior teeth) and trauma (especially in anterior teeth). A variety of chemical, physical, and microbial agents may then act on the pulp to cause irritation. Microbial invasion is by far the most serious.

Caries may advance rapidly through the thin coronal dentine of primary and young permanent teeth, and the speed of assault means that the usual protective responses of tubular sclerosis and secondary dentine deposition are frequently minimal or non-existent. Mild, local inflammatory changes may be seen in the pulp from the moment caries enters dentine, but marked inflammation is not seen until the lesion has penetrated to within 0.5 mm of the pulp. Up to this point, the tooth may give classical symptoms of reversible pulpal inflammation, namely transient sensitivity to hot, cold, and sweet stimuli. Often no symptoms are reported. Provided the pulp has not been invaded, excavation of the caries and restoration of the cavity is likely to allow the pulp to return to health.

As caries progresses more deeply, increasing numbers of micro-organisms and increasing amounts of microbial toxin enter the pulp, and the inflammatory changes become more profound. At the point of carious exposure, large-scale microbial invasion occurs and marked, acute inflammatory changes with tissue necrosis are seen in the pulp underlying the exposure site. Classically, the symptoms may now be those of irreversible pulpal inflammation, with persistent, often throbbing pain which may occur spontaneously and interrupt sleep. Again, paradoxically, it is not unusual for few or no symptoms to be reported. The affected area of the pulp is now unable to return to health, and if the tooth is to be preserved, the affected tissue must be removed and an appropriate dressing placed on the tissue which remains.

It should be noted that inflammation spreads progressively through the pulp (Fig. 8.2(a)–(b)), and that the radicular pulp has great capacity to maintain healthy function if the infected, irreversibly inflamed coronal tissue is removed (Fig. 8.2a and b).

Microbial invasion is also a significant consideration in the management of pulps exposed by trauma. Again, the radicular pulp has enormous capacity to remain healthy if all infected and inflamed coronal tissue is removed and an appropriate wound dressing applied.

The untreated infected pulp will ultimately succumb in its entirety, and inflammation will then spread through the apical foramen and through any patent lateral and accessory canals to affect the periradicular tissues (Fig. 8.2c and d). Classically, the symptoms will then be of periodontitis, with tenderness on biting, and swelling of the soft tissues adjacent to the tooth. A number of alternative reaction patterns may also be seen following pulpal irritation.

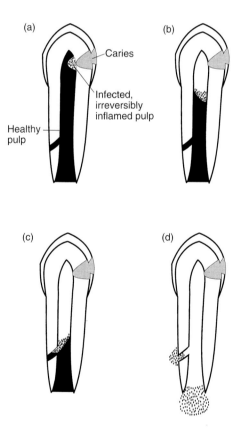

Fig. 8.2 Extension of pulpal inflammation following carious exposure and microbial infection. (a) and (b) Infection and tissue breakdown spreads progressively through the pulp. The underlying pulpal tissue may remain healthy if the overlying infected and irreversibly inflamed tissue is removed. (c) and (d) Untreated, pathological changes extend to involve the whole pulp, with extension through patent apical and lateral foramina to involve the periradicular tissues.

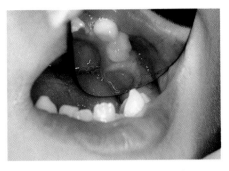

Fig. 8.3 Hyperplastic pulpitis (pulp polyp) in a primary molar caused by exuberant growth of vascular pulpal tissue through a wide pulpal exposure. The surface of the lesion is epithelialized by cells derived from the adjacent gingiva or oral mucosa.

Occasionally, the widely exposed pulp of a primary or immature permanent tooth may respond by proliferation (Fig. 8.3). Highly vascular pulp tissue may grow exuberantly through an exposure site to form a so-called pulp polyp, which often becomes epithelialized by cells derived from the gingiva or oral mucosa. Pulp polyps ultimately break down and should be considered a form of irreversible pulpitis.

Internal resorption may also be encountered in primary and permanent teeth, often following trauma, or partial removal of the pulp. A classic scenario is the resorption which arises in the pulps of primary teeth following pulp amputation (pulpotomy) where calcium hydroxide has been used to dress the radicular pulp stumps. The precise mechanisms of this response are poorly understood, although its prevalence generally rules out calcium hydroxide pulp capping and pulpotomies in primary teeth. Internal resorption typically creates few symptoms, and is usually detected as an incidental finding on routine radiographic examination (Fig. 8.4). It should be considered a form of irreversible pulpal inflammation.

Finally, the pulp of a primary or permanent tooth may undergo sudden ischaemic necrosis following tooth displacement or avulsion, which catastrophically disturbs its apical blood supply.

Key Points	Pulp pathosis:
	• microbial infection is the principal threat to pulpal health
	• control of infection is the key determinant of success in endodontic treatment

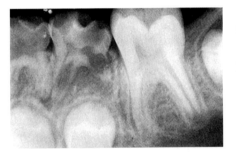

Fig. 8.4 Internal inflammatory resorption, identified as an incidental finding on routine radiographic examination.

8.4 CASE ASSESSMENT

Treatment should never be commenced before a case has been properly assessed and a clinical diagnosis made. Assessment should follow an orderly pattern and include a case history, clinical examination, and often a range of special tests.

History

A pain history can be very helpful in pulp diagnosis. Questioning should be undertaken in a calm and sympathetic manner, and directed both to the child and to an accompanying parent or carer who may provide helpful clarification. The use of leading questions or emotive terminology should be avoided.

The history should not be unduly laboured at the risk of creating further alienation and fear. The quality of information gathered depends greatly on the age and maturity of the child, in addition to their level of anxiety and distress.

1. *Primary teeth.* In the primary dentition, the pain history rarely provides very clear information, but a history of spontaneous pain does appear to correlate well with advanced, irreversible pulpitis.

2. *Permanent teeth.* Older children and adolescents may give a more discerning history, more akin to a good adult pain history.

   History of sharp, stabbing pain lasting a few seconds and brought on by hot, cold, or sweet, may indicate dentine sensitivity or reversible pulpitis. Pain lasting longer than a minute when the stimulus is removed, coming on spontaneously, or disturbing sleep may indicate an irreversible pulpitis. Swelling and tenderness on biting may indicate loss of pulp vitality and apical periodontitis.

Pain history — important information:
- area involved
- what the affected tooth feels like
- duration of the problem (days/weeks/months)
- precipitants and relieving factors
- duration of pain (seconds/minutes/hours)
- spontaneous or precipitated by external stimuli
- analgesia required

Medical history

The child's general medical history should also be reviewed with the accompanying adult to exclude systemic disorders or medications of dental relevance. Examples may include: an immunocompromised child, where it is often preferable to remove grossly carious teeth which may present a serious infection hazard; and a child with a bleeding disorder where hospital admission and expensive in-patient extraction is best avoided wherever possible. Generally, the control of local haemorrhage from pulp exposures or pulpotomy sites in such patients does not present a clinical problem, although consideration should be given to the possible dangers of local anaesthesia.

In such cases, the child's physician should be contacted for further clarification of the history and to plan co-ordinated care.

Previous dental history and attitude to tooth preservation

A brief review of the child's previous history may reveal important information on the family's general attitude to dentistry, and the likely compliance with complex restorative treatment.

Examination

During history taking, any gross facial swelling or guarding indicative of soft tissue infection will have been noted. Gentle palpation may reveal facial tenderness or the presence of enlarged lymph nodes. Individual teeth must not be viewed in isolation, but should be assessed with due regard to the general state of the mouth and the developing occlusion.

Intra-oral examination commences with a brief visual inspection of all the teeth and associated soft tissues before focusing on suspected problem areas.

Note should be made of all carious lesions, fractured and displaced restorations, discoloured and fractured teeth, in addition to areas of soft tissue swelling or erythema indicative of apical infection. Soft tissue swelling associated with pulpal breakdown in primary molars often presents over the bi- or trifurcation as micro-organisms exit via the many patent accessory communications in the pulp chamber floor (Fig. 8.5).

Other causes of pain and swelling mimicking pulpal disease should be excluded. Pericoronitis associated with partially erupted teeth may occasionally cause discomfort, which may be confused with pathology of pulpal origin.

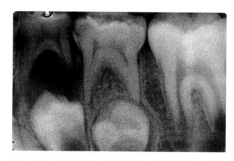

Fig. 8.5 Extension of pulpal pathosis through patent communications in the floor of the pulp chamber to present as a furcal lesion. The non-vital tooth presents with a charcteristic furcal swelling and radiolucency.

Special tests

A variety of special tests may be applied to suspect teeth in an attempt to evaluate their pulpal condition.

Pulp sensitivity tests

Thermal and electrical stimulation may excite sensory nerves in the pulp and elicit a response from healthy and pulpally inflamed teeth. While it is often possible to determine whether a tooth is vital or not, sensitivity tests will rarely give a clear picture of the extent of pulpal inflammation and the results should be interpreted with caution. Anxious children may give an exaggerated response to relatively minor stimulation of a healthy tooth, while poorly innervated, immature teeth, or teeth which have been concussed by trauma may give no response in the presence of advanced inflammation.

Methods of pulp vitality assessment which do not depend on the application of a potentially painful stimulus, or on the presence of a functional sensory nerve supply are certainly required and may ultimately be provided by refinements of non-invasive methods such as laser Doppler flowmetry.

Mobility and tenderness on percussion

Non-vital teeth with periradicular inflammation are frequently mobile and tender on biting. Suspect teeth should be tested for tenderness and mobility with a fingertip, not with a mirror handle, and the response compared with the antimere. Other causes of mobility should be excluded, including root fracture and physiological root resorption.

Radiographic examination

Case assessment is not complete without accurate radiographs. However, radiographic appearances should not be given undue weight in the absence of clinical findings. Special care should be exercised in the primary and mixed dentitions where physiological root resorption, expanded dental follicles and immature root apices may be wrongly interpreted as apical pathosis (Fig. 8.6).

An orthopantomograph is a useful screening view to assess the general state of the mouth, and the developing occlusion. Although detail may be lacking, multiple affected teeth may be rapidly screened and the viability of conservative treatment assessed.

Good quality periapical, and often bitewing radiographs can provide supplementary evidence on the presence and extent of caries, the extent of previous restora-

Fig. 8.6 Orthopantomograph in the mixed dentition. Radiolucent areas associated with the apices of immature teeth may be mistaken by the unwary as periapical pathosis.

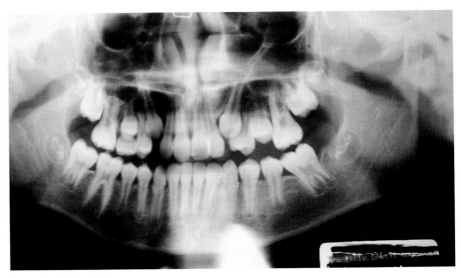

tions, and the presence of apical or furcal pathosis. They are often the only way of diagnosing with certainty the presence of a resorptive defect or a root fracture.

Direct visual inspection

It will be apparent from the foregoing account that pulp diagnosis in children is not always easy. Clinicians should therefore be prepared to review their diagnosis and treatment plan in the light of new information obtained when treatment has commenced. Caries may be found to have progressed further than anticipated when a lesion is actually excavated, and in the same way, an empty pulp chamber may be entered in a tooth which was presumed to be vital. Another situation of particular relevance in paediatric endodontics is the direct assessment of pulpal bleeding following exposure or partial amputation. Bleeding from infected, inflamed pulpal tissue is more likely to be heavy and difficult to control than that from healthy tissue. A tooth scheduled for a simple pulp cap may consequently be found to be a poor candidate for conservative treatment, and a more radical approach may be necessary if the tooth is to be preserved.

8.5 INDICATIONS AND CONTRA-INDICATIONS FOR ENDODONTIC TREATMENT

The many benefits of avoiding extraction and restoring teeth to healthy function indicate endodontic treatment for the majority of pulpally affected primary and young permanent teeth. Nevertheless, planning for individual teeth should not be considered in isolation from the overall plan for the child's mouth, which may be modified by wider behavioural, social and medical issues.

A number of circumstances may then arise when endodontic treatment is not the preferred option.

1. *The unrestorable tooth.* Teeth which are unrestorable or of doubtful prognosis should be extracted without delay. The only circumstance in which endodontic treatment can be indicated for such teeth is as a short-term, first aid measure to relieve pain or prevent flare-up prior to extraction.

2. *The uncooperative or non-compliant child.* Children who are insufficiently co-operative, or who are unwilling or unable to attend regularly for complex restorative care may be better candidates for simple treatment. Wholesale extractions, on the other hand may do little to improve attitudes to dentistry, but clearing of the worst affected teeth may allow scope for introducing the child to preventive and operative dental care.

3. *The medically compromised child.* If, for whatever reason, it is considered that a child may be at risk from the retention of a pulpally compromised tooth, arrangements should be made for its extraction.

4. *The orthodontic extraction.* Occasionally, the loss of pulpally affected but restorable primary or young permanent teeth may be considered within a broader orthodontic treatment plan. This subject will be discussed more fully elsewhere.

Endodontic treatment — contra-indications:
- unrestorable tooth
- uncooperative child
- medical considerations
- orthodontic considerations

Key Points

Operative paediatric endodontics aims to relieve pain and suffering associated with pulpal injury, prevent the extension of pulpal disease, and restore teeth to healthy function.

The following account describes common endodontic procedures for the conservative management of pulpally compromised primary and young permanent teeth.

Successful treatment demands the co-operation of a comfortable child. Effective local anaesthesia must therefore be provided wherever vital dentine or pulp is to be instrumented, or when tooth movement may elicit pain from inflamed periradicular tissues. A potent topical anaesthetic paste (e.g. benzocaine, 20 per cent) should first be applied to the injection site for 2–3 min before slow infiltration of a warmed local anaesthetic solution. Sufficient time must be allowed for anaesthesia to develop fully before commencing treatment.

The outcome of endodontic treatment even in the most compliant child is critically dependent on the control of infection. A well fitting rubber dam (Fig. 8.7) provides the most effective means of isolating the pulp canal system from the oral flora, in addition to safeguarding the oral soft tissues and airway from endodontic medicaments and instruments. The many benefits of rubber dam isolation make its use an essential component of any endodontic treatment in children or adults.

It will be assumed for each of the procedures described that whenever necessary, local anaesthesia will have been provided and that wherever possible, a well fitting rubber dam will be in place.

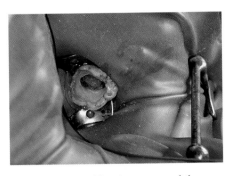

Fig. 8.7 Use of rubber dam to control the operating environment.

Key Points	Advantages of rubber dam isolation:
	• control of infection
	• protection of oral soft tissues/airway/gastrointestinal tract
	• improved visibility
	• improved patient comfort

8.6.1   Stabilization of the mouth

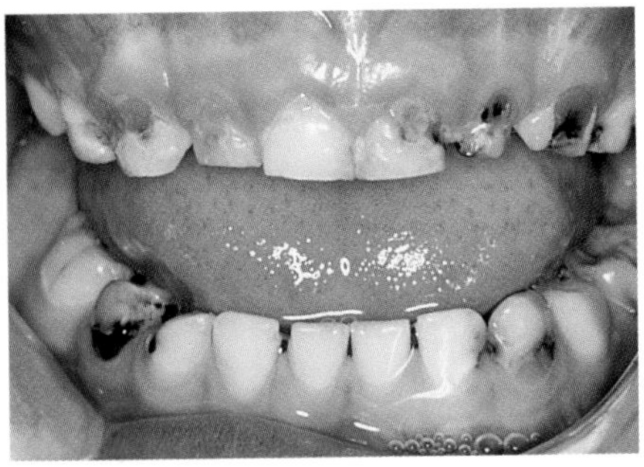

Caries progresses rapidly through the relatively thin dentine of primary and young permanent teeth and may quickly advance to endanger the pulp . When a child presents with a large number of carious teeth (Fig. 8.8), there is a real danger that one or more may become the focus of a painful flare-up if early steps are not taken to gain control of the many teeth involved.

During initial assessment, those teeth which are unrestorable and those which for other reasons are not to be preserved should be identified and extracted without delay. Similarly, those teeth which are to be preserved should be identified and temporized as a first-aid measure prior to the definitive treatment of each tooth in turn.

Gross caries excavation is undertaken either by hand, or with a large round bur running at slow speed. Effort should be made to clear caries from the periphery of each cavity and to remove as much of the softened dentine overlying the pulp as possible. It should be noted that the endurance and trust of the patient should not be tested in trying to remove all of the deep caries at this stage. Often, such gross excavation can be completed without the need for local anaesthetic.

Fig. 8.8 Rampant caries in the mixed dentition. Any of the affected teeth may become the focus of a painful flare-up if early steps are not taken to gain control of the many teeth involved.

Linings of setting calcium hydroxide cement may be placed in the deepest parts of the preparations, which are subsequently sealed with a reinforced zinc oxide/eugenol cement.

Gross caries excavation and sealing of the preparations in this way is likely to arrest or at least slow caries progression, and should reduce any thermal or osmotic sensitivity which may have been experienced.

Definitive treatment can then be planned without the immediate fear of losing control of the case. A programme of preventive care including dietary advice, oral hygiene instruction, and fluoride therapy must also be implemented.

Stabilization of the mouth — aims:

Key Points

- removal of unrestorable teeth
- arrest of restorable lesions
- prevention of painful flare-up
- introduction to preventive and operative dentistry without fear of losing control

8.6.2 Vital pulp therapy

Pulp capping

A pulp cap is a layer of lining or cement material placed on to a thin layer of dentine overlying a macroscopically unexposed pulp (indirect pulp cap), or directly on to exposed pulp tissue (direct pulp cap) with the intention of preserving pulp vitality.

Pulp caps can be applied to teeth in the primary and permanent dentitions provided that strict selection criteria are applied.

Indirect pulp capping (Fig. 8.9(a)–(d))

In the majority of circumstances, carious lesions can and should be fully excavated before tooth restoration. A clinical dilemma is presented by a deep lesion in a vital, symptom-free tooth where complete removal of softened dentine on the pulpal floor is likely to result in frank exposure. (Fig 8.9(a)) The advancing front of a carious lesion contains very few cariogenic bacteria. Provided the bulk of infected overlying dentine is removed, a small amount of softened dentine may often be left in the deepest part of the preparation without endangering the pulp. This is the basis of indirect pulp capping.

All caries is first cleared from the cavity margins with a steel round bur running at slow speed. Gentle excavation then follows on the pulpal floor, removing as much of the softened dentine as possible without exposing the pulp. Precisely how much dentine should be removed becomes a matter of experience and clinical judgement, although some have advocated the use of indicator dyes (e.g. 0.5 per cent basic fuchsin) to show when all infected dentine has been eliminated. A thin layer of setting calcium hydroxide cement is then placed on the cavity floor to destroy any remaining micro-organisms and to promote the deposition of reparative secondary dentine (Fig. 8.9b).

In its classical application, the indirect pulp cap was covered with zinc oxide–eugenol cement, and following several weeks observation, the cavity was re-entered to remove all remaining softened dentine. More commonly, the calcium hydroxide pulp cap is simply covered with a layer of hard setting cement and the tooth permanently restored at the same visit (Fig. 8.9c). Periodic clinical and radiographic review is then undertaken to monitor the pulp response (Fig. 8.9d).

Fig. 8.9 Indirect pulp capping. (a) Symptom-free molar tooth with deep proximal caries. (b) Excavation of caries to the brink of pulpal exposure, leaving a small amount of softened but uninfected dentine on the pulpal wall. A thin layer of setting calcium hydroxide cement is applied to the softened dentine as an indirect pulp cap. (c) The direct pulp cap is overlaid with a hard cement and the tooth restored with amalgam. (d) Appearance at review some months later. The pulp has remained healthy, and the deposition of irregular secondary dentine is apparent.

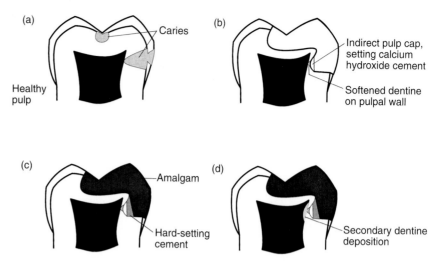

Occasionally, the pulp may be exposed during deep excavation, and the opportunity for indirect pulp capping is lost. In this circumstance, direct pulp capping or a more radical form of treatment such as pulp amputation (pulpotomy) may be considered.

Direct pulp capping
Primary teeth

Direct pulp capping is generally contra-indicated for primary teeth. Pulpal inflammation usually persists and results in total pulp necrosis or internal resorption, especially if a calcium hydroxide pulp cap has been applied. In the majority of cases, a more radical form of treatment such as pulp amputation (formocresol pulpotomy) will offer a much higher rate of success.

The only possible exception to this rule is the case of a small, mechanical exposure on a vital, symptom-free tooth which was already isolated with rubber dam. This sort of injury may follow a child biting down on a handpiece during cavity preparation. Haemorrhage from the exposure site should be minimal and should be readily controlled by the application of a moistened pledget of sterile cotton wool for 2 min. If the haemorrhage is more severe and cannot be controlled by this method, the degree of pulpal inflammation is more serious and the tooth is not a good candidate for pulp capping. Pulp amputation (formocresol pulpotomy) should once again be considered the treatment of choice.

Permanent teeth

The highly vascular pulps of immature permanent teeth have great healing capacity, and the scope of direct pulp capping is therefore greater. In addition to pulps traumatically exposed during cavity preparation, pulps exposed by coronal fracture may respond favourably provided the child is seen within 24 h of the incident. Any residual caries at the periphery of the fracture or cavity preparation should be quickly removed. No instruments should be inserted into the exposure site, and any bleeding should be controlled with sterile cotton wool, not with a blast of air from the 3 in 1 syringe which may drive debris and micro-organisms into the pulp. A layer of setting calcium hydroxide cement is gently flowed on to the exposed pulp and surrounding dentine which is covered with zinc oxide–eugenol cement, and a permanent restoration.

For anterior teeth, the calcium hydroxide pulp cap is quickly overlaid with a non-eugenol containing material such as glass ionomer cement and by a thin 'bandage' of acid etch retained composite resin pending aesthetic restoration at a later date. A successful direct pulp capping procedure will allow the remaining pulp to remain healthy and should promote the deposition of a bridge of reparative dentine to seal off the exposure site.

The patient and carer should be advised of the procedure and of the need to monitor the pulpal response. They should be advised to return if the tooth suddenly becomes sensitive to hot and cold, or if any other untoward symptoms arise.

Provided all remains well, the patient will be seen after a few weeks, and then at 6 monthly intervals for up to 4 years in order to assess pulp vitality. Periodic radiographic review should also be arranged to monitor dentine bridge formation, and to exclude the development of internal resorption or progressive pulpal obliteration which would necessitate further endodontic intervention.

Key Points

Pulp capping:

● not recommended for primary teeth

● not recommended for permanent teeth if signs and symptoms of pulp pathosis

● best prognosis within 24 h in permanent teeth exposed by trauma

---

Pulp amputation (Pulpotomy)

Pulp amputation or pulpotomy is a procedure in which a portion of exposed vital pulp is removed, usually as a means of preserving the vitality and function of the remaining portion. There are important differences in the way pulp amputation (pulpotomy) procedures are conducted for primary and young permanent teeth.

Pulp amputation (Vital or formocresol pulpotomy) — Primary teeth

Primary teeth are generally poor candidates for direct pulp capping or pulp amputation procedures involving the application of calcium hydroxide. Despite its undoubted ability to promote healing and secondary dentine deposition in the pulps of permanent teeth, calcium hydroxide application has been associated with persistent chronic inflammation and destructive internal resorption in primary teeth. The precise mechanisms of this unfavourable response are unclear.

Alternative treatments and medicaments are therefore required for the restoration of vital primary teeth pulpally exposed by caries or trauma. In most circumstances, the treatment of choice will involve amputation of the entire coronal pulp (vital pulpotomy), and application of a non-calcium hydroxide medicament to the radicular pulp stumps.

Alternatives to calcium hydroxide in primary endodontics

1. *Formocresol.* Buckley's formocresol was introduced in 1905 and welcomed as a relatively non-toxic devitalization agent in the days before local anaesthesia was in routine use for pulp treatment. Since the 1950s it has been applied with great success as a primary pulp medicament and remains the most popular agent in vital primary pulp therapy today.

In current practice, one part of the concentrated stock solution (Fig 8.10) is mixed with four parts of diluent to create a standard 1:5 dilution. There are no advantages to be gained by the use of a more concentrated preparation.

The active ingredients of formocresol are tricresol and formalin. Tricresol is a powerful, although short-acting antiseptic agent which is believed to kill micro-organisms at the pulp amputation site. The contribution made by tricresol to the efficacy of formocresol is unclear.

Formocresol	
Concentrated stock solution:	
Formaldehyde	19 ml
Tricresol	35 ml
Glycerol	15 ml
Water	31 ml
Diluent solution:	
Glycerol	3 parts
Water	1 part

Fig. 8.10 Formocresol, common formulation.

Formalin is a potent tissue fixative and without doubt the main active ingredient. When formocresol is applied to healthy, vital pulp tissue for a short period of time (e.g. 5 min), the superficial tissue is rapidly fixed, and the underlying tissue remains unaltered and healthy. Provided the tooth is subsequently restored to prevent reinfection of the treated pulp tissue, a very high rate of success is anticipated. Figures in excess of 90 per cent after 5 years have been reported.

It should be emphasiszed that superficial fixation of an infected, inflamed radicular pulp by the application of formocresol for 5 min will have no beneficial effect on the disease process in the underlying pulp. Radicular pulp breakdown will continue unchecked and signs and symptoms of apical pathosis are likely to follow. Infected and inflamed radicular pulps are therefore poor candidates for this form of treatment.

A number of reports have identified formocresol as an irritant material, capable of inducing inflammation and internal resorption when applied to healthy pulp tissue. However, it is not always possible to determine that the pulps responding in this way were in fact healthy at the outset.

Longer exposure to formocresol results in progressively deeper fixation. This property may be usefully employed in the controlled devitalization and conservative treatment of irreversibly inflamed primary radicular pulps, and will be discussed more fully on p. 157.

The clinical efficacy of formocresol in paediatric endodontics is beyond question. Nevertheless, much controversy surrounds the use of this medicament, which many now believe to be hazardous.

It has been noted that formocresol is a potent tissue fixative, and great care should be exercised in its use in the mouth. The volume of medicament applied to the tissues should be as small as possible and controlled by blotting the cotton wool pellets or paper points with which it is applied on a cotton wool roll prior to use. A well-fitting rubber dam should be in place to guard the oral soft tissues from inadvertent contact, and restoration margins should be checked to safeguard against seepage of the medicament on to the oral tissues with potentially damaging local effects. Local tissue damage may also be anticipated if formocresol is extruded into the periapical tissues, and a number of reports have suggested the possibility of injury to developing permanent tooth germs, and disorders of eruption following formocresol exposure. However, there appears to be little evidence of damaging effects if small volumes of diluted medicament are confined within the pulp chamber and root canals of primary teeth.

Other local effects which have been the focus of concern include the potential mutagenicity and carcinogenicity of formocresol demonstrated in animal and tissue culture studies following prolonged exposure to the full strength medicament. However, extrapolation cannot be made directly to the *in vivo* human situation, particularly at the concentrations currently used in primary pulp treatment.

The effects of formocresol may not only be local. Formocresol is rapidly absorbed into the systemic circulation following its application to vital tissue. Animal studies, again involving long exposure to large doses of formocresol have demonstrated wide distribution of the medicament which is able to bind with cells in the kidneys, lungs, and liver. Once again, there is little evidence of danger to humans in the concentrations routinely employed in clinical practice.

2. *Glutaraldehyde.* Another preparation which attracts interest as a primary pulp medicament is aqueous glutaraldehyde solution (2–4 per cent). Like formocresol, it is a powerful tissue fixative which may be applied with success to the vital, uninflamed pulp stumps of primary teeth following coronal pulp amputation. Inadvertent contact with the oral tissues may again cause local damage and care should always be exercised in its use.

Local toxicity of glutaraldehyde is low and it is said to have minimal carcinogenic or mutagenic potential. Unlike formocresol, it is poorly absorbed from sites of application and remains almost entirely confined within pulp tissue. The potential for systemic distribution and action at distant sites is consequently reduced.

Glutaraldehyde does not penetrate tissue as well as formocresol and the optimal concentration and exposure time for pulp treatment have not been fully established. A 4 min application has been recommended for the 4 per cent preparation, but precise data are lacking on the preferred 2 per cent solution. Problems are confounded by the instability of glutaraldehyde on storage which necessitates frequent replacement if predictable results are desired. Most importantly, success rates have generally been lower for glutaraldehyde than for formocresol even in its 1:5 diluted form.

Although research continues, it is widely held that formocresol in 1:5 dilution is an acceptably safe medicament for use in primary endodontics. Until a demonstrably more effective and less toxic material becomes available, it is likely that formocresol will remain the medicament of choice in this setting.

Operative procedure (Fig. 8.11(a)–(e))

All caries is first excavated from the tooth to assess the degree of coronal destruction and to eliminate infected tissue. A standard access cavity is then prepared, removing the whole of the pulp chamber roof to fully expose its contents. Non-end-cutting burs such as the slow-speed Batt bur (Maillefer) or the high speed Endo-Z bur (Maillefer) (Fig. 8.12) can be very helpful in removing the pulp chamber roof without fear of furcal or lateral perforation.

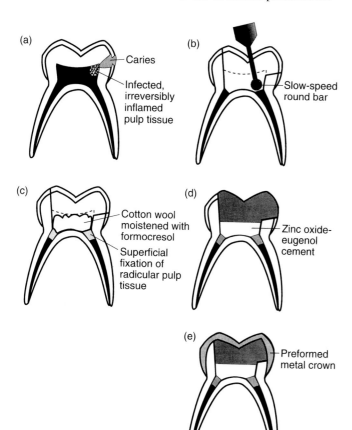

Fig. 8.11 Primary pulp amputation (vital or formocresol pulpotomy). (a) Carious primary molar with an infected, irreversibly inflamed coronal pulp. (b) Caries is excavated, the pulp chamber widely opened, and the coronal pulp removed with a sterile round bur running at slow speed. (c) A cotton-wool pellet, moistened with formocresol is laid gently on the radicular pulp stumps. Note the superficial fixation of the radicular pulp. (d) Interim restoration with zinc oxide–eugenol cement and amalgam. (e) Definitive restoration with a preformed metal crown.

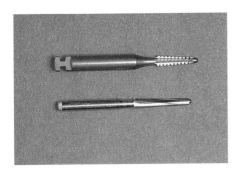

Fig. 8.12 Endo-Z and Batt burs (Maillefer): non-end-cutting burs for safe removal of the pulp chamber roof during access cavity preparation.

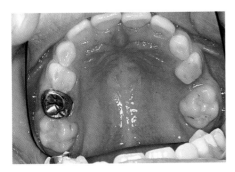

Fig. 8.13 Root treated primary molar restored with a preformed metal crown.

The contents of the pulp chamber are now removed with a sharp spoon excavator or a sterile steel round bur running at slow speed (Fig. 8.11b). Care should be taken not to damage or perforate the pulp chamber floor in posterior teeth. In anterior teeth, amputation may be taken deeper into the canal if desired by removal of the coronal two-thirds of the radicular pulp with a large file.

Following amputation, the pulp chamber is gently irrigated with sterile saline, and light pressure applied to the radicular pulp stumps with moistened cotton wool pledgets to control bleeding. If bleeding is profuse and uncontrollable after 2 min, this indicates more serious inflammation of the radicular pulp, and a devitalization procedure or pulpectomy is indicated. If bleeding is slight and readily controlled, the tooth is a good candidate for vital pulp treatment with formocresol.

For posterior teeth, a small pledget of cotton wool is moistened with formocresol and blotted free of excess on a cotton wool roll. Application to anterior teeth is often simpler with a large paper point moistened and blotted in the same way. The pledget or paper point is placed in gentle contact with the radicular pulp stumps and remains in place for 5 min (Fig. 8.11c). On removal, the pulp stumps will appear dark brown or black with minimal oozing of blood.

Preparations must now be sealed bacteria-tight to prevent the re-entry of micro-organisms to the treated pulp tissue which would result in failure. Molar pulp chambers are usually packed with a proprietary reinforced zinc oxide–eugenol cement. This may be overlaid with amalgam, or ideally with a preformed metal crown (Figs 8.11d, e and 8.13). In anterior teeth where pulp amputation was taken subgingivally, a softer material should be placed in the canal which will be absorbed as the tooth undergoes physiological resorption. This is usually a non-reinforced zinc oxide–eugenol cement produced by mixing pure zinc oxide powder with eugenol. The cement is mixed to a soft paste and spun into the preparation before sealing the access bacteria-tight with 3 mm of glass ionomer cement or composite resin.

The patient and carer should be warned that the tooth may be uncomfortable for a few days, and advice should be given on appropriate analgesia. If symptoms persist beyond a few days, the patient should return for pulp devitalization (see p. 156) or for extraction.

Review

All pulp amputations should be reviewed clinically at 6 monthly intervals, and radiographed annually to check the treated tooth and its permanent successor. If clinical signs and symptoms of pulpal breakdown are noted, non-vital pulp therapy may be considered (see p. 157). However, the extension of pulpal infection to involve the underlying dental follicle should be taken seriously and is a clear indication for extraction. Similarly, teeth undergoing internal resorption should be extracted.

Finally, special vigilance should be exercised at about the time when the treated tooth is due to be shed. Radiographic checks should be made to ensure that root resorption is proceeding normally and that the permanent successor is not being displaced into ectopic eruption.

Pulp amputation (Apexogenesis procedure, vital or calcium hydroxide pulpotomy) — Immature permanent teeth

Pulp amputation for immature permanent teeth is an extension of direct pulp capping where a portion of infected, irreversibly inflamed coronal pulp tissue is removed in order to preserve the vitality and function of the radicular pulp. Completion of apical root development (apexogenesis) and general thickening of the dentine walls of the tooth may then be allowed to proceed. This procedure may be the treatment of choice: (a) Following pulpal exposure where bleeding cannot be easily controlled, and (b) Following trauma where the pulp has been exposed to the mouth for more than 24 h.

Operative procedure (Fig. 8.14(a)–(d))

Entry is made to the exposure site and pulp tissue excised with a diamond bur running at high speed under constant water cooling (Fig. 8.14b). This method of tissue removal has been shown to cause least injury to the underlying pulp and is preferred to hand excavation or the use of slow-speed steel burs.

Microbial invasion of an exposed, vital pulp is usually superficial and as a general rule of thumb, 2 or 3 mm of pulp tissue should be removed. However, excessive bleeding from the residual pulp which cannot be controlled with moist cotton wool indicates that further excision is required to reach healthy tissue. Removal of tissue may occasionally extend deeply into the tooth in a desperate effort to preserve the apical portion of the pulp and safeguard apical closure. When all grossly inflamed tissue has been removed, the wound should be gently rinsed with sterile saline and any shredded tissue removed. The preparation above the excision should also be carefully inspected and any remaining tags of tissue which will undergo necrosis and potentially act as a nidus for reinfection should be removed.

A calcium hydroxide dressing should then be applied to destroy any remaining micro-organisms and to promote calcific repair. In superficial wounds, a setting calcium hydroxide cement may be gently flowed on to the pulp surface, but if the excision was deep, it is often easier to prepare a stiff mixture of calcium hydroxide powder (analytical grade) in sterile saline or local anaesthetic solution, which

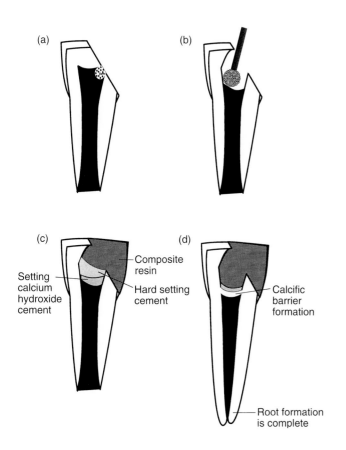

Fig. 8.14 Pulp amputation (apexogenesis procedure), permanent incisor. (a) Complicated fracture of an immature incisor with microbial invasion of the coronal pulp. The pulp has been exposed to the mouth for more than 24 h.
(b) Access to the coronal pulp and amputation of coronal pulp tissue with a diamond bur running at high speed with constant water cooling.
(c) Dressing the pulpal wound to promote calcific repair. Setting calcium hydroxide cement is flowed on to the pulp, and overlaid with a hard cement, and the tooth restored with composite resin. (d) The same tooth after 12 months showing calcific barrier formation. The calcific barrier was directly inspected in this case, and a new layer of setting calcium hydroxide cement placed on the barrier before definitive restoration. The remaining pulp has remained healthy and deposited dentine to complete root formation.

is carried to the canal in an amalgam carrier and gently packed into place with pluggers. The calcium hydroxide dressing should be overlaid with a hard cement (Fig. 8.14c) to prevent its forceful injection into the pulp by chewing forces and a restoration which will seal the preparation against the re-entry of micro-organisms.

The patient and carer should be advised that the tooth may be uncomfortable for a few days, and advice should be given on appropriate analgesia. If symptoms persist beyond a few days, the patient should return for further evaluation.

Review

The case should be reviewed with radiographs after 6 weeks. If there is evidence of continued pulp pathosis, non-vital pulp therapy should be considered (see p. 157). However, if all remains well, the patient should be recalled after a further 6 weeks, and then annually for evaluation of pulp vitality and assessment of calcific bridge formation (Fig. 8.14d). Direct visual inspection of the calcific bridge is allowable, although not always necessary. If vitality is lost, non-vital pulp therapy should be undertaken through the calcific bridge.

Pulp amputation is a highly successful procedure and should allow the radicular pulp to remain healthy *at least* until root development is complete (Fig. 8.15). Pulpectomy and root canal treatment may be considered at a later date if the pulp subsequently loses vitality, if it is feared that the canal is becoming obliterated by dentine deposition, or if the root canal is required for restorative purposes.

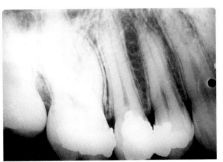

Fig. 8.15 Periapical radiograph showing a pulp amputation procedure undertaken some 10 years previously. Calcific barrier formation is apparent, and root development was completed many years ago. The pulp has remained vital.

Key Points

Pulp amputation:

- more predictable than pulp capping for primary teeth
- better prognosis than direct pulp capping for immature permanent teeth exposed for more than 24 h
- not recommended if signs and symptoms of radicular pulp pathosis

Devitalization of primary teeth

There are occasions when it is not possible to administer a local anaesthetic, or when a vital primary pulp cannot be anaesthetized for amputation. In this situation, the entire pulp may be devitalized by the application of a paraformaldehyde-containing paste. The most common formulation is Aeslick's devitalizing paste, containing paraformaldehyde (1 g), lignocaine (0.06 g), carmine (0.01 g), carbowax (1.3 g), and propylene glycol (0.5 g). Devitalizing paste may be applied to a small pulpal exposure on a tiny pledget of cotton wool and must be sealed tightly in place to prevent seepage into the mouth. The preparation is said to release formaldehyde vapour which permeates and fixes coronal and radicular pulp tissue over the course of 7–10 days. Some discomfort may be anticipated, and the parent and child should be advised that analgesia may be required. On reopening, the pulp should be non-vital, and treatment may proceed as for a non-vital tooth (p. 157). If the pulp remains vital, the procedure may be repeated.

Another situation where devitalization may be considered is in the case of the infected, bleeding pulp stump following coronal pulp amputation. In anterior teeth it is usually possible to extirpate the pulp conventionally, but the complex anatomy of posterior teeth may make this difficult. Devitalization may be achieved with paraformaldehyde paste as described above, or by the application of formocresol for a comparable length of time. Following devitalization, the tooth may once again be treated as a non-vital case.

8.6.3 Non-vital pulp therapy

The infected, necrotic contents of a non-vital pulp system are inaccessible to host defences and cannot be eliminated without operative intervention. In the endodontic management of mature permanent teeth, organic debris, and micro-organisms are removed from the canal system by chemomechanical preparation, and the space is obliterated with a non-resorbable material to prevent reinfection. A number of anatomical and physiological considerations modify this approach for the primary and young permanent tooth.

Endodontic management of non-vital primary teeth ('Non-vital pulpotomy')

The chemomechanical preparation of primary root canals with endodontic hand instruments and irrigants is controversial. Concern has been expressed that the apical canal openings of primary teeth are not always distinct and that inadvertent over-instrumentation may injure subjacent permanent tooth germs. This is illustrated by the resorbing primary molar where the canal opening may be several millimetres from the radiographic root apex and sited toward the furcal side of the root. In addition, the root canal walls, especially of molars, have been considered too thin to tolerate intracanal instrumentation without perforation, and the anatomical ramifications too complex to be reliably cleaned with instruments and irrigants. Greater emphasis has therefore been placed on the use of antimicrobial and tissue fixative medicaments, especially in posterior teeth.

Operative procedure (Fig. 8.16(a)–(e))

Treatment is conducted over two visits, the first for canal debridement and disinfection, the second for obturation.

First visit (Fig. 8.16a–c)

Caries removal and access cavity preparation is undertaken as described above for pulp amputation. Necrotic pulp debris is then removed from the coronal pulp

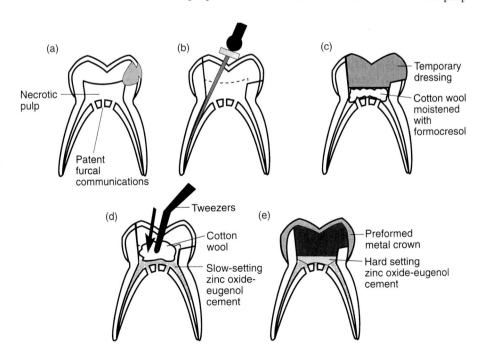

Fig. 8.16 Non-vital pulp therapy — primary tooth. (a) A carious, but restorable non-vital primary molar. (b) Caries is eliminated and access made to the pulp. Gentle canal debridement is undertaken with small files and irrigation. (c) Disinfection of the canal system. A pledget of cotton wool barely moistened in formocresol is sealed into the pulp chamber for 7–10 days. (d) The tooth is reopened at a second visit, and after irrigation and drying, a soft mixture of slow-setting zinc oxide–eugenol cement is gently packed into the canals with cotton wool pledget. (e) The pulp chamber is packed with accelerated zinc oxide–eugenol cement before definitive restoration of the tooth.

chamber with hand instruments, accompanied by copious irrigation. The antimicrobial and tissue solvent actions of a sodium hypochlorite solution (0.5–1.0 per cent) may be advantageous.

Limited canal instrumentation may then be undertaken both for anterior and posterior teeth (Fig. 8.16b). With the guidance of an accurate pre-operative radiograph, small files may be gently inserted into the canal(s) keeping them 2–3 mm short of the radiographic root apex to minimize the danger of over-instrumentation. Radiographs may be obtained to confirm working lengths.

The canal walls are then filed with a light, rasping action to remove adherent debris which is washed from the canal with irrigant. It should be noted that preparation is limited to debridement, and that extensive canal shaping by vigorous dentine removal is not required. After drying the canal(s) with premeasured paper points, a pledget of cotton wool, barely moistened with formocresol is sealed into the pulp chamber with a hard setting cement (Fig. 8.16c).

The medicated pledget of cotton wool remains in place until the next appointment, some 7–10 days later, with the intention of fixing any remaining pulpal remnants and killing micro-organisms remaining after canal preparation. It is usual for signs and symptoms of periapical or furcal pathosis to have resolved by the time of the second appointment. If they have not, further gentle canal debridement and medication may be considered.

Second visit (Fig. 8.16d,e)

After removing the temporary dressing and cotton wool pledget, the canals may be re-irrigated and dried prior to filling. The roots of primary teeth undergo physiological resorption as their permanent successors erupt, and any filling material placed in their canals must therefore be capable of resorbing at a comparable rate. A soft, slow setting zinc oxide–eugenol cement made by mixing pure zinc oxide powder with eugenol is the current material of choice. The consistency of the mixture may be adjusted to allow placement by a variety of methods. Fluid mixtures may be introduced to canals with a spiral paste filler, while stiffer mixtures may be packed with cotton wool pledgets (Fig. 8.16d) or pluggers. Dense obturation is desirable to incarcerate and destroy any remaining micro-organisms and to prevent the re-entry of oral microbes to the apical and furcal tissues, but care should be taken not to extrude material beyond the root apices which may provoke a painful postoperative response.

The tooth may now be restored in a manner appropriate to the degree of coronal breakdown (Fig. 8.16e).

Review

The treatment of non-vital primary teeth is highly successful, but periodic review should again be arranged to monitor the response of the periapical and furcal tissues. Annual radiographs are necessary to check the treated tooth and its permanent successor as described on p. 154 for primary pulp amputation.

Key Points

'Non-vital pulpotomy':

● predictable treatment if infection controlled and canal sealed bacteria-tight
● control of intracanal infection by irrigation and disinfection
● vigorous canal enlargement not required and risks perforation and failure
● resorbable material for canal obturation

Endodontic management of non-vital, immature permanent teeth

The endodontic management of non-vital, immature permanent teeth presents a number of special difficulties. Premature loss of pulp vitality results in thin and

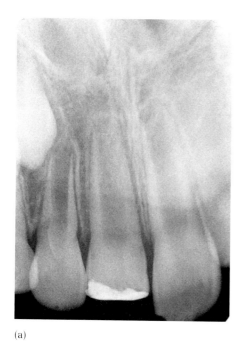

(a)

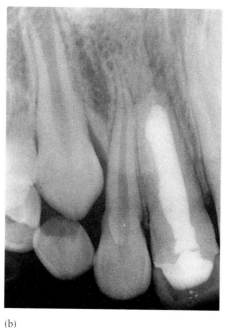

(b)

Fig. 8.17 Root-end closure (apexification). (a) Immature permanent central incisor devitalized by trauma. (b) The same tooth 18 months later. Canal debridement and calcium hydroxide therapy has allowed the development of an apical calcific barrier. The canal has been densely obturated with thermoplastic gutta percha and sealer.

relatively weak tooth structure which should not be weakened further by excessive dentine removal during canal preparation. In addition, the open and often diverging apices of immature permanent teeth create technical difficulties for the controlled condensation of root filling materials, and a root end closure (apexification) procedure is often required to produce an apical calcific barrier against which filling materials may be packed (Fig. 8.17a and b). The most important precondition for calcific barrier formation is the elimination of micro-organisms from the root canal system. This is achieved by thorough canal debridement and by the long-term application of a non-toxic, antimicrobial medicament such as non-setting calcium hydroxide.

Root end closure is a predictable although lengthy modality of treatment. Patients and carers should be advised from the outset of the need to monitor barrier formation for anything between 12 and 30 months before definitive canal obturation and restoration.

Operative procedure for root-end closure (apexification) (Fig. 8.18(a)–(d))
Access

Following caries removal, standard access is prepared with a high-speed, medium tapered fissure bur (Fig. 8.18a). On entry to the pulp chamber, safe-ended burs (Fig. 8.12) may once again be helpful in removing the entire roof without danger of overcutting or perforation. Loose debris should be removed from the pulp chamber with hand instruments, accompanied by copious, gentle irrigation with sodium hypochlorite solution (1–2 per cent).

Canal preparation

Canal preparation involves two distinct processes: *cleaning*, to free the root canal system of organic debris, micro-organisms and their toxins; and *shaping*, to modify the form of the existing canal to allow the placement of a root filling, which is well condensed throughout its length.

Cleaning is achieved primarily by the use of irrigants and dressing agents, while shaping is achieved by the controlled use of enlarging instruments. It should be emphasized that dentine removal must be restricted to that required for

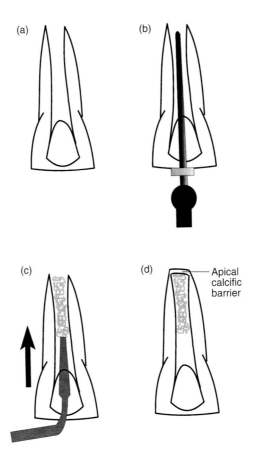

Fig. 8.18 Root-end closure (apexification): clinical procedure. (a) Access into the necrotic pulp of an immature permanent incisor. (b) Following irrigation and gentle debidement in a crown-to-apex direction, working length is determined.(c) Non-setting calcium hydroxide paste packed into the canal with premeasured pluggers. (d) The same tooth 18 months later. A calcific barrier is apparent, and the tooth is ready for definitive obturation and restoration.

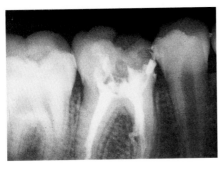

Fig. 8.19 Strip perforation on the furcal wall of an immature permanent lower molar caused by careless overcutting with Gates Glidden drills. The long-term prognosis is very poor.

satisfactory shaping, and in the case of wide, immature canals, little, if any canal enlargement is therefore indicated.

Preparation should be undertaken in a crown to apex sequence in order to optimize debridement while minimizing apical extrusion of debris.

Canal entrances are generally wide and require no enlargement, but occasionally, Gates Glidden drills may be used to improve access for instruments and irrigant. Gates Glidden drills should not be used deep in the canals of immature teeth where they may overcut and create a strip perforation (Fig. 8.19). Deeper preparation is continued with hand files. Working slowly in an apical direction, files are directed around the canal walls with a light rasping action to remove adherent debris. In the curved canals of molars, special care should be taken to avoid overcutting on the thin furcal walls which may again result in damaging strip perforation. Instrumentation is frequently punctuated by high-volume, low-pressure irrigation to flush out debris, and if the irrigant is sodium hypochlorite solution, to continue dissolving organic debris and killing micro-organisms deep in the canal. Irrigant is usually delivered by premeasured, 27 gauge needle and syringe, although the benefits of ultrasound are increasingly recognized. Ultrasonic units should be fitted with a size 15 or 20 endosonic K file, which is introduced to the desired level in the canal before activation. Irrigant is then allowed to flow in high volume over the energized file, which creates turbulence in the irrigant solution, throwing it into all ramifications and 'scrubbing' the canal walls to enhance debridement. The action of the file is simply to enhance irrigation, not to remove dentine, and care should be taken to place the file loosely into the canal, and to minimize contact with the canal walls while activated.

Preparation continues in this way until a provisional working length is reached. This is usually a point some 2 or 3 mm from the radiographic apex, estimated from an undistorted pre-operative periapical film. At this point, a working length radiograph may be exposed and a definitive working length established 1 mm short of the radiographic root apex (Fig. 8.18b). Further gentle filing and irrigation is then continued to the definitive working length.

After final irrigation, the canal is dried, first by aspiration through the irrigating needle, and then with paper points. Paper points should be premeasured to avoid inadvertent overextension and damage to the periapical tissues.

Dressing the root canal

The prepared canal is now filled with a non-setting calcium hydroxide paste, whose antimicrobial and mild tissue solvent activity will continue to cleanse the canal, and whose high pH is believed to encourage calcific root end closure.

Relatively fluid proprietary pastes such as Pulpdent paste (Pulpdent Corporation, Massachusetts, USA) may be conveniently spun into canals with a spiral paste filler, while stiff pastes created by mixing calcium hydroxide powder (analytical grade) with sterile saline or local anaesthetic may be carried to the canal with an amalgam carrier and packed incrementally with premeasured pluggers (Fig. 8.18c). The method of delivery appears to have little bearing on outcome, although with either method, care should be taken to avoid gross overfilling. A radiograph may be exposed to ensure a dense fill to each root terminus (Fig. 8.20).

It is important that the access cavity is sealed tightly between appointments to prevent the leaching of calcium hydroxide, and critically, to prevent the re-entry of micro-organisms from the mouth which would disturb the process of root end closure. A 3 mm thickness of glass ionomer cement or composite resin is adequate to provide a bacteria-tight seal.

Monitoring root-end closure

Review appointments should be arranged at 3–6 monthly intervals. At each appointment, the calcium hydroxide dressing is carefully washed from the canal, and the presence of a calcified barrier assessed by gently tapping a premeasured paper point at the working length. Radiographs should be exposed to assess the progress of barrier formation (Fig. 8.18d).

If the canal is closed, obturation may be undertaken. If calcific barrier formation is not complete, the canal should be redressed and the patient discharged for a further 3–6 months. Calcific barrier formation is usually complete within 12–18 months, although it may be up to 30 months before hope is lost in an unresponding case.

Obturation

When root-end closure is complete, the canal should be densely obturated with gutta percha and sealer to prevent the re-entry of oral micro-organisms to the apical tissues. Cold lateral condensation of gutta percha and sealer may provide satisfactory results in regular, apically converging canals, but in irregular and diverging canals, a thermoplastic gutta percha technique is required to improve adaptation. The use of single cone techniques cannot be recommended in any circumstance.

One popular technique successfully combines the thermal adaptation of gutta percha in the apical portion of the canal with cold lateral condensation more coronally.

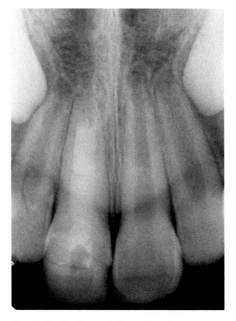

Fig. 8.20 Radiograph to confirm dense obliteration of the prepared canal with non-setting calcium hydroxide paste.

Operative procedure (Fig. 8.21(a)–(c))

A master point is first selected and tried in the canal. This is usually the widest point which will reach the canal terminus, and may be inverted in the widest canals. After drying the canal and lightly coating its walls with a slow setting sealer, the tip of the master point is softened by passage through a bunsen burner flame (Fig. 8.21a). Without delay, the point is inserted to the apical limit of the canal and pressed gently against the calcific barrier to adapt the softened gutta percha (Fig. 8.21b). Cold lateral condensation then follows by the insertion of a spreader to within 1 mm of the apical limit of the canal and the addition of accessory gutta percha cones lightly coated with sealer. Condensation continues until the spreader is able to reach no further than 2 or 3 mm into the canal (Fig. 8.21c). A check radiograph may then be exposed to assess the quality of fill before removing excess gutta percha with a hot instrument and vertically condensing the warm gutta percha at the canal entrance. Further cold or warm condensation may be undertaken at this stage if required to obtain a uniformly dense obturation.

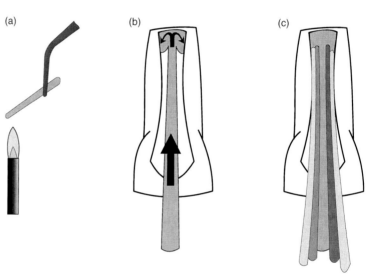

Fig. 8.21 Obturation following root-end closure in an apically diverging canal. (a) The widest gutta percha point which will reach the apical terminus of the canal is warmed by passage of its tip through a flame. (b) Without delay, the point is introduced to the canal (the canal is already lightly coated with sealer), and advanced to adapt against the apical barrier. (c) Additional points are now packed around the master point with cold or warm condensation until the canal is densely filled.

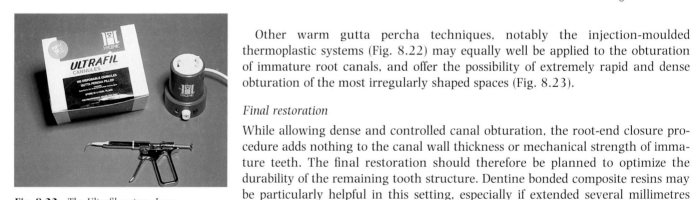

Fig. 8.22 The Ultrafil system. Low temperature injection moulded thermoplastic gutta percha.

Other warm gutta percha techniques, notably the injection-moulded thermoplastic systems (Fig. 8.22) may equally well be applied to the obturation of immature root canals, and offer the possibility of extremely rapid and dense obturation of the most irregularly shaped spaces (Fig. 8.23).

Final restoration

While allowing dense and controlled canal obturation, the root-end closure procedure adds nothing to the canal wall thickness or mechanical strength of immature teeth. The final restoration should therefore be planned to optimize the durability of the remaining tooth structure. Dentine bonded composite resins may be particularly helpful in this setting, especially if extended several millimetres into the root canal to provide internal splinting. Periodic clinical and radiographic review should be arranged.

Key Points

Root-end closure
● predictable result if infection controlled and canal sealed bacteria-tight
● infection controlled by irrigation and disinfection
● canal enlargement only to allow dense obturation
● adds nothing to strength of tooth
● coronal restoration critical to long-term success

Alternatives to the root-end closure procedure

1. *The almost complete apex.* When pulp vitality is lost in an almost fully formed tooth, it may be possible to avoid lengthy root-end closure procedures by creating an apical stop against which a root filling may be packed. Following crown to apex preparation as described above, endodontic hand files may be used in gentle watch-winding or balanced-force motion at working length to shave an apical seat for canal obturation. Alternatively, calcium hydroxide powder (analytical grade) may be packed in the apical 1–2 mm of the canal with pluggers to provide an artificial calcific barrier for obturation.

2. *Failure of the root-end closure procedure, or patient unable to undergo lengthy treatment.* In wide canals where root end closure has failed, or where the patient is unable or unwilling to attend for repeated appointments, an artificial calcific barrier may again be created by packing a stiff calcium hydroxide paste or dry calcium hydroxide powder in the apical 2 mm of the canal before obturating with gutta percha and sealer as described above. Endodontic surgery with root-end filling is becoming less popular as a means of treatment in the case of non-closure. However, it may be considered to address problems of serious, irretrievable overfill which may arise if the calcific barrier was erroneously diagnosed as complete, or if the barrier was broken by heavy-handed obturation (Fig. 8.24).

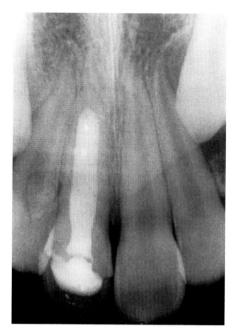

Fig. 8.23 Rapid, dense obturation of a wide and irregularly shaped canal with injection moulded thermoplastic gutta percha and sealer.

8.6.4 Some endodontic considerations in the management of traumatized teeth

Aspects of the diagnosis and treatment of traumatized primary and permanent teeth are discussed in Chapter 11. However, two common sequelae of trauma, namely root fracture and resorption may require special endodontic management and will be given further consideration in the following section.

Root fractures

More than 60 per cent of root fractured primary and permanent teeth remain vital and provided they remain firm and functional, require only periodic review. Loss of pulp vitality may be indicated by a late increase in tooth mobility, or swelling of the soft tissues overlying the root. Pulp sensitivity tests alone should not be taken as evidence of pulp death. Radiographically, the fracture line may be seen to widen due to extrusion of the coronal fragment, and a lateral lucency may be apparent. Even if the coronal portion loses vitality, the apical portion usually remains vital, but if it too becomes non-vital, a characteristic apical lucency may be noted.

Non-vital root fractured primary teeth are poor candidates for root treatment and should be extracted. The apical fragment, which is frequently vital, should not be vigorously chased at the risk of damaging the successional tooth. It will usually undergo physiological resorption as the permanent successor erupts.

Non-vital root fractured permanent teeth on the other hand respond well to conventional root canal therapy which may often be confined to the non-vital coronal portion.

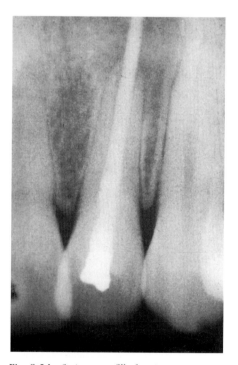

Fig. 8.24 Serious overfill of an immature incisor which may require surgical revision if orthograde retrieval is impossible.

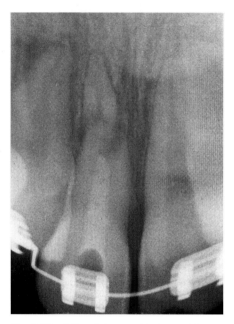

Fig. 8.25 Splinted, fractured incisor, with calcium hydroxide to the fracture line. The apical fragment usually remains vital, but may be surgically removed at a later date if required.

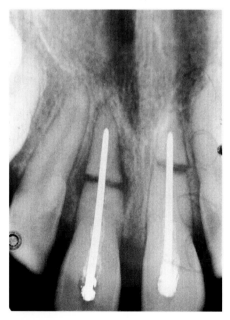

Fig. 8.26 Fractured incisors internally splinted with single, silver points. Failure is indicated by expansion of the fracture lines and lateral lucency associated with ⌐1.

Operative procedure if the apical fragment remains vital

Following conventional access preparation, the pulp chamber is flooded with irrigant, and the coronal few millimetres of the canal(s) flared with Gates Glidden drills. Working length is then determined approximately 1 mm coronal to the fracture line. In relatively narrow canals, an apical stop may be prepared by gently rotating hand files with a watch-winding motion, and the preparation completed by stepping back from the prepared apex with progressively larger files. All instrumentation is accompanied by frequent irrigation with sodium hypochlorite solution (1–2 per cent). In wide canals where it is not possible to develop an adequate apical stop, a root end closure procedure may be implemented as described on p. 159 (Fig. 8.25).

The prepared canal may then be obturated with a well condensed filling of gutta percha and sealer, and the tooth restored to prevent the access of oral micro-organisms to the fracture site and periradicular tissues. Periodic clinical and radiographic review should be arranged.

If the apical fragment subsequently loses vitality, endodontic surgery may be undertaken for its removal. However, if the coronal and apical fragments are well-aligned, endodontic retreatment may be considered with extension across the fracture line and into the apical portion.

Operative procedure if the coronal and apical portions are non-vital

If the fragments are poorly aligned, instruments cannot pass to the apical portion, and treatment should be confined to the coronal fragment as described above. Surgery may be arranged to remove the untreatable apex.

If on the other hand the fragments are well aligned, instruments may be advanced to the apex of the apical fragment and the canal prepared in the usual manner. Frequently, treatment is complicated by bleeding into the canal from the fracture line, making early obturation impossible. In this situation, the canal should be dressed with non-setting calcium hydroxide paste and reviewed at 3–6 monthly intervals to reassess the condition of the canal. The canal is usually dry within 3–6 months, although dressings are sometimes repeated for up to 12 months in an attempt to promote calcific repair of the fracture site.

When the canal is dry, obturation may be undertaken with gutta percha and sealer and the tooth restored.

Internal splinting

Fractures arising in the coronal and middle third of the root often result in mobility of the coronal fragment and techniques have been described to internally splint the coronal and apical portions together with a rigid root filling material. Internal splints have ranged from hedstroem files to nickel–chromium points, screwed and cemented into position. These approaches are in effect single cone root filling procedures, and cannot be relied upon to give a long-term safeguard against the re-entry of oral micro-organisms to the canal and fracture line. Most are doomed to failure (Fig. 8.26).

An interesting recent innovation which may find useful application in internal splinting is the Thermafil® device (Fig. 8.27), which consists of a rigid plastic or metallic core, coated on its exterior by thermoplastic gutta percha. It is likely that this type of device may offer adequate splinting, while at the same time providing dense canal obturation to prevent reinfection, although long-term evaluations are not yet available.

In general terms, internal splinting is not a reliable modality of treatment, and forced eruption (extrusion) and restoration of the apical fragment or extraction and the provision of immediate acid-etch retained bridgework are generally preferred.

Root resorption

Root resorption is a serious and destructive complication which may follow trauma to primary and permanent teeth. Primary teeth which develop pathological resorptive lesions are not good candidates for conservative treatment and should be extracted. Permanent teeth on the other hand may often be successfully treated provided tissue destruction has not advanced to an unrestorable state.

Two general forms of pathological root resorption are recognized, inflammatory and replacement.

Inflammatory root resorption

Internal and external root surfaces injured as a result of trauma are rapidly colonized by multinuclear giant cells. If giant cells are continuously stimulated, most commonly by microbial products from an infected root canal or periodontal pocket, progressive inflammatory root resorption may follow with catastrophic consequences. Inflammatory root resorption may be classified according to its site of origin as external root resorption, cervical resorption (a special form of external resorption) and internal resorption.

External inflammatory root resorption

Teeth affected by external inflammatory root resorption are invariably non vital. Resorptive activity is propagated by infected root canal contents seeping to the external root surface through patent dentinal tubules, and may be extremely aggressive. However, if the infected canal contents are removed, the propagating stimulus is lost and the lesion will predictably arrest. Depending on the size of the resorptive defect, it may be subsequently repaired by cementum deposition.

1. *Diagnosis.* External inflammatory root resorption is usually detected as a chance radiographic finding, and is characterized by change of the external contour of the root, which is often surrounded by a bony lucency (Figs 8.28 and 11.30). Sometimes it may present as a radiolucency overlying the root, and can be distinguished from internal resorption by its asymmetrical shape, and by the contour of the intact root canal walls, which are often superimposed.

2. *Treatment.* Provided the tooth is still restorable, external inflammatory root resorption should be treated without delay. Following access cavity preparation, the root canal should be cleaned and shaped, taking care not to weaken the root excessively, or to risk perforation into the resorbed area. It is common practice to dress the root canal with non-setting calcium hydroxide paste and to monitor the tooth for several months prior to definitive obturation to ensure that the lesion has arrested. Nevertheless, control of intracanal infection is the key determinant of success, and there is good evidence to suggest that if the canal is adequately prepared, it may be filled without protracted calcium hydroxide treatment.
Periodic clinical and radiographic review should be arranged.

Cervical resorption

Cervical resorption is an unusual form of external inflammatory root resorption, initiated by damage to the root surface in the cervical region, and propagated either by infected root canal contents, or by the periodontal microflora. From a

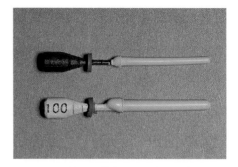

Fig. 8.27 Thermafil devices. Thermoplastic gutta percha surrounding a plastic carrier, combining control with rapid, dense obturation. The rigid core may provide satisfactory internal splinting for root-fractured teeth.

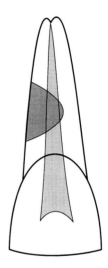

Fig. 8.28 External inflammatory root resorption. Usually presents as an assymetrical radiolucency on the lateral surface of the root. If the lesion overlies the root canal, its lateral walls are usually still visible.

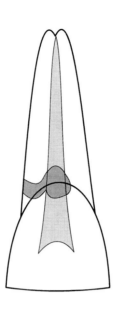

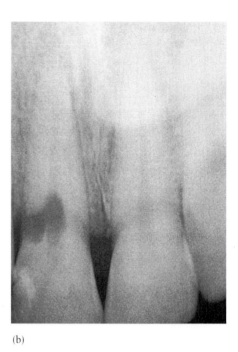

(a)   (b)

Fig. 8.29 Cervical resorption. (a) Resorption commences from a small entry point below the gingival crevice, and often spreads widely within the crown before the root canal is invaded. The lateral walls of the pulp chamber are often superimposed over the defect. (b) Periapical radiograph showing a typical clinical case.

very small entry point, the resorptive process may extend widely before penetrating the pulp chamber (Fig. 8.29a and b).

1. *Diagnosis.* Extensive intracoronal extension may occasionally present cervical resorption as a clinically visible pink spot. More commonly, it is identified on routine radiographs as a characteristically sited radiolucency (Fig. 8.29).

2. *Treatment.* If the tooth is non-vital, conventional root canal therapy should be undertaken to eliminate the propagating stimulus. Arrangements should then be made to open the resorptive defect in a similar manner to cavity preparation, and to curette away all traces of inflammatory tissue before restoring the resultant defect (Fig. 8.30). Often, a flap must be raised to adequately eliminate resorptive tissue and contour the restoration.

If the tooth is vital, and the pulp has not been invaded, treatment may be limited to opening and curetting the resorption lacuna before placing a setting calcium hydroxide lining and restoring the defect with an appropriate material.

Periodic clinical and radiographic review should again be arranged.

Internal inflammatory root resorption

Internal inflammatory root resorption is seen in the canals of traumatized teeth which are undergoing progressive pulp necrosis. Infected material in the non-vital, coronal part of the canal is believed to propagate resorption by the underlying vital tissue, and rapid tissue destruction follows.

1. *Diagnosis.* Large resorptive defects affecting the coronal third of the canal may present as a pink discoloration of the affected tooth. More commonly, it is detected as a chance finding on routine radiographic examination. Radiographically internal resorption presents as a rounded, symmetrical radiolucency, centred on the root canal. The contours of the root canal walls are rarely superimposed (Fig. 8.31a and b).

2. *Treatment.* Internal resorption should be considered to be a form of irreversible pulpitis and treated without delay.

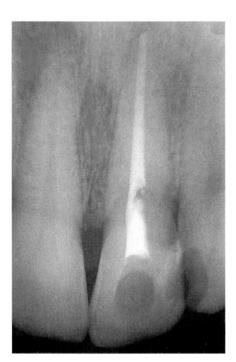

Fig. 8.30 Cervical resorption, following endodontic treatment of the necrotic pulp, and surgical repair of the external defect.

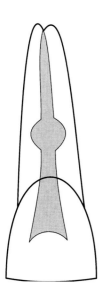

(a)

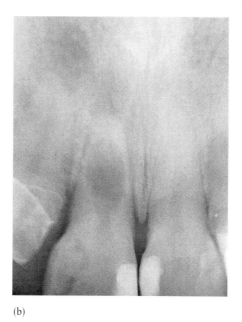

(b)

Fig. 8.31 Internal inflammatory root resorption. (a) Symmmetrical expansion of the root canal walls in a permanent central incisor. (b) Periapical radiograph showing a typical clinical case.

Following standard access cavity preparation, the pulp chamber and coronal portion of the canal is usually found to contain necrotic debris. However, deeper penetration of the canal often provokes torrential haemorrhage as the vascular, resorptive tissue is entered.

Root canal preparation is undertaken in the usual manner, and following apical enlargement, haemorrhage from the canal is greatly reduced as the blood supply to the resorptive tissue is severed. Instrumentation of the expanded, resorbed area is difficult, and can be greatly enhanced by the use of sonic or ultrasonic devices which are able to throw irrigant into uninstrumented areas. The antimicrobial and tissue solvent actions of sodium hypochlorite make it the irrigant of choice in such cases.

As in the case of external inflammatory resorption, it is usual to dress the canal with non-setting calcium hydroxide following debridement. This may be highly advantageous in the internal resorption case where the antimicrobial and mild tissue solvent actions of calcium hydroxide may be exploited further to clean the resorbed area.

Obturation may then be undertaken with gutta percha and sealer, usually employing a thermoplastic technique to allow satisfactory condensation and adaptation in the resorbed area (Fig. 8.32).

Replacement resorption

Replacement resorption is a distinct form of root resorption which follows serious luxation or avulsion injury that has caused damage to the investing periodontal ligament. A classic scenario is the avulsed tooth which has been stored dry, or scrubbed before replantation, with resultant death of periodontal fibroblasts on much of the root surface. If more than 20 per cent of the periodontal ligament is damaged or lost and the tooth is subsequently reimplanted, bone cells are able to grow into contact with the root surface more quickly than the remaining periodontal fibroblasts are able to recolonize the root surface and intervene between tooth and bone. The consequence is that the root now becomes involved in the normal remodelling process of the bone in which it is implanted, and is gradually replaced by bone over the course of the following years. In young children where

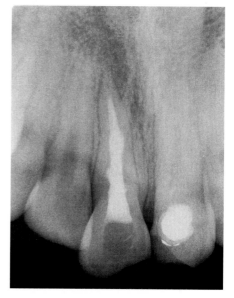

Fig. 8.32 Internal inflammatory root resorption. Maxillary central incisor demonstrating internal resorptive defects at two levels. The canal was cleaned, shaped and obturated with thermoplasticized gutta pecha and sealer.

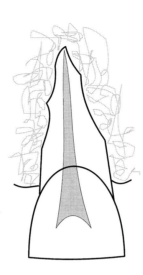

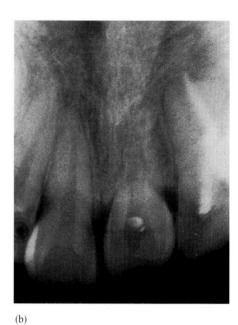

(a)　　　　　　　　　　　　　　　　　　　　　　(b)

Fig. 8.33 Replacement resorption. (a) Roots affected by replacement resorption have ragged outlines, and merge with the surrounding bone to which they are fused. (b) Periapical radiograph showing advanced replacement resorption. Clinically, the tooth is rock solid.

the rate of bone remodelling is high, the root may be entirely lost within 3–4 years. In adolescents, it may be 10 years or more before the tooth is lost.

1. *Diagnosis.* The absence of a ligamentous joint between the tooth and its supporting bone (ankylosis) means that even when root resorption is advanced, the tooth will appear rock solid. A bright, metallic tone will also be noted if the tooth is percussed. Radiographically, the root will appear ragged in outline, with no obvious periodontal ligament space separating it from the surrounding bone (Fig. 8.33(a) and (b)).

2. *Treatment.* There is no effective treatment for established replacement resorption and parents and carers should be advised of the inevitable course of events. Prevention is the only effective form of management, and the need to minimize periodontal ligament injury and secure early replantation is discussed in Chapter 11. From an endodontic point of view, it is important to note that if pulp extirpation is undertaken within 2 weeks of reimplantation, calcium hydroxide paste should not be used to dress the canal as apical extrusion of this medicament into the periapical tissues may cause further periodontal injury and actually encourage replacement resorption. The initial root canal dressing should therefore be a polyantibiotic or antibiotic/steroid (Ledermix, Lederle) preparation which should be replaced subsequently with non-setting calcium hydroxide, no sooner than 2 weeks after tooth reimplantation.

If endodontic treatment was not undertaken soon after reimplantation and the tooth subsequently loses vitality, conventional root canal therapy may be undertaken in order to address any painful periapical pathosis and to avoid the additional insult of inflammatory resorption which would lead to more rapid loss of root substance. A resorbable root filling material may be preferred to gutta percha and sealer in such cases. Most commonly, this would be a non-setting calcium hydroxide paste, replaced at 6 monthly intervals, although resorbable zinc oxide–eugenol or calcium hydroxide-based root canal sealers applied without gutta percha may be acceptable alternatives.

8.7 SUMMARY

1. Endodontic procedures can predictably restore the majority of pulpally compromised primary and young permanent teeth to healthy function. Unplanned extractions in the primary and mixed dentitions should be avoided wherever possible.

2. Unrestorable teeth should not be considered for endodontic therapy. Extraction may also be preferred for uncooperative and certain medically compromised children.

3. Successful endodontics demands the co-operation of a comfortable child. Effective local anaesthesia should be provided if there is any risk of pain during treatment.

5. From indirect pulp capping to non-vital pulp therapy, control of microbial infection is the key determinant of endodontic treatment success. A well-fitting rubber dam should be in place wherever possible, and all stages of all endodontic procedures should be conducted with due regard to the elimination of infection and the prevention of its recurrence.

6. Root canal systems are cleaned principally by antimicrobial and tissue-solvent irrigants and medicaments, not by exuberant dentine removal. Dentine removal, especially in fragile primary and young permanent teeth, should be rational and restricted to that required for successful obturation only.

7. Potent medicaments still have a place in primary endodontics. Formocresol (1:5 dilution) remains the medicament of choice in vital and non-vital primary pulp therapy but there is no justification for the use of a more concentrated and potentially more toxic solution. Calcium hydroxide cannot be currently recommended as a primary pulp medicament.

8. All endodontic procedures should be conducted with deliberate, gentle instrumentation, with meticulous attention to detail, and with respect for the tooth under treatment and the child to whom it belongs.

8.8 FURTHER READING

Cohen, S. and Burns, R. C. (1994). *Pathways of the pulp* (6th edn). Mosby, St Louis. (*The definitive endodontic reference book.*)

European Society of Endodontology (1994). Consensus Report of the European Society of Endodontology on quality guidelines for endodontic treatment. *International Endodontic Journal*, **27**, 115–24. (*A synopsis of current terminology and good practice in endodontics.*)

Ketley, C. E. and Goodman, J. R. (1991). Formocresol toxicity: is there a suitable alternative? *International Journal of Paediatric Dentistry*, **2**, 67–72. (*A good review of primary pulp medicaments.*)

Nunn J. H., Smeaton I., and Gilroy J. (1996). The development of formocresol as a medicament for primary molar pulpotomy procedures. *Journal of Dentistry for Children* **63**, 51–53. (*A review of formocresol as a pulpotomy medicament together with consideration of the interpretation of the formula in current use*)

9 Advanced restorative dentistry

9 Advanced restorative dentistry
N. M. KILPATRICK and R. R. WELBURY

9.1 INTRODUCTION

The aim of this chapter is to cover the management of more complicated clinical problems associated with children and adolescents; tooth discoloration, inherited enamel and dentine defects, and tooth surface loss. There is considerable overlap in the application of the various restorative techniques; therefore, the chapter is divided into two parts: the first outlines the clinical steps involved in the various procedures while the second covers the more general principles of management of the particular dental problems.

9.2 ADVANCED RESTORATIVE TECHNIQUES

It is not the remit of this chapter to cover advanced restorative dentistry in detail, but many of the techniques used in children are the same as those for adults (Tables 9.1 and 9.2).

Seven of the restorative procedures will be described in simple stages with the aid of some clinical examples. Omitted from this list are the stages involved in the provision of full crown restorations and bridgework, which are the specific

Table 9.1 Advanced restorative techniques

Hydrochloric acid — pumice microabrasion technique
Non-vital bleaching
Vital bleaching — chairside and nightguard
Localized composite resin restorations
Composite veneers — direct and indirect
Porcelain veneers
Adhesive metal castings
Full crowns
Bridgework — adhesive and fixed

Table 9.2 **Ideal features of restorative treatments**

Resolve sensitivity
Restore function
Aesthetic
Have proven durability
Cause insignificant loss of tooth structure
Preserve dental hard tissues
Enhance periodontal health
Simple, quick and tolerable to the patient

remit of a restorative dentistry textbook. However, the provision of porcelain veneers, more commonly associated with adult patients, will be mentioned briefly.

9.2.1 The hydrochloric acid pumice microabrasion technique

This is a controlled method of removal of surface enamel in order to improve discolorations that are *limited to the outer enamel layer*. It is achieved by a combination of abrasion and erosion and the term 'abrosion' is sometimes used. In the clinical technique that will be described no more than 100 μm of enamel are removed. Once completed the procedure should not be repeated again in the future. Too much enamel removal is potentially damaging to the pulp and cosmetically the underlying dentine colour will become more evident.

Indications:

(1) fluorosis;
(2) idiopathic speckling;
(3) post-orthodontic treatment demineralization;
(4) prior to veneer placement for well demarcated stains;
(5) white/brown surface staining, e.g. secondary to primary predecessor infection or trauma (Turner teeth).

Armamentarium:

(1) bicarbonate of soda/water;
(2) copalite varnish;
(3) fluoridated toothpaste;
(4) Non-acidulated fluoride (0–2 years: drops);
(5) pumice;
(6) rubber dam;
(7) rubber prophylaxis cup;
(8) soflex discs;
(9) 18 per cent hydrochloric acid;
(10) a complete kit for the acid-pumice microabrasion can be purchased commercially as PREMA (Premier Dental Products).

Technique:

1. Pre-operative vitality tests, radiographs and photographs (Fig. 9.1a).
2. Clean teeth with pumice and water, wash, and dry.
3. Isolate teeth to be treated with rubber dam and paint Copalite varnish around necks of the dam.
4. Place a mixture of sodium bicarbonate and water on the dam behind the teeth to protect in case of spillage (Fig. 9.1b).
5. Mix 18 per cent hydrochloric acid with pumice into a slurry and apply a small amount to the labial surface on either a rubber cup rotating slowly for 5 s or a woodenstick rubbed over the surface for 5 s (Fig. 9.1c), before washing for 5 s directly into an aspirator tip. Repeat until the stain has reduced, up to a maximum of 10 × 5 second applications per tooth. Any improvement that is going to occur will have done so by this time.
6. Apply the fluoride drops to the teeth for 3 min.
7. Remove the rubber dam.
8. Polish the teeth with the finest Soflex discs.
9. Polish the teeth with fluoridated toothpaste for 1 min.

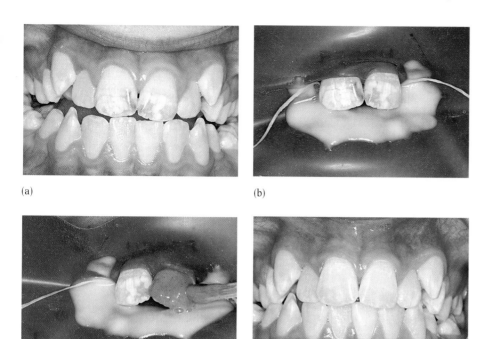

(a)

(b)

(c)

(d)

Fig. 9.1 (a) Characteristic appearance of fluorotic discoloration. (b) Rubber dam isolation with bicarbonate of soda in position. (c) Application of hydrochloric acid/pumice slurry with wooden stick. (d) Appearance 2 years post-treatment.

10. Review in 1 month for vitality tests and clinical photographs (Fig. 9.1d).
11. Review biannually checking pulpal status.

Critical analysis of the effectiveness of the technique should not be made immediately, but delayed for at least 1 month as the appearance of the teeth will continue to improve over this time. Experience has shown that brown mottling is removed more easily than white, but even where white mottling is incompletely removed it nevertheless becomes less perceptible. This phenomenon has been attributed to the relatively prismless layer of compacted surface enamel produced by the 'abrosion' technique, which alters the optical properties of the tooth surface.

Long-term studies of the technique have found no association with pulpal damage, increased caries susceptibility, or significant prolonged thermal sensitivity. Patient compliance and satisfaction is good and any dissatisfaction is usually due to inadequate pre-operative explanation. The technique is easy to perform for operator and patient, and is not time consuming. Removal of any mottled area is permanent and has been achieved with an insignificant loss of surface enamel. Failure to improve the appearance by the HCl–pumice microabrasion technique does not have any harmful effects and may make it easier to mask some lesions with veneers.

9.2.2   Non-vital bleaching

This technique describes the bleaching of teeth that have become discoloured by the diffusion into the dentinal tubules of haemoglobin breakdown products from necrotic pulp tissue.

Indications:

(1) discoloured non-vital teeth;

(2) well condensed gutta percha root filling;

(3) no clinical or radiological signs of periapical disease.

Contra-indications:

(1) heavily restored teeth;
(2) staining due to amalgam.

Armamentarium:

(1) rubber dam;
(2) zinc phosphate cement;
(3) 37 per cent phosphoric acid;
(4) 30 volume hydrogen peroxide;
(5) sodium perborate powder (Bocasan);
(6) cotton wool;
(7) glass ionomer cement;
(8) white gutta percha;
(9) composite resin.

Technique:

1. Pre-operative periapical radiographs are essential to check for an adequate root filling (Fig. 9.2a).
2. Clean teeth with pumice and make a note of the shade of discoloured tooth.
3. Place rubber dam isolating the single tooth. Ensure adequate eye and clothing protection for the patient, operator and dental nurse
4. Remove palatal restoration and pulp chamber restoration.
5. Remove root filling to the level of the dentogingival junction — may need to use adult burs in a mini-head (Fig. 9.2b and c).
6. Place 1 mm of zinc phosphate cement over the gutta percha.
7. Freshen dentine with a round bur. Do not remove excessively.

Fig. 9.2   (a) Radiograph of upper right central incisor with well condensed root filling. (b) Standard bur in a contra-angled head may not reach the dentogingival junction. (c) Correct depth achieved using a standard bur in a miniature head.

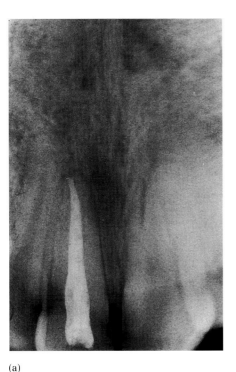

(a)

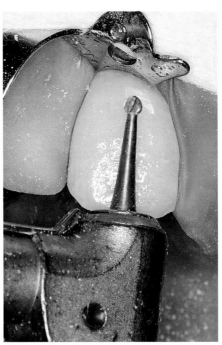

(b)

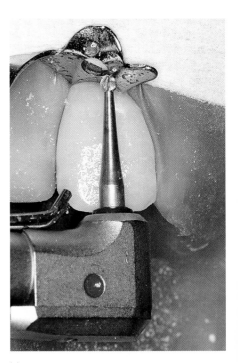

(c)

8. Etch the pulp chamber with 37 per cent phosphoric acid for 30–60 s, wash, and dry — this will facilitate the ingress of the hydrogen peroxide.

9. Mix the hydrogen peroxide and the sodium perborate into a thick paste. This should be done immediately before placement. Place into tooth either alone with a flat plastic instrument or on a cotton wool pledget.

10. Place a dry piece of cotton wool over the perborate mixture.

11. Seal the cavity with glass ionomer cement.

12. Repeat process at weekly intervals until the tooth is slightly over bleached.

13. Place non-setting calcium hydroxide into the pulp chamber for 2 weeks. Seal with glass ionomer cement.

14. Finally, restore the tooth with white gutta percha (to facilitate reopening pulp chamber again if necessary at a later date) and composite resin.

Figure 9.3a and b is an example of a highly successful result. If the colour of a tooth has not significantly improved after three changes of bleach then it is unlikely to do so and further bleaching should be abandoned. The maximum amount of bleach applications is usually accepted as 10. Failure of a tooth to bleach could be due to either inadequate removal of filling materials from the pulp chamber or to 'time expired' hydrogen peroxide. Both these factors should be checked before abandoning a procedure.

Slight over-bleaching is desirable but the patient should be instructed to attend the surgery before the next appointment if marked over-bleaching has occurred.

Non-vital bleaching has a reputation for causing brittleness of the tooth. This may be the result of previous injudicious removal of dentine, (which only needs to be 'freshened' with a round bur), rather than a direct effect of the bleaching procedure itself.

This method of bleaching has been associated with the later occurrence of external cervical resorption. The exact mechanism of this association is unclear but it is thought that the hydrogen peroxide diffuses through the dentinal tubules to set up an inflammatory reaction in the periodontal ligament around the cervical region of the tooth. In a small number of teeth there is a gap between the end of the enamel and the beginning of the cementum, and in these cases the above explanation is tenable. The purpose of the 1 mm layer of zinc phosphate cement is to cover the openings of the dentinal tubules at the level where there may be a communication to the periodontal ligament. In the same way non-setting calcium hydroxide is placed in the pulp chamber for 2 weeks prior to final restoration in order to eradicate any inflammation in the periodontal ligament that may have been initiated.

Clinical studies have demonstrated that regression can be expected with this technique. The longest study after 8 years gave a 21 per cent failure rate. However, if white gutta percha has been placed within the pulp chamber then it is readily removed and the tooth easily rebleached.

The advantages of the technique are many: easy for operator and patient; conserving of tooth tissue and maintenance of the original crown morphology; no irritation to gingival tissues; no problems with changing gingival level in young patients compared to veneers or crowns; no technical assistance required.

The use of perborate and water only has recently been reported but long term clinical results have yet to be published.

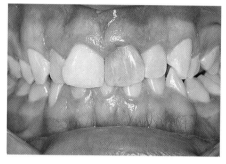

(a)

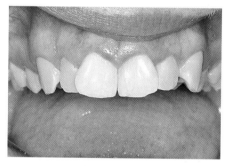

(b)

Fig. 9.3 (a) and (b) Intensely darkened non-vital upper left central incisor treated by four changes of bleach.

9.2.3 Vital bleaching — chairside

This technique involves the external application of hydrogen peroxide to the surface of the tooth followed by its activation with a heat source. The technique has

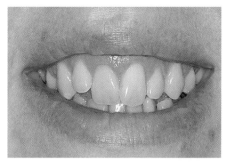

(a)

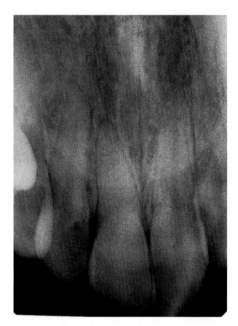

(b)

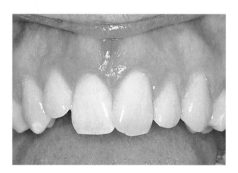

(c)

Fig. 9.4 (a) and (b) A discoloured upper right central incisor with radiograph confirming sclerosis of pulp chamber and root canal. (c) Appearance of upper right central incisor after four chairside bleaching treatments.

achieved considerable success in the United States but is a lengthy and time consuming procedure that requires a high degree of patient compliance and motivation.

Indications:

(1) very mild tetracycline staining without obvious banding;
(2) mild fluorosis;
(3) yellowing due to ageing;
(4) single teeth with sclerosed pulp chambers and canals.

Armamentarium:

(1) rubber dam with clamps and floss ligatures;
(2) orabase gel;
(3) topical anaesthetic;
(4) gauze;
(5) 37 per cent phosphoric acid;
(6) heating light with rheostat;
(7) 30 volume hydrogen peroxide;
(8) polishing stones;
(9) fluoride drops (0–2 years: drops).

Technique:

1. Pre-operative periapical radiographs and vitality tests. Any leaking restorations should be replaced.
2. Clean teeth with pumice and water to remove extrinsic staining. Pre-operative photographs should be taken with a tooth from a 'Vita' shade guide registering the shade, adjacent to the patient's teeth.
3. Apply topical anaesthetic to gingival margins.
4. Coat the buccal and palatal gingivae with Orabase gel as extra protection from bleaching solution.
5. Isolate each tooth to be bleached using individual ligatures. The end teeth should be clamped (usually from second premolar to second premolar).
6. Cover the metal rubber dam clamps with damp strips of gauze in order to prevent them from getting hot under the influence of the heat source.
7. Etch the labial and a third of the palatal surfaces of the teeth with the phosphoric acid for 60 s, wash, and dry. Thoroughly soak a strip of gauze in the 35 per cent hydrogen peroxide and cover the teeth to be bleached.
8. Position the heat lamp 13–15 inches from the patient's teeth. Set the rheostat to a mid-temperature range and then increase it until the patient can just feel the warmth in their teeth and then reduce it slightly until no sensation is felt.
9. Keep the gauze damp by reapplying the hydrogen peroxide every 3–5 min using a cotton bud. The bottle should be closed between applications as the hydrogen peroxide deactivates on exposure to air.
10. After 30 min remove the rubber dam, clean off the Orabase gel and polish the teeth using the shofu stones. Apply the fluoride drops for 2–3 min.
11. Postoperative sensitivity may occur and should be relieved with paracetamol.
12. Assess the change — it may be necessary to repeat the process three to 10 times per arch. Treat one arch at a time. Keep the patient under review as rebleaching may be required after 1 or more years.
13. Take postoperative photographs with the original 'Vita' shade tooth included.

This technique is very time consuming and retreatment may be necessary so the patient must be highly motivated. The technique can be used in the treatment of discoloration caused by pulp chamber sclerosis (Fig. 9.4a–c). These cases require isolation of the single tooth.

9.2.4 Vital bleaching — nightguard

This technique involves the daily placement of carbamide peroxide gel into a custom fitted tray of either the upper or the lower arch. As the name suggests it is carried out by the patient at home and is initially done on a daily basis.

Indications:

(1) mild fluorosis;

(2) moderate fluorosis as an adjunct to hydrogen chloride–pumice micro-abrasion;

(3) yellowing of ageing.

Armamentarium:

(1) upper impression and working model;

(2) soft mouthguard — avoiding the gingivae;

(3) 10 per cent carbamide peroxide gel: Opalescence (Ultradent, Optident UK), Rembrandt (Den Mat UK), White and Brite (Omnii UK).

Technique:

1. Take an alginate impression of the arch to be treated and cast a working model in stone.

2. Relieve the labial surfaces of the teeth by about 0.5 mm (Opalescence include resin with the kit for this purpose) and make a soft pull down vacuum formed splint as a mouthguard (Fig. 9.5a). The splint should be no more than 2 mm in thickness and should not cover the gingivae. It is only a vehicle for the bleaching gel and not to protect the gingivae.

3. Instruct the patient on how to floss their teeth thoroughly. Perform a full mouth prophylaxis and instruct them how to apply the gel into the mouthguard (Fig. 9.5b).

4. The length of time the guard should be worn depends on the product used; Rembrandt recommends a maximum of 2 h a day while White and Brite and Opalescence recommend throughout the night, with White and Brite in particular needing to be topped up as it has a very low viscosity.

5. Review the patient about 2 weeks later to check that they are not experiencing any sensitivity, and then at 6 weeks, by which time 80 per cent of any colour change should have occurred.

Ten per cent carbamide peroxide gel breaks down in the mouth into 3 per cent hydrogen peroxide and 7 per cent urea. Both urea and hydrogen peroxide have low molecular weights which allow them to diffuse rapidly through enamel and dentine and thus explain the transient pulpal sensitivity occasionally experienced with home bleaching systems.

Pulpal histology with regard to these materials has not been assessed but no clinical significance has been attributed to the changes seen with 35 per cent hydrogen peroxide over 75 years of usage except where teeth have been over-heated or traumatized. By extrapolation 3 per cent hydrogen peroxide in the home systems should therefore be safe.

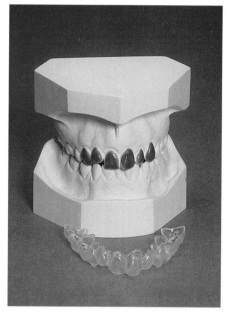

(a)

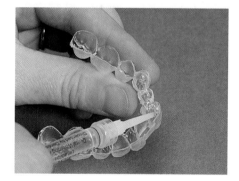

(b)

Fig. 9.5 (a) Model of upper arch with wax relief for construction of night guard.
(b) Mouthguard being loaded with carbamide peroxide gel.

Although most carbamide peroxide materials contain trace amounts of phosphoric and citric acids as stabilizers and preservatives, there is no indication of etching or significant change in surface morphology of enamel by scanning electron microscopy analysis. There was early concern that bleaching solutions with a low pH would cause demineralization of enamel when the pH fell below the 'critical' pH of 5.2–5.8. However, no evidence of this process has been noted to date in any clinical trials or laboratory tests and this may be due to the urea (and subsequently the ammonia) and carbon dioxide released on degradation of the carbamide peroxide, elevating the pH.

There is an initial decrease in bond strengths of enamel to composite resins immediately after home bleaching but this returns to normal within 7 days. This effect has been attributed to the residual oxygen in the bleached tooth surface which inhibits polymerization of the composite resin. The home bleaching systems do not affect the colour of restorative materials. Any perceived effect is probably due to superficial cleansing.

Minor ulceration or irritation may occur during the initial treatment. It is important to check that the mouth guard does not extend on to the gingivae and the edges of the guard are smooth. If ulceration persists a decreased exposure time may be necessary. If there is still a problem then allergy is a possibility.

There are no biological concerns regarding the short-term use of carbamide peroxide. It has a similar cytotoxicity on mouse fibroblasts as zinc phosphate cement and Crest toothpaste, and it has been used for a number of years in the United States to reduce plaque and promote wound healing. However, there are no long-term studies on its safety and laboratory studies have shown that carbamide peroxide has a mutagenic potential on vascular endothelium and there may be harmful effects on the periodontium, together with delayed wound healing.

In the European Community all externally applied bleaching systems (Vital Bleach and Home Bleach Systems) with hydrogen peroxide in concentration greater than 0.1 per cent are currently banned while the Department of Trade and Industry awaits evidence of their long-term safety.

Published clinical studies of 1–2 years duration prior to their ban have shown that the yellowing of ageing responds best to treatment. Although this would appear to take home bleaching out of the remit of paediatric dentistry it may well still have a part to play in the preliminary lightening of tetracycline-stained teeth prior to veneer placement, and also in cases of mild fluorosis. Irrespective of the clinical application, evidence suggests that annual retreatment may be necessary to maintain any effective lightening. This highlights further the importance of more research into the long-term effects of this treatment on the teeth, the mucosa, and the periodontium.

The exact mechanism of bleaching in any of the three methods described is unknown. Theories of oxidation, photo-oxidation, and ion exchange have been suggested. Conversely, the cause of rediscoloration is also unknown. This may be a combination of chemical reduction of the oxidation products previously formed, marginal leakage of restorations allowing ingress of bacterial and chemical by-products, and salivary or tissue fluid contamination via permeable tooth structure.

9.2.5 Localized composite resin restorations

This restorative technique uses recent advances in dental materials science to replace defective enamel with a restoration that bonds to and blends with enamel.

Indications: well demarcated white, yellow or brown hypoplastic enamel.

Armamentarium:

(1) rubber dam/contoured matrix strips (Vivadent);
(2) round and fissure diamond burs;
(3) enamel/dentine bonding kit;
(4) new generation highly polishable hybrid composite resin;
(5) soflex discs and interproximal polishing strips.

Technique:

1. Pre-operative photographs and shade selection (Fig. 9.6a).
2. Apply rubber dam or contoured matrix strips.
3. Remove demarcated lesion with round diamond bur down to amelodentinal junction (ADJ).
4. Chamfer enamel margins with diamond fissure bur to increase surface area available for retention.
5. Etch enamel margins — wash and dry.
6. Apply dentine primer to dentine and dry.
7. Apply enamel and dentine bonding agent and light cure.
8. Apply chosen shade of composite using a brush lubricated with the bonding agent to smooth and shape, and light cure for the recommended time.
9. Remove matrix strip/rubber dam.
10. Polish with graded Soflex discs (3M), finishing burs and interproximal strips if required. Add characterization to surface of composite.
11. Postoperative photographs (Fig. 9.6b).

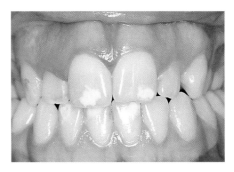

(a)

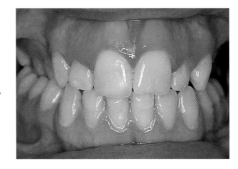

(b)

Fig. 9.6 (a) and (b) Well demarcated white opacities on the upper central incisors treated by localized composite restorations.

The localized restoration is quick and easy to complete. Despite the removal of defective enamel down to the ADJ there is often no significant sensitivity and therefore no need for local anaesthesia. If the hypoplastic enamel has become carious and extends into dentine then a liner of glass ionomer cement (correct shade) prior to placement of composite resin will be necessary. In these cases local anaesthesia will probably be required. Advances in bonding and resin technology make these restorations simple and obviate the need for a full labial veneer. Disadvantages are marginal staining, accurate colour match, and reduced composite translucency when lined by a glass ionomer cement.

9.2.6 Composite resin veneers

Although the porcelain jacket crown (PJC) may be the most satisfactory long-term restoration for a severely hypoplastic or discoloured tooth it is not an appropriate solution for children for two reasons: (a) the large size of the young pulp horns and chamber, and (b) the immature gingival contour.

Composite veneers may be direct (placed at initial appointment) or indirect (placed at a subsequent appointment having been fabricated in the laboratory). The conservative veneering methods may not just offer a temporary solution, but a satisfactory long-term alternative to the PJC. Most composite veneers placed in children and adolescents are of the 'direct' type as the durability of the indirect composite veneers is as yet unknown.

Before proceeding with any veneering technique, the decision must be made whether to reduce the thickness of labial enamel before placing the veneer. Certain factors should be considered:

1. Increased labiopalatal bulk makes it harder to maintain good oral hygiene. This may be courting disaster in the adolescent with dubious oral hygiene technique.

2. Composite resin has a better bond strength to enamel when the surface layer of 200–300 μm is removed.

3. If a tooth is very discoloured some sort of reduction will be desirable as a thicker layer of composite will be required to mask the intense stain.

4. If a tooth is already instanding or rotated its appearance can be enhanced by a thicker labial veneer.

New generation highly polishable hybrid composite resins can replace relatively large amounts of missing tooth tissue as well as being used in thin sections as a veneer. Combinations of shades can be used to simulate natural colour gradations and hues.

Indications:

(1) discoloration;
(2) enamel defects;
(3) diastemata;
(4) malpositioned teeth;
(5) large restorations.

Contra-indications:

(1) insufficient available enamel for bonding;
(2) oral habits, e.g. woodwind musicians.

Armamentarium:

(1) rubber dam/contoured matrix strips (Vivadent);
(2) preparation and finishing burs;
(3) new generation, highly polishable hybrid composite resin;
(4) Soflex discs (3M) and interproximal polishing strips.

Technique:

1. Use a tapered diamond bur to reduce labial enamel by 0.3–0.5 mm. Identify finish line at the gingival margin and also mesially and distally just labial to the contact points.

2. Clean tooth with a slurry of pumice in water. Wash and dry and select shade (Fig. 9.7a).

3. Isolate the tooth either with rubber dam or a contoured matrix strip. Hold this in place by applying unfilled resin to its gingival side against the gingiva and curing for 10 s (Fig. 9.7b).

4. Etch the enamel for 60 s, wash, and dry.

5. Where dentine is exposed apply dentine primer.

6. Apply a thin layer of bonding resin to the labial surface with a brush and cure for 15 s. It may be necessary to use an opaquer at this stage if the discoloration is intense.

7. Apply composite resin of the desired shade to the labial surface and roughly shape it into all areas with a plastic instrument before using a brush lubricated with unfilled resin to 'paddle' and smooth it into the desired shape. Cure 60 s gingivally, 60 s mesio-incisally, 60 s disto-incisally, and 60 s from the palatal aspect if incisal coverage has been used. Different shades of composite can be combined to achieve good matches with adjacent teeth and a transition from a relatively dark gingival area to a lighter more translucent incisal region (Fig. 9.7c).

8. Flick away the unfilled resin holding the contour strip and remove the strip.

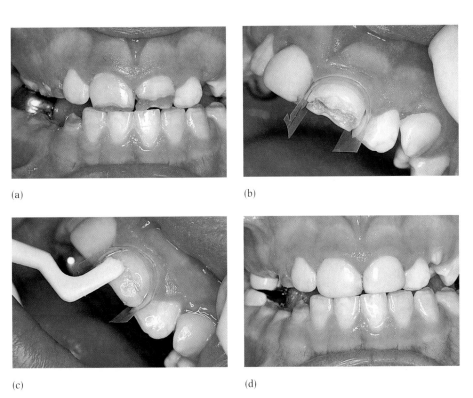

(a)

(b)

(c)

(d)

Fig. 9.7 (a) A young patient with amelogenesis imperfecta. (b) Contoured matrix strip in position. (c) Incremental placement of dentine shade composite. (d) Post-operative view showing final composite veneers.

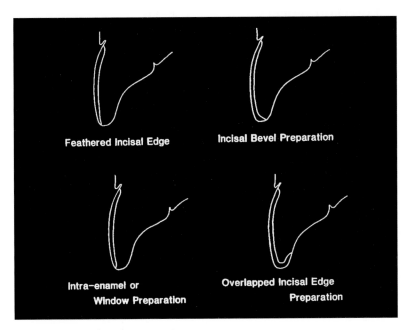

Fig. 9.8 Types of veneer preparation.

9. Finish the margins with diamond finishing burs and interproximal strips and the labial surface with graded sandpaper discs. Characterization should be added to improve light reflection properties (Fig 9.7d).

The exact design of the composite veneer will be dependent upon each clinical case, but will usually be one of four types: intra-enamel or window preparation; incisal bevel; overlapped incisal edge or feathered incisal edge (Fig. 9.8).

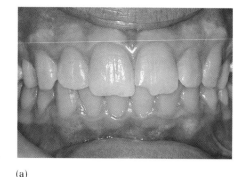

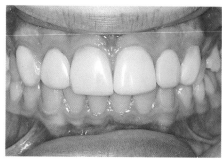

Fig. 9.9 (a) Teenage girl with dark tetracycline discoloration and an enamel fracture. (b) 5 years post-placement of composite veneers.

(a)

(b)

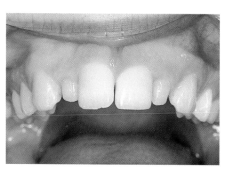

(a)

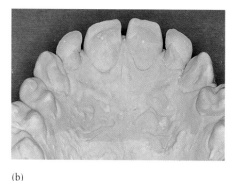

(b)

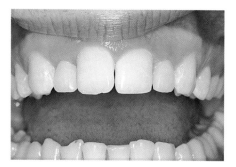

(c)

Fig. 9.10 (a) Peg-shaped lateral incisors in a 15 year old. (b) Laboratory model showing 3/4 wrap around porcelain veneers on the upper laterals. (c) Final restorations on the upper laterals 2 years post-cementation.

Tooth preparation will not normally expose dentine, but this will be unavoidable in some cases of localized hypoplasia or with caries. Sound dentine may need to be covered by glass ionomer cement prior to placement of the composite veneer.

Figure 9.9a and b show an example of successful composite veneers that have been in place for 5 years. Studies have shown that composite veneers are durable enough to last through adolescence until a more aesthetic porcelain veneer can be placed. This is normally only considered at about the age of 18–20 when the gingival margin has achieved an adult level and the standard of oral hygiene and dental motivation are acceptable

9.2.7 Porcelain veneers

Porcelain has several advantages over composite as a veneering material: its appearance is superior, it has a better resistance to abrasion and it is well tolerated by the gingival tissues. However, it is vital that the fit of the porcelain is exact and that the film thickness of the luting cement is kept to a minimum. These luting cements are only moderately filled composite resins and absorb water, hydrolyse, and stain. This coupled with the apical migration of the gingival margin in young patients can result in an unacceptable aesthetic appearance in a relatively short period of time.

Instruction in standard porcelain veneer preparation is covered in restorative dentistry textbooks. If there are occasions when they are used at an earlier age then the same principles apply. However, a non-standard application that is being used more frequently at a younger age is the restoration of the peg lateral incisor (Fig. 9.10a). This utilizes a no-preparation technique and the technician is asked to produce a three-quarter wrap around veneer finished to a knife edge at the gingival margin (Fig. 9.10b). An elastomeric impression is taken after gingival retraction to obtain the maximum length of crown and cementation should be under rubber dam (Fig. 9.10c).

9.2.8 Adhesive metal castings

The development of acid-etched retained cast restorations has allowed the fabrication of cast occlusal onlays for posterior teeth and palatal veneers for incisors and canines. These restorations are manufactured with minimal or no tooth preparation and are ideal for cases where there is a risk of tooth tissue loss.

Indications:

(1) amelogenesis imperfecta;

(2) dentinogenesis imperfecta;

(3) dental erosion, attrition, or abrasion;

(4) enamel hypoplasia.

Armamentarium:

(1) gingival retraction cord;

(2) elastomeric impression material;

(3) facebow system;

(4) semi-adjustable articulator;

(5) rubber dam;

(6) Panavia Ex (Kuraray).

Technique:

1. Study models are essential and photographs if possible.

2. Full mouth prophylaxis

3. Ensure good moisture isolation

4. Place retraction cord into the gingival crevices of the teeth to be treated and remove immediately prior to taking the impression.

5. Take an impression using an elastomeric impression material — a putty/wash system is the best and check the margins are easily distinguishable.

6. Take a facebow transfer and inter-occlusal record in the retruded axis position.

7. Mount the casts on a semi-adjustable articulator.

8. Construct cast onlays, a maximum of 1.5 mm thick occlusally in either nickel/chrome or gold.

9. Grit blast the fitting surfaces of the occlusal onlays.

10. Return to the mouth and check the fit of the onlays.

11. Polish teeth with pumice and isolate under rubber dam where possible

12. Cement onlays using Panavia Ex.

13. Check occlusion.

14. Review in 1 week for problems and regularly thereafter.

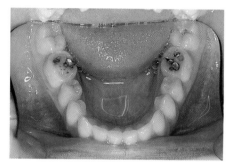

(a)

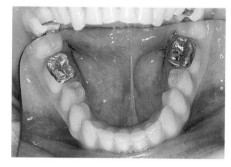

(b)

Fig. 9.11 (a) Marked occlusal enamel loss of lower first permanent molars. (b) Cast occlusal onlays *in situ* after replacement of amalgam restorations with composite resin.

Figures 9.11a and b show gold onlays cemented on to the lower first permanent molars of a 16 year old boy with erosive tooth surface loss. Such cast restorations may be provided for both posterior and anterior teeth with very little or no tooth preparation. Nevertheless, some children may find this treatment challenging as it demands high levels of patient co-operation. Local anaesthesia may be needed as the hypoplastic teeth are often sensitive to the etching and washing procedure and the placement of gingival retraction cord can be uncomfortable. Furthermore moisture control can be difficult and, while preferable, rubber dam is not always feasible.

When used to protect the palatal aspect of upper anterior teeth there may be an aesthetic problem as the metal may 'shine through' the translucent incisal tip of young teeth. Long-term evaluation is still awaited but initial results have been encouraging.

9.3   TOOTH DISCOLORATION

The colour of a child's teeth can be of great importance. Peer group pressure can be very strong and teasing about size, position, and colour of teeth can be very harmful to a child or adolescent.

Table 9.3 The aetiology of tooth discoloration

Extrinsic staining	
Beverages/food	
Smoking	
Poor oral hygiene (chromogenic bacteria): green/orange stain	
Drugs	
Iron supplements: black stain	
Minocycline: black stain	
Chlorhexidine: brown/black stain	
Intrinsic discoloration	
Enamel	
Local causes	caries
	idiopathic
	injury/infection of primary prececessor
	internal resorption
Systemic causes	amelogenesis imperfecta
	drugs, e.g. tetracyclines
	fluorosis
	idiopathic
	systemic illness during tooth formation
Dentine	
Local causes	caries
	internal resorption
	metallic restorative materials
	necrotic pulp tissue
	root canal filling materials
Systemic causes	bilirubin (haemolytic disease of newborn)
	congenital porphyria
	dentinogenesis imperfecta
	drugs, e.g. tetracyclines

The causes of discoloured teeth may be classified in a number of ways: congenital/acquired; enamel/dentine; extrinsic/intrinsic; systemic/local. The most useful method of classification for the clinical management of discoloration is one which identifies the main site of discoloration (Table 9.3). Once the aetiology of the discoloration had been identified the most appropriate method of treatment can be chosen. Ideal and permanent results may not be realistic in the young patient; however, significant improvements are achievable which do not compromise the teeth in the long term.

The approach to treatment for all forms of discoloration should be cautious with the emphasis on minimal tooth preparation. For example in a case of fluorosis the microabrasion technique may produce some improvement but the patient/parent may still be dissatisfied. Composite veneers can then be placed, although if the child requires subsequent fixed appliance treatment these may be damaged and require replacement before placing porcelain veneers as the definitive restoration in the late teenage years.

Key Points

- Microabrasion should be the first line of treatment in all cases of enamel opacities.
- Composite should be used in preference to porcelain in children.

Discoloration originating in the dentine is often difficult to treat. The single non-vital dark incisor presents particular problems. In the young patient, the

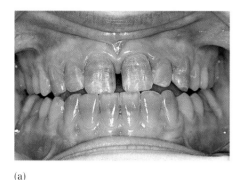

(a)

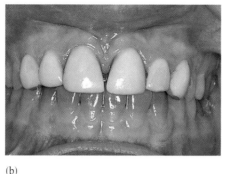

(b)

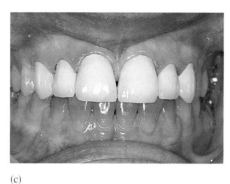

(c)

apex may be immature, root canal therapy incomplete, and non-vital bleaching therefore precluded. A composite veneer can improve the aesthetics but may fail to adequately disguise the discoloration even with the use of opaqueing agents. Ultimately a jacket crown may be the best option in the older patient. Similarly, moderate to severe tetracycline discoloration, which fortunately is less common today, is very difficult to treat in the young patient. Long-term full crowns or porcelain veneers often provide definitive treatment, but composite veneers can be acceptable in the adolescent without completely masking the underlying discoloration (Fig. 9.12a–c). Indirect composite veneers, placed with minimal tooth preparation, may be useful in the management of this problem but this technique has yet to be evaluated.

Finally, it is very important to bear in mind the expectations of the patient and often more importantly the parent. An unrealistically high expectation of brilliant white 'film star' teeth will result in postoperative disappointment. For instance, in fluorosis cases it is the excessively white, mottled areas which will be removed by the microabrasion technique resulting in a uniform colour that is the same as the original background colour and some patients will feel their treated teeth are 'too yellow'. Adequate pre-operative explanation, preferably with photographic examples, may help to minimize this problem. Nevertheless, there will remain a group of dissatisfied patients and for medico-legal reasons careful documentation of all cases of cosmetic treatment should be kept.

Fig. 9.12 (a) Severe tetracycline discoloration in a 14 year old. (b) Composite veneers placed using opaqueing agents to mask discoloration. (c) Porcelain jacket crowns were provided at 20 years of age.

9.4 TOOTH SURFACE LOSS

Dentists have been aware of the problem of tooth wear or non-carious loss of tooth tissue for a long time. However, it is only more recently that it has been associated increasingly with our younger population. There are three processes that make up the phenomenon of tooth wear:

(1) *attrition* — wear of tooth as a result of tooth to tooth contact;
(2) *erosion* — irreversible loss of tooth substance brought about by a chemical process that does not involve bacterial action;
(3) *abrasion* — physical wear of tooth substance produced by something other than tooth to tooth contact.

In children abrasion is relatively uncommon. The most frequent cause of abrasion is over-zealous tooth brushing which tends to develop with increasing age. Attrition during mastication is common particularly in the primary dentition where almost all upper incisors show some signs of attrition by the time they exfoliate (Fig. 9.13). However, over the past decade the contribution of erosion to the overall process of tooth wear in the younger population has been highlighted.

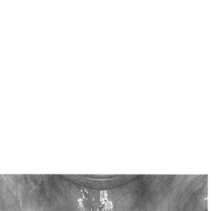

Fig. 9.13 Primary incisors showing physiological wear.

Table 9.4   Clinical signs of tooth wear (Smith and Knight 1984)

Pulp exposure
Loss of vitality attributable to tooth wear
Exposure of secondary dentine
Exposure of dentine on buccal or lingual surfaces
Cupped occlusal or incisal surfaces
Wear in one arch more than the other
Restorations projecting above the surface of the tooth
Wear producing sensitivity
Reduction in length of incisal teeth so that the length is out of proportion to the width

While erosion may be the predominant process, attrition and abrasion may be compounding factors, e.g. toothbrush abrasion may be increased if brushing is carried out immediately after the consumption of erosive foodstuffs or drinks. It is often difficult to identify a single causative agent in a case of tooth wear so the general term *tooth surface loss* may be more appropriate.

9.4.1   Prevalence

The problem with trying to assess the prevalence of tooth wear is that a degree of tooth tissue loss is a part of the normal physiological process of ageing; however, when it is likely to prejudice the survival of the teeth it can be said to be pathological. Smith and Knight in 1984 described a Tooth Wear Index (TWI) that included certain features that they felt were diagnostic of pathological tooth wear. These features are shown in Table 9.4.

There is very little published evidence on the prevalence or severity of tooth wear in children. In 1993 the National Child Dental Health Survey included assessment of the prevalence of erosion of both primary and permanent incisor teeth for the first time. The survey reported that 52 per cent of 5 year olds had erosion of the palatal surfaces of their primary incisors with 24 per cent showing progression in to the pulp (Fig. 9.14). The prevalence of erosion of the palatal surfaces of permanent incisors was also alarmingly high — 27 per cent of 15 year olds; however, only 2 per cent showed progression into the pulp. What is unclear at the present time is whether the problem of tooth surface loss is actually increasing or whether these figures reflect an increased awareness.

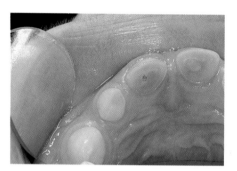

Fig. 9.14   Primary incisors showing pathological wear and pulp exposure.

9.4.2   Aetiology

In young patients there are three main causes of tooth surface loss:

(1) dietary
(2) gastric regurgitation
(3) parafunctional activity.

In addition to these three factors certain environmental factors have been linked to tooth wear. However, with the exception of frequent use of chlorinated swimming pools, most environmental and occupational hazards do not apply to children.

Dietary causes of tooth surface loss

The most common cause of erosive tooth surface loss is excessive intake of acidic food or drink. Table 9.5 shows the types of foodstuffs implicated in erosive tooth surface loss in young patients.

Table 9.5 Examples of foods and drinks with erosive potential

Citrus fruits e.g. lemons, oranges, grapefruits
Tart apples
Vinegar and pickles
Yoghurt
Fruit juices
Carbonated drinks including low calorie varieties, sparkling mineral water, and 'sports' drinks
Vitamin C tablets

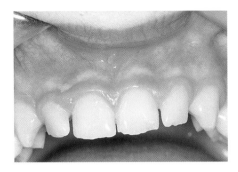

(a)

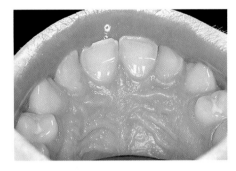

(b)

Fig. 9.15 (a) and (b) Teeth of a teenager who consumed considerable amounts of carbonated drinks. Note chipping of incisal edges and characteristic palatal tooth surface loss.

Acidic drinks, in particular, are available to all age groups of children. Pure 'baby' fruit juices are marketed for consumption by infants and these have been shown to have pH values below the critical pH for the dissolution of enamel (pH = 5.5). Many of these drinks are given to infants in a feeding bottle and the combination of the highly acidic nature of the drink and the prolonged exposure of the teeth to the acidic substrate may result in excessive tooth surface loss as well as dental caries. While a wide range of foods and drinks are implicated in the aetiology of tooth surface loss, soft drinks make up the bulk of the problem. Soft drink consumption has increased dramatically over the past 40 years to a staggering 151 litres per capita of the population in the United Kingdom in 1991 with adolescents accounting for up to 65 per cent of these purchases. Pure fruit juices do contribute to this figure but, increasingly, carbonated drinks make up a large part of the younger population's intake and are now widely available in vending machines located in schools, sports centres, and other public areas. Both normal and so-called 'diet' carbonated drinks have very low pH values and are associated with tooth surface loss. While there is no *direct* relationship between the pH of a substrate and the degree of tooth surface loss, pH does give a useful indication as to the potential to cause damage. Other factors such as titrateable acidity, the influence on plaque pH, and the buffering capacity of saliva will all influence the erosive potential of a given substrate. In addition it has been shown that erosive tooth surface loss tends to be more severe if the volume of drink consumed is high or if the intake occurs at bedtime.

Key Points

The degree of erosive tooth surface loss may be related to:
- the frequency of intake
- the timing of intake
- tooth-brushing habits

The pattern of dietary erosive tooth surface loss depends on the manner in which the substrate is consumed. Carbonated drinks are not uncommonly held in the mouth for some time as the child 'enjoys' the sensation of the bubbles around the mouth. This habit may result in a generalized loss of surface enamel (Fig. 9.15a and b). Note the chipping of the incisal edges of the upper anterior teeth — this is an example of attrition contributing to the overall pattern of tooth surface loss. Generalized loss of surface enamel of posterior teeth is often evident particularly on the first permanent molars and characteristic saucer shaped lesions develop on the cusps of the molars. This phenomenon is known as *perimolysis*. More peculiar habits are not uncommon; Fig. 9.16 shows the dentition of a young cyclist who consumed a lemon drink very frequently via a straw from his bicycle drink bottle. Fig. 9.17 is an example of a young adult who, for many years, daily consumed 2 lbs of raw Bramley cooking apples. The extent of tooth surface loss has left his amalgam restorations 'proud'.

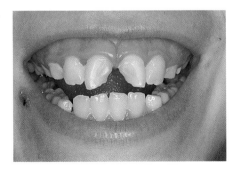

Fig. 9.16 A 12 year old with an unusual pattern of tooth surface loss.

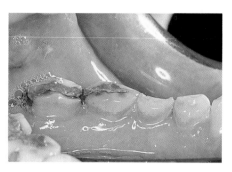

Fig. 9.17 Marked tooth surface loss may eventually leave amalgam restorations 'proud'.

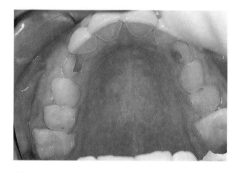

(a)

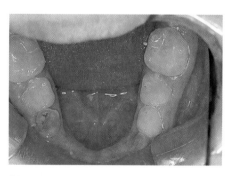

(b)

Fig. 9.18 (a) and (b) Upper and lower arch of a 10 year old boy with chronic gastro-oesophageal reflux.

Gastric regurgitation and tooth surface loss

The acidity of the stomach contents is below pH 1.0 and therefore any regurgitation or vomiting is potentially damaging to the teeth. As many as 50 per cent of adults with signs of tooth surface loss have a history of gastric reflux. The aetiology of gastric regurgitation may be divided into two categories: (a) those with upper gastrointestinal disorders, and (b) those with eating disorders.

In young patients long-term regurgitation is associated with a variety of underlying problems (Table 9.6).

Table 9.6 Conditions in children associated with chronic regurgitation

Gastro-oesophageal reflux
Oesophageal strictures
Chronic respiratory disease
Disease of the liver/pancreas/biliary tree
Over-feeding
Feeding problems/failure to thrive conditions
Children with mental handicap
Reye's syndrome
Rumination

In addition there are a group of patients that suffer from gastro-oesophageal reflux disease (GORD). This may be either symptomatic in which case the individual knows what provokes the reflux, or more insidiously asymptomatic GORD in which the patient is unaware of the problem and continues to ingest reflux provoking foods.

Unexplained erosive tooth surface loss is one of the principle signs of an eating disorder. There are three such disorders to be aware of: anorexia nervosa, bulimia nervosa, and more rarely rumination (this is a condition of unknown aetiology in which food is voluntarily regurgitated into the oral cavity and either expelled or swallowed again).

Anorexia nervosa is a socio-cultural disease mainly affecting middle class, intelligent, females between 12 and 30 years of age. Like bulimia nervosa it is a secretive disease with sufferers denying illness and refusing therapy. Anorectics exhibit considerable weight loss (up to 25 per cent of their body weight in severe cases), have a fear of growing fat, and a distorted view of their body shape. Bulimics suffer characteristic binges on 'junk foodstuffs' and follow this with self-induced vomiting, over-zealous exercise, and use of laxatives to prevent weight gain. Bulimics may subsequently develop GORD which causes typical signs of heartburn and oesophagitis.

The pattern of erosive tooth loss seen in all patients who suffer from chronic gastric regurgitation is similar with marked erosion of the palatal surface of upper incisors and premolars. There is a surprising lack of tooth sensitivity. Over a period of time the buccal and occlusal surfaces of the lower molars and premolars also become affected (Fig. 9.18a and b).

As a result of the asymptomatic nature of some of the gastrointestinal disorders and the secretive nature of the eating disorders, dentists may well be the first professionals to see the signs of gastric regurgitation. The presence of erosive tooth surface loss may be the only sign of an underlying disorder and such a finding should be taken seriously and handled carefully in communication with medical colleagues.

Parafunctional activity

Localized tooth surface loss frequently occurs in patients who exhibit abnormal parafunctional habits. The excessive grinding that is a feature of this problem is not always apparent to the patient; however, apart from the marked tooth tissue loss, other signs of bruxism may be evident including hypertrophy of the muscles of mastication, cheek biting, and tongue faceting. An example of erosion and parafunction having a disastrous effect on the dentition may be seen (and heard) in children who have cerebral palsy. These children often have chronic gastric regurgitation and also severe bruxism resulting in excessive tooth surface loss.

9.4.3 Management

Immediate

The most important aspect of the management of tooth surface loss is early diagnosis. While it is important to treat any dental sensitivity resulting from the tooth surface loss it is essential to establish the aetiology and where possible to eliminate the cause. This may not always be possible — the existence of an underlying eating disorder cannot be resolved quickly or simply. Indeed, as with all forms of behaviour modification, the elimination of dietary causes of erosion will often be difficult, particularly in young adolescents who are no longer under parental control and who often find it hard to adjust to alternative life-styles and dietary habits. Ideally, the cause of the tooth surface loss should be eliminated before restorative treatment is started. In order to achieve this, all patients and parents should be given dietary counselling which should be personal, practical, and positive. It is important not to simply advise against all carbonated drinks but to offer positive alternatives, and to suggest that such drinks may be taken as a treat occasionally and that intake should be limited to meal times. Table 9.7 gives some practical suggestions that may be made to patients depending on the aetiology of the problem.

In young patients dental sensitivity may be a problem. Erosive tooth loss may be rapid and with the large pulp chambers pulpal inflammation is common and secondary dentine does not have time to form. The use of glass ionomer cements or resin-based composites as temporary coverage may resolve the sensitivity and also act as a diagnostic aid.

Definitive treatment

In many cases, if the tooth surface loss is diagnosed early, preventive counselling may be sufficient. It is a good idea to make study casts of all patients with signs

Table 9.7 Practical prevention of erosion

Inform patients of types of foods and drinks that have greatest erosive potential (see Table 9.5)
Consumption of still/non-carbonated drinks as an alternative
Limiting the intake of acidic foods/drinks to meal times
Advocate consumption of a neutral food immediately after a meal, e.g. cheese
Advise use of neutral fluoride mouthwash or gel for daily use to try and minimize the effect of the acids
Encourage use of bicarbonate of soda mouthrinse in cases of recurrent gastric reflux
Where attrition is marked neutral fluoride gel can be placed into an occlusal guard during the night or during episodes of vomiting

Table 9.8 Treatment techniques for tooth surface loss

Technique	Advantages	Disadvantages
Cast metal (nickel/chrome or gold)	Fabricated in thin section — require only 0.5 mm space	May be cosmetically unacceptable due to 'shine through' of metallic grey
	Very accurate fit possible	Cannot be simply repaired or added to intra-orally
	Very durable	
	Suitable for posterior restorations in parafunction	
	Does not abrade opposing dentition	
Composite		
Direct	Adequately durable for labial veneers only	Technically difficult for palatal veneers
	Least expensive	Limited control over occlusal and interproximal contour
	May be used as a diagnostic tool	Inadequate as a posterior restoration
Indirect	Can be added to and repaired relatively simply intra-orally	Requires more space — minimum of 1.0 mm
	Aesthetically superior to cast metal	Unproven durability
	Control over occlusal contour and vertical dimension	
Porcelain	Best aesthetics	Potentially abrasive to opposing dentition
	Good abrasion resistance	Inferior marginal fit
	Well tolerated by gingival tissues	Very brittle — has to be used in bulk section
		Hard to repair

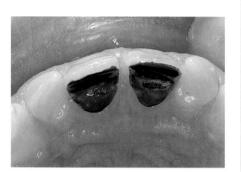

(a)

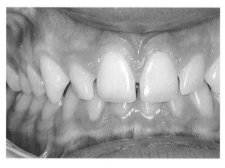

(b)

Fig. 9.19 (a) and (b) Cast palatal veneers on upper central incisors. Note the 'shine through' despite placement of labial composite veneers.

of tooth surface loss and to give these to the patient to keep. The rate of progression of the wear can then be monitored. However, in more advanced cases, where there is sensitivity or cosmetic problems active intervention is required. Table 9.8 shows the relative merits of the options available.

Key Points

Main treatment objectives for tooth surface loss:

- resolve sensitivity
- restore missing tooth structure
- prevent further tooth tissue loss
- maintain a balanced occlusion

In some cases there will be only localized tooth wear and an incomplete overbite, leaving enough space to place the restorations. Figure 9.19a and b shows the same patient as shown earlier in Fig. 9.15a and b who consumed considerable quantities of carbonated drinks in association with sporting activities. This habit caused considerable palatal wear of his upper incisors with characteristic chipping of the incisal edges. Cast adhesive veneers may be placed on the palatal aspect of the upper incisors to protect from further wear and direct resin-based composite labial veneers were used to restore the aesthetics. Note in this case the slight grey 'shine through' effect on the incisal tips due to the cast restorations.

In many other cases compensatory growth, which will help to maintain the occlusal vertical dimension, or the presence of a significant malocclusion, may

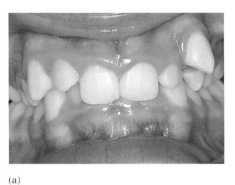

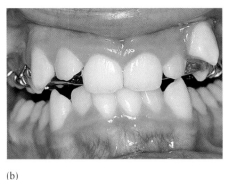

(a)   (b)

Fig. 9.20 (a) Skeletal pattern II with deep overbite compounding palatal erosion in a 12 year old boy. (b) An upper removable appliance in position to reduce the overbite.

result in inadequate space for the necessary restorations. Figure 9.20a shows a case of a 12 year old boy who has a class II division 2 malocclusion and who consumed three cans of carbonated drinks everyday. The combination of the erosive drink and the attrition brought about by the close tooth to tooth contact has resulted in loss of palatal tooth tissue from the upper central incisors. There is insufficient space palatally to place any form of restoration and simple removable orthodontic appliance with a flat anterior bite plane can be used to reduce the overbite (Fig. 9.20b). In children this occurs relatively quickly (within 6 weeks) principally by compensatory overeruption of the posterior segments. Once sufficient space has been created cast metal palatal veneers can be placed.

Alternatively, if there has been marked wear of the posterior teeth as shown in (Fig. 9.21a) it will be necessary to restore the occlusal surfaces and protect them from further wear prior to placing anterior restorations. Cast adhesive occlusal onlays are recommended in these cases (Fig. 9.21b). Young patients will accommodate the increase in vertical dimension easily, providing a balanced occlusal contact is achieved. The use of a facebow record facilitates this. The main advantage of using cast metal onlays is the minimal thickness of material needed and its resistance to abrasive wear. Indirect composite veneers are a recent addition to our armamentarium and they offer considerable advantages particularly in cases where the aetiology is unclear or the patient cannot cease the habit/problem. These restorations facilitate future additions and repairs (using direct composite) if the erosion continues or restarts. However, if there is an element of attrition or signs of parafunction composite onlays will not be adequately durable in the posterior segments and cast restorations are recommended.

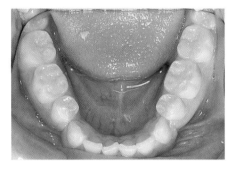

(a)

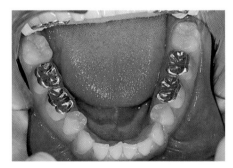

(b)

Fig. 9.21 (a) A 16 year old boy with marked tooth surface loss of lower permanent molars. Note the perimolysis of the first molars. (b) Post-cementation of gold onlays on the permanent molars.

Long-term review

All patients with tooth surface loss should be reviewed regularly for three reasons:

(1) to monitor future tooth surface loss;
(2) to maintain the existing restorations;
(3) to provide support for the patient.

Patients with eating disorders in particular are prone to periods of relapse and the dentist is in an ideal position to diagnose these periods. The dentist can develop a special and trusting relationship with the young patient over the longer term which is based not simply on seeing the patient when they are 'ill' and therefore to admonish them, but also when they are well to support and encourage them. Likewise in patients with dietary erosion, continual reinforcement of good dietary habits is needed throughout the child's life and into adulthood. People change their diet as they get older — one example is the young adolescent who manages to cease drinking Coca Cola but starts drinking lager to excess instead and the erosion continues!

9.5 INHERITED ANOMALIES OF ENAMEL AND DENTINE

Chapter 12 covers the whole range of dental anomalies; however, the treatment of amelogenesis imperfecta and dentinogenesis imperfecta poses specific challenges to the dentist. In view of the wide variety of presentations and degree to which each individual case is affected, it is difficult to make generalizations. Early diagnosis of these conditions is important to their long-term prognosis; parents need to be educated in the implications of the condition; monitoring of the amount of tooth wear can start, and, where necessary, teeth can be protected. There are four main clinical problems associated with inherited enamel and dentine defects:

(1) poor aesthetics;

(2) chipping and attrition of the enamel;

(3) exposure and attrition of the dentine causing sensitivity;

(4) poor oral hygiene, gingivitis, and caries.

While it is not possible to draw up a definitive treatment plan for all cases it is possible to define the principles of treatment planning for this group of patients. It is important to realize that not all children with amelogenesis imperfecta or dentinogenesis imperfecta are affected equally. Many will not have marked tooth wear or symptoms, and will not require advanced intervention. Table 9.9 describes the principles of treatment in terms of the age of the child/adolescent and with regard to the three aspects of care: prevention, restoration, and aesthetics.

Key Points   Main treatment objectives for dental anomalies:

- alleviate symptoms
- maintain/restore occlusal height
- improve aesthetics

Table 9.9 Principles of treatment for amelogenesis and dentinogenesis imperfecta

	Prevention	Restoration	Aesthetics
Primary dentition (0–5 years)	Diet advice Fluoride supplements Oral hygiene instruction	Glass ionomer cement (GIC) Stainless steel crowns (SSCs) (particularly on E's)	Minimal intervention GICs
Mixed dentition (6–16 years)	Diet advice Fluoride supplements Oral hygiene instruction ± chlorhexidine	SSCs on primary molars Adhesive castings on first permanent molars Localized composite/GIC	Direct }Composite veneers Indirect
Permanent dentition (16+ years)	Oral hygiene instruction Topical fluoride	Adhesive castings on premolars Full mouth rehabilitation	Porcelain veneers Full crowns Over dentures Complete dentures

Prevention

Prevention is an essential part of the management of children with anomalies of enamel and dentine. Oral hygiene in these children is often poor, due in part to the rough enamel surface which promotes plaque retention and to the sensitivity of the tooth to brushing. As a result there may be marked gingival inflammation and bleeding. The combination of gingival swelling and enamel hypoplasia can result in areas of food stagnation and a generally low level of oral health. Oral hygiene instruction must be given sympathetically, with plenty of encouragement, and should be continually reinforced. In some cases it may be necessary to carry out some restorative/cosmetic treatment before good oral hygiene measures can be practised. For example, the placement of anterior composite veneers may reduce dentine sensitivity and improve the enamel surface so that the patient can brush their teeth more effectively. Conventional caries prevention with diet advice, fluoride supplements, and topical fluoride applications is mandatory. In this group of children it is particularly important to preserve tooth tissue and not allow caries to compromise further the dental hard tissues.

Restoration

Restorative treatment varies considerably depending on the age of the child and extent of the problem. The basic principle of treatment is that of minimal intervention. If there is sensitivity or signs of enamel chipping, techniques to cover and protect the teeth should be considered. In the very young child it is often not possible to carry out extensive operative treatment, but the placement of glass ionomer cement over areas of enamel hypoplasia is simple and effective. In older/more co-operative children stainless steel (or nickel chrome) preformed crowns should be placed on the second primary molars to minimize further wear due to tooth on tooth contact (Chapter 7). It is advisable (and usually possible) to place such restorations with minimum tooth preparation because of the pre-existing tooth tissue loss.

Young children with dentinogenesis imperfecta often pose the greatest problems. The teeth undergo such excessive wear that they become worn down to gingival level and are unrestorable. Teeth affected by dentinogenesis imperfecta are also prone to spontaneous abscesses due to the progressive obliteration of the pulp chambers. In these cases pulp therapy is not successful and extraction of the affected teeth is necessary.

As the permanent dentition develops close monitoring of the rate of tooth wear will guide the decision about what intervention is needed. Cast occlusal onlays on the first permanent molars not only protect the underlying tooth structure but also maintain function and control symptoms. The resulting increase in the vertical dimension is associated with a decrease in the vertical overlap of the incisors. Within a few weeks full occlusion is usually re-established, the whole procedure being well tolerated by young patients. As the premolars erupt similar castings may be placed if wear is marked (Fig. 9.22a–c). Alternatively, localized composite or glass ionomer cement restorations may be placed over areas of hypoplasia.

The emphasis should remain on minimal tooth preparation until the child gains adulthood. At this point, if clinically indicated, full mouth rehabilitation may be considered and should have a good prognosis in view of the conservative approach that has been adopted throughout the early years (Fig. 9.23a and b). Patients with dentinogenesis imperfecta should be treated with caution. The characteristic form of the teeth in this condition is unfavourable for crowning; the teeth being supported by short, thin roots. The permanent dentition, like the

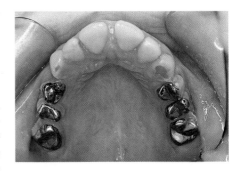

(a)

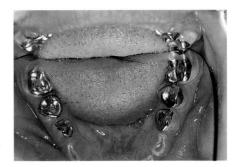

(b)

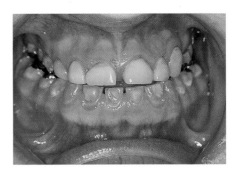

(c)

Fig. 9.22 (a)–(c) Upper and lower arches of a 14 year girl with dentinogenesis imperfecta showing cast onlays on the second permanent molars and the premolars and labial and palatal composite veneers on the upper incisors.

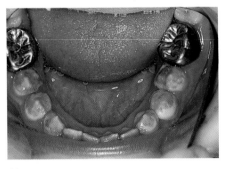

(a)

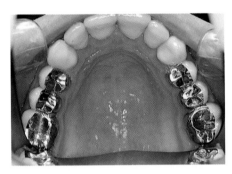

(b)

Fig. 9.23 (a) A 14 year old boy with severe hypocalcified amelogenesis imperfecta. Stainless steel crowns were placed on the first permanent molars at 9 years of age (lower arch).
(b) At 20 years of age a full mouth rehabilitation was completed (upper arch).

primary dentition, is prone to spontaneous abscesses and the prognosis for endodontic treatment very poor. The long-term plan for these patients is often some form of removable prosthesis, either an overdenture placed over the worn permanent teeth or a more conventional complete denture. The role of implants in these patients has yet to be defined fully.

Aesthetics

Aesthetics is not usually a problem in the primary dentition. Where the child is sufficiently co-operative the use of glass ionomer cements to restore and improve the appearance of primary incisors can be useful in gaining the respect and support from the patient and parent. In a few exceptional cases the loss of primary teeth may cause upset and can be compensated by constructing dentures. In cases of dentinogenesis imperfecta where the teeth are very worn but remain asymptomatic, overdentures can be constructed to which young children adapt remarkably well. These will need to be remade regularly as the child grows.

As the permanent incisors erupt they must be protected from chipping of the enamel. The placement of composite veneers not only improves the appearance but also promotes better gingival health and protects the teeth from further wear. In a few cases the quality of the enamel is so poor that the bond between composite and tooth will be unsuccessful. It should be noted that in these cases porcelain veneers are also likely to be unsuccessful. In such cases full coronal restorations are the only option.

Early consultation with an orthodontist is advisable in order to keep the orthodontic requirements simple. Treatment for these patients is possible and in many cases proceeds without problems. The use of removable appliances where appropriate and orthodontic bands rather than brackets will minimize the risk of damage to the abnormal enamel. The problem is twofold: there may be frequent bond failure during active treatment or the enamel may be further damaged during debonding. Some orthodontists prefer to use bands even for anterior teeth while others will use glass ionomer cement as the bonding agent in preference to more conventional resin-based agents. In other instances cosmetic restorative techniques (veneers and crowns) may be more appropriate than orthodontic treatment.

9.6   SUMMARY

1. The management of children with advanced restorative problems should be viewed as a long-term commitment.
2. Advanced restorative problems in children should be treated as conservatively as possible.
3. Identification of the aetiology of tooth discoloration is essential for selection of the most appropriate treatment technique.
4. Microabrasion should be the first treatment option in all cases of enamel surface discoloration.
5. Porcelain veneers should be delayed until a mature gingival contour is attained.
6. Nearly 30 per cent of all 15 year olds have experience of erosive tooth surface loss.
7. The cause of tooth surface loss should be determined and prevention eliminated before active treatment is started.

8. Maintenance of occlusal face height is essential in patients with amelogenesis or dentinogenesis imperfecta.

9.7 FURTHER READING

Bishop, K., Briggs, P., and Kelleher, M. (1994). The aetiology and management of localized anterior tooth wear in the young adult. *Dental Update*, **21**, 153–60. (*A good review with alot of references and clinical examples.*)

Harley, K. E. and Ibbetson, R. J. (1993). Dental anomalies — are adhesive casting the solution? *British Dental Journal*, **174**, 15–22. (*A well written study covering the clinical technique and the follow up of 12 children with amelogenesis or dentinogenesis imperfecta.*)

Haywood, van B. (1992). History, safety and effectiveness of current bleaching techniques and applications of the nightguard vital bleaching technique. *Quintessance International* **23**, 471–88. (*An extensive review of this technique with many references.*)

Kilpatrick, N. M. and Welbury, R. R. (1993). Hydrochloric acid–pumice microabrasion technique for the removal of enamel pigmentation. *Dental Update*, **20**, 105–7. (*A clinical study assessing the effectiveness of the microabrasion technique*).

Millward, A., Shaw, L., Rippin, J. W., and Harrington, E. (1994). The distribution and severity of tooth wear and the relationship between erosion and dietary constituents in a group of children. *International Journal of Paediatric Dentistry*, **4**, 151–7. (*One of the first epidemiological surveys assessing the extent of the problems of dental erosion in children.*)

Welbury, R. R. (1991). A clinical study of a microfilled composite resin for labial veneers. *International Journal of Paediatric Dentistry*, **1**, 9–15. (*A longitudinal clinical study evaluating composite veneers in adolescents.*)

10 Periodontal diseases in children

10 Periodontal diseases in children

P. A. HEASMAN and J. J. MURRAY

10.1 INTRODUCTION

Periodontal diseases comprise a group of infections that affect the supporting structures of the teeth: marginal and attached gingiva, periodontal ligament, cementum, and alveolar bone.

Acute gingival diseases, primarily herpetic gingivostomatitis and necrotizing gingivitis are ulcerative conditions that result from specific viral and bacterial infection. Chronic gingivitis, however, is a non-specific inflammatory lesion of the marginal gingiva which reflects the bacterial challenge to the host when dental plaque accumulates in the gingival crevice. The development of chronic gingivitis is enhanced when routine oral hygiene practices are impaired. Chronic gingivitis is reversible if effective plaque control measures are introduced. If left untreated the condition invariably converts to chronic periodontitis that is characterized by resorption of the supporting connective tissue attachment and apical migration of the junctional epithelia. Slowly progressing, chronic periodontitis affects most of the adult population to a greater or lesser extent, although the early stages of the disease are detected in adolescents.

Children are also susceptible to aggressive periodontal conditions, the so-called early-onset diseases. Prepubertal and juvenile periodontitis involve the primary and permanent dentitions, respectively, and present in localized or generalized forms. These conditions, which are distinct clinical entities affecting otherwise healthy children, must be differentiated from the extensive periodontal destruction that is associated with certain systemic diseases, degenerative disorders, and congenital syndromes.

Periodontal tissues are also susceptible to changes that are not, primarily, of an infectious nature. Factitious stomatitis is characterized by self-inflicted trauma to oral soft tissues and the gingiva are invariably involved. Drug-induced gingival overgrowth is becoming increasingly more prevalent with the widespread use of organ transplant procedures and the use of long-term immunosuppressant therapy. Localized overgrowth may occur as a gingival complication of orthodontic treatment.

A classification of periodontal diseases in children is given in Table 10.1.

10.2 ANATOMY OF THE PERIODONTIUM IN CHILDREN

Marginal gingival tissues around the primary dentition are more highly vascular and contain fewer connective tissue fibres than tissues around the permanent teeth. The epithelia are thinner with a lesser degree of keratinization, giving an appearance of increased redness that may be interpreted as mild inflammation.

Table 10.1   A classification of periodontal diseases in children

Gingival conditions without loss of connective tissue attachment	Periodontal conditions with loss of connective tissue attachment
Acute gingivitis	Chronic periodontitis
herpetic gingivostomatitis	plaque induced
necrotizing ulcerative gingivitis	complication of orthodontic treatment.
Chronic gingivitis	Early-onset periodontitis
plaque induced	prepubertal
puberty gingivitis	juvenile
Gingival overgrowth	Prepubertal periodontitis associated with
drug induced (generalized)	systemic disease
	Papillon Lefèvre syndrome
	Ehlers-Danlos syndrome
Factitious gingivitis	hypophosphatasia
	Chediak-Higashi syndrome
	leukocyte adhesion deficiency syndrome
Mucogingival problems	neutropenias
	histiocytosis

Furthermore, the localized hyperaemia that accompanies eruption of the primary dentition can persist, leading to swollen and rounded interproximal papillae and a depth of gingival sulcus exceeding 3 mm.

During eruption of the permanent teeth the junctional epithelium migrates apically from the incisal or occlusal surface towards the cemento-enamel junction (CEJ). While the epithelial attachment is above the line of maximum crown convexity, the gingival sulcus depth often exceeds 6 or 7 mm, which favours the accumulation of plaque. When the teeth are fully erupted, there continues to be an apical shift of junctional epithelium and the free gingival margins. Stability of the gingiva is achieved at about 12 years for mandibular incisors, canines, second premolars, and first molars. The tissues around the remaining teeth continue to recede slowly until about 16 years. The gingival margins are thus frequently at different levels on adjacent teeth that are at different stages of eruption. This sometimes gives an erroneous appearance that gingival recession has occurred around those teeth that have been in the mouth longest.

A variation in sulcus depths around posterior teeth in the mixed dentition is common. For example, sulcus depths on the mesial aspects of Es and 6s are greater than those on the distal of Ds and Es, respectively. This is accountable to the discrepancy in the horizontal position of adjacent CEJs due to the difference in occluso-apical widths of adjacent molar crowns.

The attached gingiva extends from the free gingival margin to the mucogingival line minus the sulcus depth in the absence of inflammation. Attached gingiva is necessary to maintain sulcus depth, to resist functional stresses during mastication, and to resist tensional stress by acting as a buffer between the mobile gingival margin and the loosely structured alveolar mucosa. The width of attached gingiva is less variable in the primary than in the permanent dentition. This may in part account for the scarcity of mucogingival problems in the primary dentition.

The periodontal ligament space is wider in children, partly as a consequence of thinner cementum and alveolar cortical plates. The ligament is less fibrous and more vascular. Alveolar bone has larger marrow spaces, greater vascularity, and fewer trabeculae than adult tissues, features that may enhance the rate of progression of periodontal disease when it affects the primary dentition.

The radiographic distance between the CEJ and the healthy alveolar bone crest for primary canine and molar teeth is in the range 0–2 mm. Individual surfaces display distances of up to 4 mm when adjacent permanent or primary teeth are erupting or exfoliating, respectively, and eruptive and maturation changes must be considered when radiographs are used to diagnose periodontal disease in children. When such changes are excluded, a CEJ–alveolar crest distance of >2 mm should arouse suspicion of pathological bone loss in the primary dentition.

Key Points

Anatomy:
- junctional epithelium
- marginal gingiva
- attached gingiva
- alveolar bone

10.3   ACUTE GINGIVAL CONDITIONS

The principal acute gingival conditions that affect children are primary herpetic gingivostomatitis and acute ulcerative necrotizing gingivitis. The latter is most frequently seen in young adults, but it also affects teenagers.

10.3.1   Primary herpetic gingivostomatitis

Herpetic gingivostomatitis is an acute infectious disease caused by the herpesvirus hominis. The primary infection is most frequently seen in children between 2 and 5 years of age, although older age groups can be affected. A degree of immunity is transferred to the newborn from circulating maternal antibodies so an infection in the first 12 months of life is rare. Almost 100 per cent of urban adult populations are carriers of, and have neutralizing antibodies to, the virus. This acquired immunity suggests that the majority of childhood infections are subclinical.

Transmission of the virus is by droplet infection and the incubation period is about 1 week. The child develops a febrile illness with a raised temperature of 100–102°F. Headaches, malaise, oral pain, mild dysphagia, and cervical lymphadenopathy are the common symptoms that accompany the fever and precede the onset of a severe, oedematous marginal gingivitis. Characteristic, fluid-filled vesicles appear on the gingiva and other areas such as the tongue, lips, buccal, and palatal mucosa. The vesicles, which have a grey, membranous covering, rupture spontaneously after a few hours to leave extremely painful yelllowish ulcers with red, inflamed margins (Fig. 10.1(a) and (b)). The clinical episode runs a course of about 14 days and the oral lesions heal without scarring. Very rare but severe complications of the infection are aseptic meningitis and encephalitis.

The clinical features, history, and age group of the affected children are so characteristic that diagnosis is rarely problematic. If in doubt, however, smears from recently ruptured vesicles reveal degenerating epithelial cells with intranuclear inclusions. The virus protein also tends to displace the nuclear chromatin to produce enlarged and irregular nuclei.

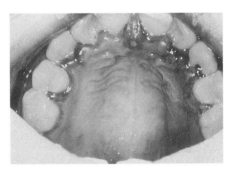

(a)

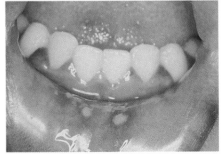

(b)

Fig. 10.1 Ulcerative stage of primary herpetic gingivostomatitis: (a) palatal gingiva; (b) lower lip mucosa.

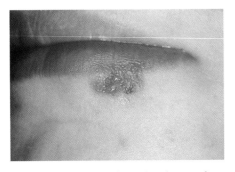

Fig. 10.2 Herpetic 'cold sore' at the vermilion border of the lower lip.

Herpetic gingivostomatitis does not respond well to active treatment. Bed rest and a soft diet are recommended during the febrile stage and the child should be kept well hydrated. Pyrexia is reduced using a paracetamol suspension and secondary infection of ulcers may be prevented using chlorhexidine. A mouthrinse (0.2 per cent, two to three times a day) may be used in older children who are able to expectorate, but in younger children (<6 years) a chlorhexidine spray can be used (twice daily) or the solution applied using a sponge swab. In severe cases of herpes simplex, systemic acyclovir can be prescribed as a suspension (200 mg) and swallowed, five times daily for 5 days. In children under 2 years the dose is halved. Acyclovir is active against the herpesvirus but is unable to eradicate it completely. The drug is most effective when given at the onset of the infection.

Key Points

Herpetic gingivostomatitis:

● primary/recurrent
● viral
● vesicular lesions
● symptomatic treatment

After the primary infection the herpesvirus remains dormant in epithelial cells of the host. Reactivation of the latent virus or reinfection in subjects with acquired immunity occurs in adults. Recurrent disease presents as an attenuated intra-oral form of the primary infection or as herpes labialis, the common 'cold sore' on the mucocutaneous border of the lips (Fig. 10.2). Cold sores are treated by applying acyclovir cream (5%, five times daily for about 5 days).

10.3.2   Acute necrotizing ulcerative gingivitis

Acute necrotizing ulcerative gingivitis (ANUG) is one of the commonest acute diseases of the gingiva. In the United States and Europe, ANUG affects young adults in the 16–30 age range with reported incidence figures of 0.7–7 per cent. In developing countries ANUG is prevalent in children as young as 1 or 2 years of age when the infection can be very aggressive leading to extensive destruction of soft and hard tissues (Fig. 10.3). Epidemic-like occurrences of ANUG have been reported in groups such as army recruits and first year college students. These outbreaks are more likely a consequence of the prevalence of common predisposing factors rather than communicability of infection between subjects.

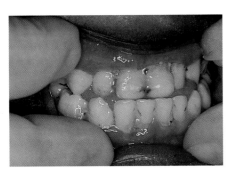

Fig. 10.3   A 5 year old Ethiopian boy with acute necrotizing ulcerative gingivitis.

Clinical features

ANUG is characterized by necrosis and ulceration which first affects the interdental papillae and then spreads to the labial and lingual marginal gingiva. The ulcers are 'punched out', covered by a yellowish-grey pseudomembranous slough, and extremely painful to touch (Fig. 10.3). The acute exacerbation is often superimposed upon a pre-existing gingivitis, and the tissues bleed profusely on gentle probing. The standard of oral hygiene is usually very poor. A distinctive halitosis is common in established cases of ANUG, although fever and lymphadenopathy are less common than in herpetic gingivostomatitis.

The clinical course of ANUG is such that the acute stage enters a chronic phase of remission after 5–7 days. Recurrence of the acute condition is inevitable, however, and if this acute–chronic cycle is allowed to continue then the marginal tissues lose their contour and appear rounded. Eventually, the inflammation and necrosis involve the alveolar crest and the subsequent necrotizing periodontitis leads to rapid bone resorption and gingival recession. Progressive changes are also a consequence of inadequate or incomplete treatment.

Aetiology

A smear taken from an area of necrosis or the surface of an ulcer will reveal numerous dead cells, polymorphonuclear leukocytes, and a sample of the micro-organisms that are frequently associated with ANUG. Fusiform bacteria and spirochaetes are both numerous and easy to detect. A fusospirochaetal complex has been strongly implicated as the causative organisms in ANUG. Other Gram-negative anaerobic organisms including *Porphyromonas gingivalis*, *Veillonella*, and *Selenomonas* species have been detected, which suggests that ANUG could be a broad anaerobic infection.

A viral aetiology has also been suggested primarily because of the similarity between ANUG and known viral diseases. The restriction of the disease to children and young adults for example, may infer that older subjects have undergone seroconversion (and are thus immune) as a consequence of clinical or subclinical viral infection in earlier life. The recurring episodes of the disease may also be explained by a viral hypothesis. The ability to undergo latent infection that is subject to reactivation is a characteristic of the herpesvirus. The argument for the implication of a virus in ANUG is therefore valid and novel, although a specific virus has yet to be isolated from oral lesions.

Predisposing factors

Poor oral hygiene and a pre-existing gingivitis invariably reflect the patient's attitude to oral care. Many young adults with ANUG are heavy smokers. The effect of smoking on the gingiva may be mediated through a local irritation or by the vasoconstrictive action of nicotine, thus reducing tissue resistance and making the host more susceptible to anaerobic infection. Smoking is obviously not a predisposing factor in young children. In underdeveloped countries, however, children are often undernourished and debilitated, which may predispose to infection. Outbreaks of ANUG in groups of subjects who are under stress has implicated emotional status as an important predisposing factor. Elevated plasma levels of corticosteroids as a response to an emotional upset are thought to be a possible mechanism.

It is conceivable that all the predisposing factors have a common action to initiate or potentiate a specific change in the host such as lowering the cell-mediated response. Indeed, patients with ANUG have depressed phagocytic activity and chemotactic response of their polymorphonuclear leukocytes.

Treatment

It is important at the outset that the patient is informed of the nature of ANUG and the likelihood of recurrence of the condition if the treatment is not completed. Smokers should be advised to reduce the number of cigarettes smoked. A soft multitufted brush is recommended when a medium-textured brush is too painful.

Mouthrinses may be recommended but only for short-term use (7–10 days). Rinsing with chlorhexidine (0.2 per cent for about 1 min) reduces plaque formation, while the use of a hydrogen peroxide or sodium hydroxyperborate mouthrinse oxygenates and cleanses the necrotic tissues.

Mechanical debridement should be undertaken at the initial visit. An ultrasonic scaler with its accompanying water spray can be effective with minimal discomfort for the patient. Further, if ANUG is localized to one part of the mouth, local anaesthesia of the soft tissues can allow some subgingival scaling to be undertaken.

In severe cases of ANUG, a 3 day course of metronidazole (200 mg three times a day) alleviates the symptoms, but the patients must be informed that they are required to reattend for further visits.

Key Points	Acute necrotizing ulcerative gingivitis:
	• yellow-grey ulcers
	• fusospirochaetal
	• predisposing factors
	• aggressive treatment

Occasionally, it is necessary to surgically recontour the gingival margin (gingivoplasty) to improve tissue architecture and facilitate subgingival cleaning.

10.4   CHRONIC GINGIVITIS

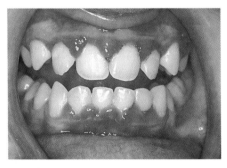

Fig. 10.4 Chronic marginal gingivitis in a 10 year old girl.

National Surveys (1973, 1983, and 1993) of children's dental health in the United Kingdom show that the prevalence of chronic gingivitis increases steadily between the ages of 5 and 9 years and is closely associated with the amount of plaque, debris, and calculus present (Fig. 10.4). For example, in 1993, 26% of 5 year olds had some signs of gingivitis, and the proportion increased to 62 per cent at the age of 9. Prevalence of gingivitis peaks at about 11 years and then decreases slightly with age to 15 years. In terms of gingivitis, there has been no improvement over the decades between surveys. Indeed, in 1993, between 11 and 14 per cent more children of all ages between 6 and 12 years had signs of gingivitis when compared with 1983. These differences were not maintained with increasing age, however, as 52 per cent of 15 year olds had gingivitis in 1993 compared with 48 per cent in 1983. Furthermore, there were no differences between 1983 and 1993, in the proportion of 15 year olds with pockets between 3.5 and 5.5 mm (9 and 10 per cent, respectively). These data suggest that the gingival condition of children in the United Kingdom has deteriorated over the 10 years between 1983 and 1993, whereas the periodontal status of 15 year olds has not changed. Certainly, changes in gingival health do not mirror the dramatic improvement in the prevalence of caries over the same period. Children's mouths tended to be cleaner in 1983 than in 1973. This trend was reversed by 1993 when between 10 and 20 per cent more children of all ages had plaque deposits. Levels of calculus were similar in both surveys.

The onset of puberty and the increase in circulating levels of sex hormones is one explanation for the increase in gingivitis seen in 11 year olds. Oestrogen increases the cellularity of tissues and progesterone increases the permeability of the gingival vasculature. Oestradiol also provides suitable growth conditions for species of black pigmenting organisms which are associated with established gingivitis.

Histopathology

The inflammatory infiltrate associated with marginal gingivitis in children is analogous to that seen in adults during the early stages of gingival inflammation. The dominant cell is the lymphocyte, although small numbers of plasma cells, macrophages, and neutrophils are in evidence. Research findings have not yet determined unequivocally whether the lymphocyte population is one of unactivated B cells or is T-cell dominated. The relative absence of plasma cells, which are found in abundance in more established and advanced lesions in adults, confirms that gingivitis in children is quiescent and does not progress inexorably to involve the deeper periodontal tissues.

Chronic gingivitis:
- plaque-associated
- lymphocyte dominated
- complex flora

Microbiology

The first organisms to colonize clean tooth surfaces are the periodontally harmless, Gram-positive cocci that predominate in plaque after 4–7 days. After 2 weeks, a more complex flora of filamentous and fusiform organisms indicate a conversion to a Gram-negative infection, which when established, comprises significant numbers of Capnocytophaga, Selenomonas, Leptotrichia, Bacteroides, and Spirochaetes. These species are cultivable from established and advanced periodontal lesions in cases of adult periodontitis. This suggests that the host response (rather than the subgingival flora) confers a degree of immunity to the development of periodontal disease in children, thus preventing spread of the contained gingivitis to deeper tissues.

10.5 DRUG-INDUCED GINGIVAL OVERGROWTH

Overgrowth of the gingiva is a well-recognized unwanted effect of a number of drugs. The most frequently implicated are phenytoin, cyclosporin, and nifedipine (Fig. 10.5).

10.5.1 Phenytoin

Phenytoin is an anticonvulsant used in the management of epilepsy. Gingival overgrowth occurs in about 50 per cent of dentate subjects who are taking the drug, and is most severe in teenagers and those who are cared for in institutions. The exact mechanism by which phenytoin induces overgrowth is not clear. The gingival enlargement reflects an overproduction of collagen (rather than a decrease in degradation) and this may be brought about by the action of the drug on phenotypically distinct groups of fibroblasts that have the potential to synthesize large amounts of protein. Phenytoin-induced overgrowth has been associated with a deficiency of folic acid which may lead to impaired maturation of oral epithelia.

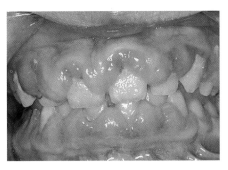

Fig. 10.5 Drug (Epanutin)-induced gingival overgrowth in a 12 year old boy.

10.5.2 Cyclosporin

Cyclosporin is an immunosuppressant drug that is used widely in post-organ transplant patients to prevent graft rejection. Approximately 30 per cent of patients taking the drug demonstrate gingival overgrowth and children are more susceptible than adults. The exact mechanism of the drug in causing overgrowth is not known. There is evidence to suggest both a stimulatory effect on fibroblast proliferation and collagen production as well as an inhibitory effect on collagen breakdown by the enzyme collagenase.

10.5.3 Nifedipine

Nifedipine is a calcium channel blocker that is used in adults for the control of cardiovascular problems. It is also given to post-transplant patients to reduce the nephrotoxic effects of cyclosporin. The incidence of gingival overgrowth in dentate subjects taking nifedipine is 10–15 per cent. The drug blocks the calcium channels in cell membranes and intracellular calcium ions are a prerequisite for the production of collagenases by fibroblasts. The lack of the enzymes could be responsible for the accumulation of collagen in the gingiva.

Clinical features of gingival overgrowth

The clinical changes of drug-induced overgrowth are very similar irrespective of the drug involved. The first signs of change are seen after 3–4 months of drug administration. The interdental papillae become nodular before enlarging more diffusely to encroach upon the labial tissues. The anterior part of the mouth is most severely and frequently involved so that the patient's appearance is compromised. The tissues can become so abundant that oral functions, particularly eating and speaking, are impaired.

Overgrown gingiva is pink, firm, and stippled in subjects with a good standard of oral hygiene. When there is a pre-existing gingivitis the enlarged tissues compromise an already poor standard of plaque control. The gingiva then exhibit the classical signs of gingivitis (Fig. 10.5).

Key Points	Gingival overgrowth: ● drug-induced ● collagen ● surgical treatment

Management of gingival overgrowth

A strict programme of oral hygiene instruction, scaling, and polishing, must be implemented. Severe cases of gingival overgrowth inevitably need to be surgically excised (gingivectomy) and then recontoured (gingivoplasty) to produce an architecture that allows adequate access for cleaning.

A follow-up programme is essential to ensure a high standard of plaque control and to detect any recurrence of the overgrowth. As the causative drugs need to be taken on a long term basis, recurrence is common. When a phenytoin-induced overgrowth is refractory to long-term treatment, the patient's physician may be requested to modify or change the anticonvulsant therapy to drugs such as sodium valproate or carbamazapine, which do not cause gingival problems. There is no alternative medication to cyclosporin, however, and the patients inevitably require indefinite oral care.

10.6 FACTITIOUS GINGIVITIS (GINGIVITIS ARTEFACTA)

Gingivitis artefacta has minor and major variants. The minor form results from rubbing or picking the gingiva using the finger nail, or perhaps abrasive foods such as crisps, and the habit is usually provoked by a locus of irritation such as an area of persistent food packing, or an already inflamed papilla (Fig. 10.6). The lesions resolve when the habit is corrected and the source of irritation is removed.

The injuries in gingivitis artefacta major are more severe and widespread and can involve the deeper periodontal tissues (Fig. 10.7(a)). Other areas of the mouth such as the lips and tongue may be involved and extra- oral injuries may be found on the scalp, limbs, or face (factitious dermatitis) (Fig. 10.7(b)). The lesions are usually viewed with complete indifference by the patient who is unable to forward details of their time of onset or possible cause.

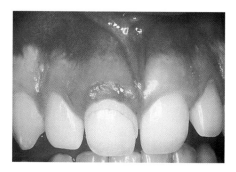

Fig. 10.6 Gingival injury inflicted by the fingernail that has been teased from the gingival crevice of 1|. (Reproduced with kind permission of the Editor, *British Dental Journal* and Mr P. R. Greene, General Dental Practitioner, Manchester.)

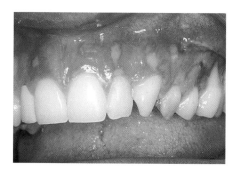

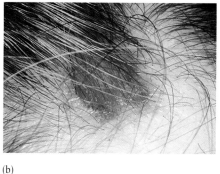

(a)   (b)

Fig. 10.7 (a) Generalized, self-inflicted ulceration of the attached gingiva and extensive loss of attachment around |6. (b) Ulcerative lesion at the hairline on the scalp. The lesions were produced by rubbing with a fingernail. (Reproduced by kind permission of the Editor, *Journal of Periodontology*.)

The treatment of these patients, other than the dressing and protection of oral wounds, does not lie with the dentist. Psychological reasons for inflicting the lesions may be complex and obscure. A psychological or psychiatric consultation, rarely welcomed either by older children or their parents, is necessary if the patient is to be prevented from ultimately inflicting serious damage upon themselves.

Gingivitis artefacta: ● minor/major ● self-inflicted ● habitual ● psychological	**Key Points**

10.7 MUCOGINGIVAL PROBLEMS IN CHILDREN

In adults much attention has focused on whether recession is more likely to occur locally where there is a reduced width of keratinized gingiva (KG). Conversely, of course, gingival recession inevitably leads to a narrowing of the zone of KG. It is, therefore, often difficult to determine unequivocally whether a narrow zone of KG is the cause or the effect of recession. A narrow or finite width of KG is compatible with gingival health providing the tissues are maintained free of inflammation and chronic, traumatic insult. A wider zone of KG is considered more desirable to withstand gingival inflammation, trauma from mastication, toothbrushing, and forces from muscle pull.

Anterior teeth with narrow zones of KG are frequently encountered in children, as the width of KG varies greatly during the mixed dentition. For example, when permanent teeth erupt labially to their predecessors they frequently appear

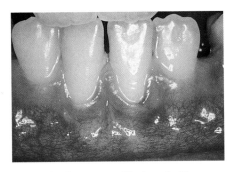

Fig. 10.8 Lower central incisors that have erupted somewhat labially to $\overline{2|2}$. There is only a minimal width of keratinized gingiva buccal to the $\overline{1|1}$.

to erupt through alveolar mucosa with a complete absence of KG (Fig. 10.8). When the tooth has fully erupted an obvious width of KG is present.

The width of KG alone should not be the sole indicator of potential sites of gingival recession in children. The position of a tooth in the arch is a better guide as studies have shown that, of those permanent incisors with recession, about 80 per cent are displaced labially. Aggravating factors such as gingivitis or mechanical irritation from excessive and incorrect toothbrushing further increase the likelihood of recession.

Gingival recession is also a common periodontal complication of orthodontic therapy when labial tipping of incisors is undertaken. When roots move labially through the supporting envelope of alveolar bone the potential for recession increases.

When gingival recession occurs in children, a conservative approach to treatment should be adopted. The maximum distance from the gingival margin to the CEJ should be recorded. Over-enthusiastic toothbrushing practices are modified and a scale and polish given. The recession must then be monitored carefully until the permanent dentition is complete. Longitudinal studies of individual cases have shown that, as the supporting tissues mature, the gingival attachment tends to creep spontaneously in a coronal direction to cover at least part of the previously denuded root surface. This cautious approach is preferred to corrective surgical intervention to increase the width of KG.

Key Points	Gingival recession:
	• narrow keratinized gingiva
	• local trauma
	• post-orthodontics
	• conservative treatment

10.8   CHRONIC PERIODONTITIS

A number of epidemiological studies (Table 10.2) have investigated the prevalence of chronic periodontitis in children. The variation in prevalence between studies is considerable and attributable to different methods of diagnosing attachment loss and the use of different cut-off levels to determine disease presence. Some workers use intra oral radiographs to measure from the CEJ to the alveolar crest while others use a periodontal probe to determine clinically the distance from the CEJ to the base of the periodontal crevice or pocket. Radiographic studies on children with a primary or a mixed dentition indicate that loss of attachment is uncommon under the age of 9 years. A microscopic examination of root surfaces of 200 extracted molars, however, demonstrated a mean attachment loss of 0.26 mm on two-thirds of the surfaces on 94 per cent of teeth. Clinically, such small changes are insignificant and difficult to detect.

Cut-off levels at which disease is diagnosed in adolescents have been set at 1, 2, or 3 mm. Larger cut-off values provide more stringent criteria for the detection of attachment loss and consequently the disease appears less prevalent. An exception to this trend was seen in a study of 602, 14–15 year olds in the United Kingdom; 51.5 per cent of subjects were diagnosed as having periodontal disease determined by a CEJ–alveolar crest distance of 3 mm. Additional radiographic features were also used, namely an irregular contour of the alveolar crest and a widened, coronal periodontal ligament space. Such observations may result from minor tooth movements following

Table 10.2 Key studies to determine the prevalence of periodontal disease (ALOSS) in children

Country of study (year)	Subjects	Method of diagnosis of ALOSS	Periodontal disease prevalence	Observations
UK (1974)	590 15 year olds	Probing from CEJ ≥1 mm ≥2 mm	46% 11%	Evidence of social class gradient; lower class higher disease prevalence
UK (1975)	602 14 year olds	Radiographs CEJ–AC > 3 mm	51.5%	Disease also diagnosed by irregular AC and widened ligament space
Norway (1984)	2409 15 year olds	Radiographs CEJ–AC > 2 mm	11%	Maxillary first molars primarily affected
USA (1987)	2264 children with primary molars	Radiographs Reduced AC height	< 1%	No evaluation of the extent of periodontal disease
Hungary (1987)	200 extracted primary molars	Microscopic examination of root surface	Mean ALOSS 0.26 mm on two-thirds surfaces of 94% teeth	More ALOSS on maxillary (than mandibular) molars and adjacent to carious tooth surfaces
Norway (1988)	2767 14 year olds	Radiographs CEJ–AC > 2 mm	4.5%	Previous orthodontic treatment may increase prevalence of ALOSS
UK (1990)	167 14 year olds	Probing from CEJ ≥1 mm ≥2 mm	3% 0%	Subgingival calculus closely correlates with future ALOSS
New Zealand (1994)	317 5 year olds	Radiographs CEJ–AC > 2 mm	2.1% Definite bone loss	Bone loss more likely with higher dmft
Sweden (1994)	8666 7–9 year olds	Radiographs CEJ-AC > 2 mm	2–5%	Children with bone loss had more calculus and higher dfs

CEJ, cemento-enamel junction; ALOSS, attachment loss;
AC alveolar crest; DMFT/S decayed, missing, filled teeth/surfaces

eruption of the second molars and consolidation of the occlusion, or from remodelling of bone after orthodontic treatment. It is, therefore, likely that 51.5 per cent is a considerable overestimate of disease prevalence in this age group. If a cut-off value of 2 mm is deemed acceptable, the majority of studies put the prevalence of disease in adolescents at 1–11 per cent. This suggests that chronic adult periodontitis initiates and progresses during the early teenage years.

Observations made with respect to periodontal disease in children include:

1. When loss of attachment occurs at interproximal sites it is a consequence of pathological change and correlates closely with the presence of subgingival calculus.

2. The prevalence of periodontal destruction correlates positively with DMF (decayed, missing, and filled) teeth or surfaces. This suggests either, that carious or broken down surfaces predispose to plaque accumulation, or perhaps more likely, that in the absence of oral health care, periodontal disease and caries progress independently.

3. When the loss of attachment occurs on buccal or palatal surfaces, it is more often associated with trauma from an incorrect toothbrushing technique than with an inflammatory response.

10.9   PERIODONTAL COMPLICATIONS OF ORTHODONTIC TREATMENT

Orthodontic treatment in adolescents, particularly with fixed appliances, can predispose to a deterioration in periodontal health and a number of well recognized complications.

10.9.1   Gingivitis

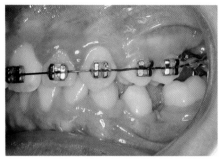

Fig. 10.9 Chronic marginal gingivitis associated with fixed appliance therapy.

Access for interproximal toothbrushing is reduced considerably during fixed appliance therapy and the accumulation of plaque induces gingivitis (Fig. 10.9). The problem is compounded when teeth are banded rather than bonded as periodontal health is more easily maintained when the gingival sulcus is not encroached upon by metal bands.

When supragingival plaque deposits are present on teeth that are being repositioned orthodontically, the type of movement used may play an important part in the development of periodontal problems. Supragingival plaque deposits are shifted into a subgingival location by tipping movements. Conversely, bodily movements are less likely to induce a relocation of supragingival plaque.

10.9.2   Gingival hyperplasia

The anterior palatal gingiva and mucosa have a propensity to hyperplastic change when tissues are 'rolled up' between incisors that are being retracted and the fixed anterior margin of the acrylic plate of a removable appliance (Fig. 10.10 (a) and (b)). Generally, however, hyperplastic changes tend to be transient and resolve when appliances are removed.

10.9.3   Attachment and bone loss

The mean, annual rate of rate of coronal attachment loss during appliance therapy is in the range of 0.05–0.30 mm, which compares favourably with figures for mean annual attachment loss in untreated populations. A well-recognized complication of orthodontic tooth movement is apical root resorption particularly when excessive forces are used (Fig. 10.11). Such changes must also be regarded as loss of attachment, albeit at an apical rather than a coronal site.

10.9.4   Gingival recession

The response of the facial periodontal tissues to labial tooth movement in anterior segments is unpredictable. Labial movement of incisors is sometimes associated with gingival recession. The risk of recession is greater when the alveolar bone plate is thin or where dehiscences or fenestrations in the bone exist.

10.9.5   Trauma

Direct local irritation of the soft tissues by components of a fixed appliance can be minimized if due care and attention is exercised during bonding, banding, and

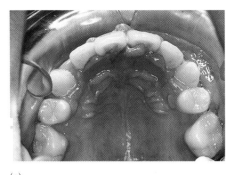

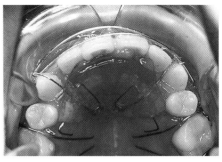

(a)   (b)

Fig. 10.10 (a) Gingival hyperplasia on the palatal aspect of retracted maxillary incisors. (b) appliance *in situ*. (Reproduced by kind permission of Mr N. E. Carter, Consultant in Orthodontics, Newcastle.)

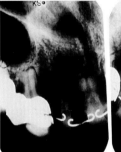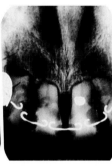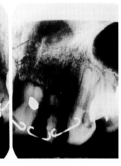

Fig. 10.11 Apical root resorption of 321 | 123 following orthodontic treatment. (Reproduced by kind permission of Dr I. L. Chapple, Lecturer in Periodontology, Birmingham, UK.)

placement of wires and elastics. If chronic irritation of the gingiva does occur then a localized, acute inflammatory reaction will quickly follow. This may develop further into a region of chronic hyperplastic tissue or a fibrous epulis that is superimposed upon a burrowing infrabony lesion.

Orthodontic problems:	**Key Points**
• gingivitis	
• hyperplasia	
• root resorption	
• gingival trauma	

10.10 EARLY-ONSET PERIODONTAL DISEASES

Early-onset diseases comprise a group of rare, but very aggressive and rapidly progressing infections that affect the primary and permanent dentitions. The disorders are associated with a more specific microbial challenge and an inherent defect in the host's immunological response. The nature of these diseases can lead to premature tooth loss at an early age. Prompt diagnosis is essential if treatment is to be successful, and the periodontal status must be monitored regularly to ensure that the treated disease remains quiescent.

Early-onset diseases are classified as prepubertal periodontitis (PP) and juvenile periodontitis (JP), both of which have localized and generalized forms. These disorders occur in the absence of underlying medical conditions that also predispose to an early onset of periodontitis.

10.10.1 Prepubertal periodontitis

This disease affects the primary dentition and may present immediately after the teeth have erupted. In the generalized form the gingiva appear fiery red, swollen, and haemorrhagic. The tissues become hyperplastic with granular or nodular proliferations that precede gingival clefting and extensive areas of recession. Gross deposits of plaque are inevitable as the soft tissue changes make it difficult to maintain oral hygiene. The disease progresses extremely rapidly, with primary tooth loss occurring as early as 3–4 years of age. The entire dentition need not be affected, however, as the bone loss may be restricted to one arch. Children with generalized PP are susceptible to recurrent general infections, principally otitis media and upper respiratory tract infections.

Localized PP progresses more slowly than the generalized form and bone loss characteristically affects only incisor-molar teeth. Plaque levels are usually low, consequently soft tissue changes are minimal with gingivitis and proliferation involving only the marginal tissues.

The predominant micro-organisms that have been identified in cases of PP are aggressive periodontopathogens: *Actinobacillus actinomycetemcomitans*, *Porphyromonas gingivalis*, *Fusobacterium nucleatum*, and *Eikenella corrodens*. This suggests that there is an infective component to the disease, although defects in the hosts' response have also been identified. Profound abnormalities in chemotaxis and phagocytosis of polymorphonuclear neutrophils and monocytes are frequently reported in these patients. These immunological defects are heritable risk factors that help to define phenotypically PP as a disease entity. Conversely, they may also be associated with more serious and life-threatening conditions, and thus a full medical screen is indicated for children suffering from PP.

Prepubertal periodontitis demands an intense treatment. Oral hygiene instruction, scaling and root planing should be undertaken at frequent (2–3 month) intervals. Bacterial culturing of the pocket flora identifies specific periodontopathogens. If pathogens persist after oral debridement, an antibiotic such as metronidazole or amoxycillin should be given systemically after sensitivity testing, as a short course over 1–2 weeks. Generalized disease responds poorly to treatment. Some improvement has been achieved following a granulocyte transfusion in a patient with a defect in neutrophil function. Extraction of involved teeth has also produced an improvement in neutrophil chemotaxis, which suggests that the defect may be induced by certain organisms in the periodontal flora. Furthermore, in severe cases of generalized periodontitis, extraction of all primary teeth (and the provision of a removable prosthesis) can limit the disease to the primary dentition. Presumably, anaerobic pathogens are unable to thrive in the absence of teeth. When the permanent teeth erupt, bacterial culturing of the subgingival flora ensures that reinfection is detected early.

10.10.2   Juvenile periodontitis

JP involves severe periodontal destruction with an onset around puberty. The localized form (LJP) occurs in otherwise healthy individuals with destruction classically localized and around first permanent molars and incisors, and not involving more than two other teeth. Generalized juvenile periodontitis (GJP) also occurs in otherwise healthy individuals but involves more than 14 teeth, that is, being generalized to an arch or the entire dentition. Some reports have monitored children suffering from PP to find that, at around puberty, they also suffered from LJP which became generalized to involve the entire dentition. Longitudinal observations suggest that PP, LJP and GPP are simply different manifestations of the same disease. Other studies describe both LJP patients who did not suffer previously with PP as well as adolescents who have GJP without suffering from LJP. Such cases are quoted by those who believe that PP, LJP, and GJP are quite distinct clinical entities while acknowledging that some rare and unfortunate individuals are susceptible to all three disorders.

Epidemiology of JP

Studies show a prevalence for JP of about 0.1 per cent in developed countries and about 5 per cent in underdeveloped nations, although some variation may be due to different methods of screening and different criteria used to define the disease. JP is clearly more prevalent in certain ethnic groups. In the United Kingdom an epidemiological study of 7266 school children in Coventry and Birmingham showed an overall prevalence for JP of 0.02 per cent in Caucasians, 0.2% in Asians, and 0.8 per cent in the Afro-Caribbean population. There was no difference in prevalence between males and females, which does not concur with the data of many earlier epidemiological studies of the disease which reported a female to male ratio of 3:1.

Clinical and radiographic features of JP

The age of onset of LJP is between 11 and 15 years. The clinical features are pocket formation and loss of attachment associated with the permanent incisors and first molar teeth. The radiographic pattern of bone loss is quite distinctive. Bilateral angular bone defects are identified on the mesial and, or distal surfaces of molars (Fig. 10.12 (a) and (b)). Angular defects are sometimes seen around the incisors, although the very thin interproximal bone is resorbed more evenly to give a horizontal pattern of resorption. The bone loss around the molars can be detected on routine bitewing radiographs. The interpretation of the films must be made with a sound knowledge of the patient's dental history, however, as localized angular defects are found adjacent to teeth with overhanging or deficient interproximal restorations, and teeth that have tilted slightly (Fig. 10.13). The gingiva can appear healthy when the levels of plaque are low, but a marginal gingivitis will be present if a good standard of plaque control is not evident.

GJP also presents at puberty. Severe generalized bone loss is the characteristic feature (Fig. 10.14). The pattern may be a combination of angular and horizontal resorption producing an irregular alveolar crest. When patients have good plaque control the degree of bone resorption is not commensurate with the level of oral hygiene. The more generalized nature of the disease predisposes to multiple and recurrent abscess formation which is a common presenting feature.

Invariably, one of the presenting signs of both LJP and GJP is tooth migration or drifting of incisors. Tooth movement is not necessarily a consequence of advanced disease as drifting may occur when only a fraction of a tooth's periodontal support is lost. Conversely, extensive bone loss can occur with no spontaneous movement of teeth and the subject may only have alerted to the problem when a minor traumatic episode, such as a blow to the mouth during a sporting activity, causes unexpected loosening of teeth.

Bacteriology and pathogenesis of JP

The subgingival microflora comprises loosely adherent, Gram-negative anaerobes including *Eikenella corrodens*, *Capnocytophaga*, and *Prevotella intermedia*. The most frequently implicated organism is *Actinobacillus actinomycetemcomitans*, which has been found in over 90 per cent of JP patients. JP sufferers also have raised IgG titres to *A. actinomycetemcomitans*, and levels of the bacteria fall significantly following successful treatment of the condition.

The extreme pathogenicity of *A. actinomycetemcomitans* is due to its ability to invade connective tissues and the wide range of virulence factors that it produces. These include a potent lipopolysaccharide that induces bone resorption, collagenase, an epitheliotoxin, a fibroblast-inhibiting factor, and a leukotoxin

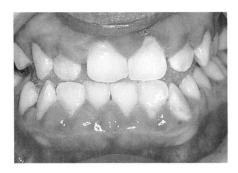

(a)

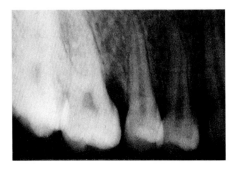

(b)

Fig. 10.12 (a) Clinical appearance of a 13 year old girl with localized juvenile periodontitis. (b) radiographic appearance of vertical bone loss on the mesial aspect of 6⌋. (Reproduced by kind permission of Mr D. G. Smith, Consultant in Restorative Dentistry, Newcastle.)

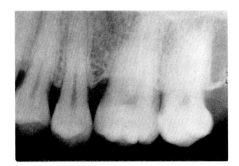

Fig. 10.13 Radiographic view of ⌊7 that has erupted and tipped mesially into ⌊6 extraction site. The contour of the bone crest on the mesial of ⌊7 gives the impression of a vertical bony defect.

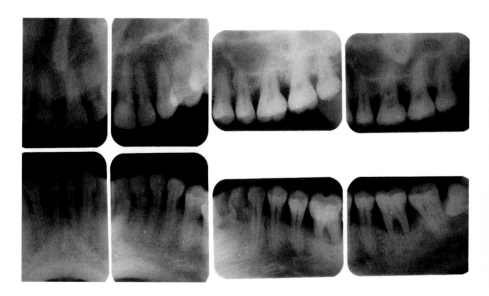

Fig. 10.14 Juvenile periodontitis with generalized bone loss in a 16 year old male.

which kills neutrophils and so dampens the host's first line of defence against bacterial challenge.

About 70 per cent of patients with JP have defects in neutrophil chemotaxis and phagocytosis. The chemotactic defect is linked to reduced amounts of cell surface glycoproteins and is transmitted as a dominant trait. About 50 per cent of siblings of patients who have both LJP and chemotactic defects, also demonstrate impaired neutrophil function.

Treatment of JP

A combined regimen of regular scaling and root planing with a 2 week course of systemic tetracycline therapy (250 mg, four times daily) has been used extensively in the management of JP. *A. actinomycetemcomitans* is sensitive to tetracycline, which also has the ability to be concentrated up to 10 times in gingival crevicular fluid when compared with serum. More recently, a combination of metronidazole (250 mg) and amoxycillin (375 mg), three times a day for 1 week, in association with subgingival scaling, has also been found to be effective.

Key Points

Early-onset diseases:
- localized/generalized
- specific flora
- immune defects
- genetic link

A more radical approach is to undertake flap surgery so that better access is achieved for root cleaning and the superficial, infected connective tissues are excised. An antimicrobial regimen can also be implemented in conjunction with a surgical approach.

10.10.3 Genetic factors in early-onset diseases

The increased prevalence of early-onset periodontal diseases in certain ethnic groups and within families suggests strongly that susceptibility to these diseases may be influenced by a number of genetic determinants. Furthermore, genetic factors are implicated in the pathogenesis of the diseases as many affected patients have functionally defective neutrophils.

The mode of transmission has not been determined unequivocally. The apparent increased incidence of JP in females suggests an X-linked dominant mode of inheritance with reduced penetrance. The association with females, however, may reflect epidemiological bias as females are more likely to seek dental attention. Large family studies of subjects with JP suggest an autosomal recessive pattern of inheritance. It is conceivable that the different forms of PP and JP are specific genotypes that are expressed as a common clinical phenotype.

The role of hereditary components in periodontal diseases has been supported by the link with specific tissue markers. The major histocompatibility complex (MHC) determines the susceptibility of subjects to certain diseases. Class I and II genes in the MHC encode for specific human leukocyte antigens (HLA I and II), which account for individual variation in immunoresponsiveness. There are clear associations between HLA serotypes and diabetes mellitus and rheumatoid arthritis. A strong link between an HLA serotype and early-onset diseases has still to be determined, although a mild association between the HLA-A9 antigen and JP has been found.

Genetic components of periodontitis:

- family associations
- ethnic associations
- major histocompatibility complex link
- link with syndromes

Key Points

10.11 PREPUBERTAL PERIODONTITIS AS A MANIFESTATION OF SYSTEMIC DISEASE

The genetic basis for PP is substantiated by the definite association between the condition and a number of rare inherited medical conditions and syndromes (Table 10.1). The pattern of inheritance reflects a single gene disorder, commonly involving inherited defects of neutrophils, enzyme reactions, or collagen synthesis.

10.11.1 Papillon Lefèvre syndrome (PLS)

This syndrome is characterized by palmar–plantar hyperkeratosis, premature loss of primary and permanent dentitions and ectopic calcifications of the falx cerebri. Some patients show an increased susceptibility to infection. The syndrome is an autosomal recessive trait with a prevalence of about 1–4/million. Consanguinity of parents is evident in about one-third of cases.

Rapid and progressive periodontal destruction affects the primary dentition with an onset at about 2 years (Fig. 10.15). Exfoliation of all primary teeth is usual before the permanent successors erupt and patients may be edentulous by the mid to late teens. Cases of a late-onset variant of PLS have also been described in which the palmar–plantar and periodontal lesions are relatively mild and only become evident in the permanent dentition. An extensive family dental history supported by clinical, laboratory, and radiographic examinations confirm a diagnosis.

10.11.2 Neutropenias

The neutropenias comprise a heterogeneous group of blood disorders that are characterized by a periodic or persistent reduction in the number of circulating polymorphonuclear neutrophils. Neutropenias can be drug-induced or be

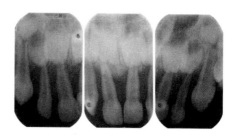

(a)

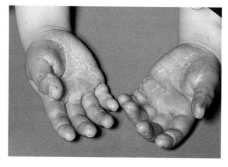

(b)

Fig. 10.15 Papillon Lefèvre syndrome in a 3 year old boy: (a) radiographic appearance showing almost total bone loss around maxillary anterior teeth; (b) hyperkeratosis of the palms of the hands.

secondary to severe bacterial or viral infections or autoimmune diseases such as lupus erythematosus. Cyclic neutropenia, benign familial and severe familial neutropenias are all heritable conditions transmitted as autosomal dominant traits and diagnoses are often made during early childhood. The chronic benign neutropenia of childhood is diagnosed between 6 and 24 months of age and is characterized by frequent and multiple pyogenic infections of the skin and mucous membranes.

The periodontal problems that are associated with the neutropenias are very similar and in many cases the patient presents with a localized or generalized early-onset periodontitis. Occasionally, the primary dentition may not be involved, and clinical signs do not appear until the permanent dentition has erupted. The gingiva are inflamed and oedematous, gingival recession, ulceration, and desquamation can also occur.

The treatment of a neutropenic-induced periodontitis involves local removal of plaque and calculus. Strict plaque control measures are difficult to achieve in younger children, so use of an antibacterial mouthrinse may prove useful.

10.11.3 Chediak-Higashi syndrome

This is a rare and very often fatal disease inherited as an autosomal recessive trait. Clinical features include partial albinism, photophobia, and nystagmus. The patients suffer from recurrent pyogenic infections and malignant lymphoma which is accompanied by neutropenia, anaemia, and a thrombocytopenia. The neutrophils show defects in migration, chemotaxis, and phagocytosis producing a diminished bactericidal capacity.

Periodontal changes that are associated with the syndrome include severe gingival inflammation and rapid, and extensive alveolar bone resorption that can lead to premature exfoliation. The nature of the changes has not been fully established and they may be plaque-induced, secondary to infection or related to the underlying defect in neutrophil function.

10.11.4 Leukocyte adhesion deficiency syndrome (LAD)

This autosomal recessive trait is characterized clinically by a delayed separation of the umbilical cord, severe recurrent bacterial infections, impaired wound healing, formation of pus, and severe PP with an aggressive gingivitis, which may be the presenting sign of the disorder. Consanguinity between the parents of affected children confirms the mode of the inheritance as autosomal recessive.

The syndrome demonstrates the important role of leukocytes (and other white blood cells) in protecting the host against periodontal disease. Moderate phenotypes, however, may appear relatively disease free, but then develop symptoms and progress 'downhill' extremely rapidly. The majority of patients do not survive beyond 30 years. The progressive periodontal condition is very difficult to control and is often of secondary importance to other life-threatening infections. Recent evidence suggests that LAD and GPP are phenotypically identical conditions.

10.11.5 Ehlers-Danlos syndrome

The syndrome is an autosomal dominant trait with nine variants that display defects in the synthesis, secretion, or polymerization of collagen. The variants of the syndrome exhibit extensive clinical heterogeneity and collectively represent the most common of the heritable disorders of connective tissues. The clinical findings are principally excessive joint mobility, skin hyperextensibility, and susceptibility to scarring and bruising of the skin, and oral mucous membranes (Fig. 10.16). Defective type IV collagen supporting the walls of small blood vessels predisposes to persistent post-extraction haemorrhage.

Gingival tissues are fragile and have a tendency to bleed on toothbrushing. The type VIII syndrome is associated with advanced periodontal disease. Periodontitis has also been linked with type IV variant, although other variants do not appear to be affected. Ultrastructural changes also occur in the teeth with abnormalities of the amelodentinal junction, vascular inclusions in dentine, fibrous degeneration of the pulp, and disorganization of cementum.

Type VIII patients require a thorough preventative periodontal programme as root debridement can cause extensive trauma to the fragile soft tissues. Periodontal surgery should be avoided because of the risk of haemorrhage and the potential problems encountered with suturing soft tissue flaps.

10.11.6 Langerhans cell histiocytosis

Langerhans cell histiocytosis (LCH) is a non-malignant granulomatous, childhood disorder that is characterized pathologically by uncontrolled proliferation and accumulation of Langerhans cells, mixed with varying proportions of eosinophils and multinucleated giant cells. LCH replaced the term histiocytosis X and the closely related syndromes eosinophilic granuloma, Hand–Schuller–Christian disease, and Letterer–Siwe disease. The clinical hallmark of LCH is the presence of lytic bone lesions that may be single or multiple. When lesions are widespread they can affect the pituitary gland and retro-orbital region, thus causing diabetes insipidus and exophthalmos, respectively. The disseminated form of LCH is extremely aggressive and has a poor prognosis. It is often diagnosed in the first 6 months of life before becoming widespread by about 3 years of age.

The periodontal manifestations of LCH may be the presenting signs and include a marginal gingivitis, bleeding gingiva, abscess formation, pain, and drifting and mobility of the teeth. Radiographs show localized or generalized bone loss, characteristic osteolytic lesions, and 'floating teeth' with no alveolar bone support (Fig. 10.17).

A biopsy will confirm the diagnosis and a full radiographic screening determines the severity of the syndrome. Local lesions that are confined to bone respond well to curettage and excision. The mortality rate increases in the more widely disseminated forms of the syndrome and when overlying soft tissues are involved. Treatment is by radiotherapy and chemotherapy.

10.11.7 Hypophosphatasia

Hypophosphatasia is a rare, inborn error or metabolism that is characterized by defective bone mineralization, a deficiency of alkaline photphatase (ALP) activity, and an increased excretion of phosphoethanolamine in the urine. ALP plays a major part in mineralization of hard tissues and so the absence of the enzyme predisposes to a range of bone and cartilage defects. The condition is an autosomal recessive trait, although the inheritance pattern of some milder forms of hypophosphatasia may be autosomal dominant.

The lesions of juvenile or childhood hypophosphatasia become apparent before 2 years of age. Bone defects are usually quite mild with bowing of the legs, proptosis, and wide open fontanelles being prominent signs. Dental features are resorption of alveolar bone (in the absence of marked gingivitis), premature exfoliation of anterior deciduous teeth, hypoplasia or complete absence of cementum, and the presence of 'small teeth' that have enlarged pulp chambers as a conse-

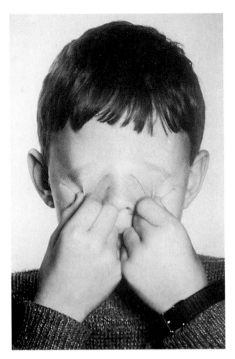

Fig. 10.16 Cutaneous hyperextensibility of the upper eyelids in a 9 year old child with Ehlers–Danlos syndrome.

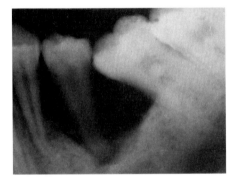

Fig. 10.17 Extensive bone loss around mandibular left premolars in a 15 year old child with Langerhans cell histiocytosis. (Reproduced by kind permission of Dr I. L. Chapple, Lecturer in Periodontology, Birmingham, UK.)

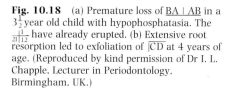

Fig. 10.18 (a) Premature loss of BA | AB in a 3½ year old child with hypophosphatasia. The ‾1|1‾ have already erupted. (b) Extensive root resorption led to exfoliation of |CD at 4 years of age. (Reproduced by kind permission of Dr I. L. Chapple, Lecturer in Periodontology, Birmingham, UK.)

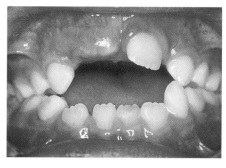

(a)

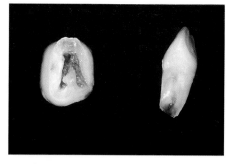

(b)

quence of defective mineralization (Fig. 10.18 (a) and (b)). The aplastic or hypoplastic cementum and a weakened periodontal attachment is thought to render the patients susceptible to infection with periodontopathogens.

The diagnosis of hypophosphatasia is confirmed biochemically by low activity of serum ALP and a raised level of phosphoethanolamine in a 24 h urine sample.

10.12 SUMMARY

1. Anatomical variation which occurs during the eruption of the teeth, and the maturation of the periodontal tissues can mimick signs of gingivitis, recession and bone loss.

2. Herpetic gingivostomatitis is most frequently seen in children under 5 years of age, whereas acute necrotising ulcerative gingivitis is more prevalent in young adults.

3. Although the prevalence of dental caries has declined in the UK and other European countries, the prevalence of plaque-induced gingivitis in children has not reduced over the last 20 years.

4. Chronic gingivitis in children appears to be in relatively stable lesion which does not necessarily progress to periodontal destruction.

5. Gingival changes can also occur in children who are prescribed drugs to control epilepsy or following transplant surgery, during orthodontic therapy, as well as at sites of self-inflicted trauma.

6. Early signs of chronic periodontitis are sometimes seen during adolescence and targeting this age group with a primary prevention strategy may help to reduce tooth loss in later life.

7. Extreme vigilance is necessary to diagnose early-onset periodontal diseases and those pre-pubertal conditions which may be associated with systemic disease. Bleeding after gentle probing in the presence of apparently healthy gingivae indicates the need for further investigation.

10.13 FURTHER READING

O'Brien, M. (1993). *Children's Dental Health in the UK, 1993*. Office of Population Censuses and Surveys, HMSO, London.

Sabiston, Jr, C. B. (1986) A review and proposal for the etiology of acute necrotising gingivitis. *Journal of Clinical Periodontology*, **13**, 727–34. (*An overview of the epidemiology of ANUG with an emphasis on a viral rather than a bacterial aetiology.*)

Schenkein, H. A. (1994) Genetics of early-onset periodontal diseases. In *Molecular pathogenesis of periodontal disease*, (ed. R. Genco, S. Hamada, T. Lehner, J. McGhee, and S.

Mergenhagen, pp. 373–86, ASM Press, Washington. (*An appraisal of the role that genetic factors play in the pathogenesis of juvenile and prepubertal periodontitis.*)

Seymour, R. A. (1993) Drug-induced gingival overgrowth. *Adverse Drug Reactions and Toxicology Review*, **12**, 215–32. (*A general account of the drugs that induce gingival overgrowth.*)

Seymour, R. A. and Heasman, P. A. (1992). *Drugs, diseases and the periodontium.* Oxford Medical Publications, Oxford University Press, Oxford. (*Comprehensive accounts of early-onset diseases, systemic disease and the periodontium, and gingival overgrowth.*)

11 Traumatic injuries to the teeth

11 Traumatic injuries to the teeth
R. R. WELBURY

11.1 EPIDEMIOLOGY

Dental trauma in childhood and adolescence is common (Fig. 11.1). At 5 years of age 31–40 per cent of boys and 16–30 per cent of girls, and at 12 years of age 12–33 per cent of boys and 4–19 per cent of girls will have suffered some dental trauma. Boys are affected almost twice as often as girls in both the primary and the permanent dentitions.

The majority of dental injuries in the primary and permanent dentitions involve the anterior teeth, especially the maxillary central incisors. The mandibular central incisors and maxillary lateral incisors are less frequently involved. Concussion, subluxation, and luxation are the commonest in the primary dentition (Fig. 11.2), while uncomplicated crown fractures are the commonest in the permanent teeth (Fig. 11.3).

11.2 AETIOLOGY

The most accident prone times are between 2 and 4 years for the primary dentition and 7 and 10 years for the permanent dentition. In the primary dentition co-ordination and judgement are incompletely developed and the majority of injuries are due to falls in and around the home as the child becomes more adventurous and explores its surroundings. In the permanent dentition most injuries are caused by falls and collisions while playing and running, although bicycles are a common accessory. The place of injury varies in different countries according to local customs but accidents in the school yard remain common.

Sports injuries usually occur in teenage years and are commonly associated with contact sports such as soccer, rugby, ice-hockey, and basketball.

Injuries due to road traffic accidents and assaults are most commonly associated with the late teenage years and adulthood and are often closely related to alcohol abuse.

One form of injury in childhood that must never be forgotten is child physical abuse or non-accident injury (NAI). Up to 50 per cent of these children will have orofacial injuries (Fig. 11.4).

The exact mechanisms of dental injuries are largely unknown and without experimental evidence, but injuries can be the result of either direct or indirect trauma. Direct trauma occurs when the tooth itself is struck. Indirect trauma is seen when the lower dental arch is forcefully closed against the upper, e.g. blow to chin. Direct trauma implies injuries to the anterior region while indirect trauma favours crown or crown–root fractures in the premolar and molar regions as well as the possibility of jaw fractures in the condylar regions and symphysis. The factors which influence the outcome or type of injury are a

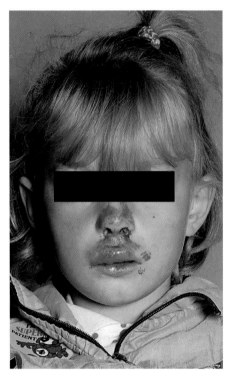

Fig. 11.1 A 7 year old girl who fell off her bicycle and sustained orofacial injuries.

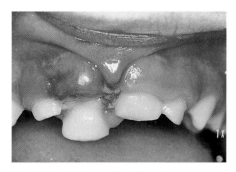

Fig. 11.2 A 3 year old child with a combination of injuries to her upper anterior teeth.

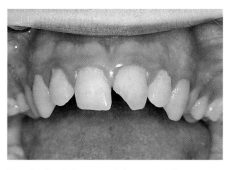

Fig. 11.3 A fracture of the upper left permanent central incisor involving enamel and dentine.

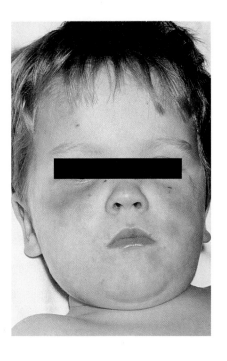

Fig. 11.4 A 3 year old boy with bruises and abrasions resulting from non-accidental injury. (Kind permission of Munskgaard.)

combination of: (a) energy impact; (b) resilience of impacting object; (c) shape of impacting object and; (d) angle of direction of the impacting force.

Increased overjet with protrusion of upper incisors and insufficient lip closure are significant predisposing factors to traumatic dental injuries. Injuries are almost twice as frequent among children with protruding incisors and the number of teeth affected in a particular incident for an individual patient also increase.

The second major group of children with predisposition to traumatic injuries are the accident-prone. They sustain repeated trauma to their teeth and frequencies have been reported to range from 4 to 30 per cent.

11.3   CLASSIFICATION

Table 11.1 summarizes the classification of dento-alveolar injuries based on the World Health Organization (WHO) system.

11.4   HISTORY AND EXAMINATION

A history of the injury followed by a thorough examination should be completed in any situation.

11.4.1   Dental history

1. *When did injury occur?* The time interval between injury and treatment significantly influences the prognosis of avulsions, luxations, crown fractures with or without pulpal exposures, and dento-alveolar fractures.
2. *Where did injury occur?* May indicate the need for tetanus prophylaxis.
3. *How did injury occur?* The nature of the accident can yield information on the type of injury expected. Discrepancy between history and clinical findings raises suspicion of NAI.
4. *Lost teeth/fragments?* If a tooth or fractured piece cannot be accounted for when there has been a history of loss of consciousness then a chest radiograph should be obtained to exclude inhalation.
5. *Concussion, headache, vomiting or amnesia?* Brain damage must be excluded and referral to a hospital for further investigation organized.

Table 11.1 Classification of the nature of dento-alveolar injuries

Injuries to the hard dental tissues and the pulp	
Enamel infraction	Incomplete fracture (crack) of enamel without loss of tooth substance
Enamel fracture	Loss of tooth substance confined to enamel
Enamel–dentine fracture	Loss of tooth substance confined to enamel and dentine not involving the pulp
Complicated crown fracture	Fracture of enamel and dentine exposing the pulp
Uncomplicated crown–root fracture	Fracture of enamel, dentine, and cementum but not involving the pulp
Complicated crown–root fracture	Fracture of enamel, dentine, and cementum and exposing the pulp
Root fracture	Fracture involving dentine, cementum, and pulp. Can be subclassified into; apical, middle and coronal third
Injuries to the periodontal tissues	
Concussion	No abnormal loosening or displacement but marked reaction to percussion
Subluxation (loosening)	Abnormal loosening but no displacement
Extrusive luxation (partial avulsion)	Partial displacement of tooth from socket
Lateral luxation	Displacement other than axially with comminution or fracture of alveolar socket
Intrusive luxation	Displacement into alveolar bone with comminution or fracture of alveolar socket
Avulsion	Complete displacement of tooth from socket
Injuries to supporting bone	
Comminution of mandibular or maxillary alveolar socket wall	Crushing and compression of alveolar socket. Found in intrusive and lateral luxation injuries
Fracture of mandibular or maxillary alveolar socket wall	Fracture confined to facial or lingual/palatal socket wall
Fracture of mandibular or maxillary alveolar process	Fracture of the alveolar process which may or may not involve the tooth sockets
Fracture of mandible or maxilla	May or may not involve the alveolar socket
Injuries to gingiva or oral mucosa	
Laceration of gingiva or oral mucosa	Wound in the mucosa resulting from a tear
Contusion of gingiva or oral mucosa	Bruise not accompanied by a break in the mucosa, usually causing submucosal haemorrhage
Abrasion of gingiva or oral mucosa	Superficial wound produced by rubbing or scraping the mucosal surface

6. *Previous dental history?* Previous trauma can affect pulpal sensibility tests and the recuperative capacity of the pulp and/or periodontium. In addition, is the child injury prone or are there suspicions of NAI? Previous treatment experience, age, and parental/child attitude will affect the choice of treatment.

11.4.2 Medical history

1. *Congenital heart disease, a history of rheumatic fever or severe immunosuppression?* These are contra-indications to any procedure that is likely to require prolonged endodontic treatment with a persistent necrotic focus. Any endodontic treatment should be under antibiotic cover. All congenital heart defects do not carry the same risks of bacterial endocarditis and the child's paediatrician/cardiologist should be consulted before a decision regarding endodontic treatment is made.

2. *Bleeding disorders?* Very important if soft tissues are lacerated or teeth are to be extracted.

3. *Allergies?* Penicillin allergy requires alternative antibiotics.

4. *Tetanus immunization status?* Referral for tetanus toxoid injection is necessary if there is soil contamination of the wound and the child has not had a 'booster' injection within the last 5 years.

11.4.3   Extra oral examination

When there are associated severe injuries a general examination is made with respect to signs of shock (pallor, cold skin, irregular pulse, hypotension), symptoms of head injury suggesting brain concussion, or maxillofacial fractures.

Facial swelling, bruises, or lacerations may indicate underlying bony and tooth injury. Lacerations will require careful debridement to remove all foreign material and suturing. Antibiotics and/or tetanus toxoid may be required if wounds are contaminated. Limitation of mandibular movement or mandibular deviation on opening or closing the mouth indicate either jaw fracture or dislocation.

Crown fracture with associated swollen lip and evidence of a penetrating wound suggests retention of tooth fragments within the lip. Clinical and radiographic examination should be undertaken (Fig. 11.5a–d).

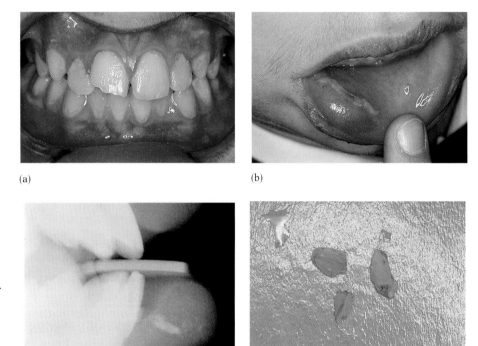

(a)

(b)

(c)

(d)

Fig. 11.5 (a) A 12 year old child presented with a enamel and dentine fracture of the upper right permanent central incisor. (b) The lower lip was swollen with a mucosal laceration. (c) Lateral radiograph confirmed presence of tooth fragments in lip. (d) Fragments retrieved under local anaesthesia from lip.

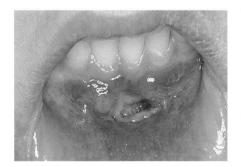

Fig. 11.6 Degloving injury to lower labial sulcus that required exploration to remove grit.

11.4.4   Intra-oral examination

This must be systematic and include the recording of:

1. Laceration, haemorrhage, and swelling of the oral mucosa and gingiva (Fig. 11.6). Any lacerations should be examined for tooth fragments or other foreign material. Lacerations of lips or tongue require suturing but those of the oral mucosa heal very quickly and may not need suturing. Orofacial signs of NAI may be present and will be discussed later.

2. Abnormalities of occlusion, tooth displacement, fractured crowns or cracks in the enamel.

The following signs and reactions to tests are particularly helpful:

1. *Mobility.* Degree of mobility is estimated in a horizontal and a vertical direction. When several teeth move together 'enblock' a fracture of the alveolar process is suspected. Excessive mobility may also suggest root fracture or tooth displacement.

2. *Reaction to percussion.* In a horizontal and vertical direction and compared against a contralateral uninjured tooth. A duller note may indicate root fracture.

3. *Colour of tooth.* Early colour change is visible on the palatal surface of the gingival third of the crown.

4. *Reaction to sensitivity tests.* Thermal tests with warm gutta percha or ethyl chloride are widely used. However, an electric pulp tester (e.p.t.) in the hands of an experienced operator is more reliable. Nevertheless, vitality testing, especially in children is notoriously unreliable and should never be assessed in isolation from the other clinical and radiographic information. Neither negative nor positive responses should be trusted immediately after trauma. A positive response does not rule out later pulpal necrosis and a negative response while indicating pulpal damage does not necessarily indicate a necrotic pulp. The negative reaction is often due to a 'shock wave' effect damaging apical nerve supply. The pulp in such cases may have a normal blood supply. In all vitality testing always include and document the reaction of uninjured contralateral teeth for comparison. In addition, all neighbouring teeth to the obviously injured teeth should be regularly assessed as they have probably suffered concussion injuries.

11.4.5   Radiographic examination

Periapical

Reproducible 'long cone technique' periapicals are the best for accurate diagnosis and clinical audit. Two radiographs at different angles may be essential to detect a root fracture. However, if access and co-operation are difficult then one anterior occlusal radiograph rarely misses a root fracture.

Occlusal

To detect root fractures and foreign bodies within the soft tissues:

(1) upper lip — lateral view using an occlusal film held by patient/helper at side of mouth (see Fig. 11.5c);

(2) lower lip — occlusal view using an 'occlusal' film held between teeth.

Orthopantomogram

Essential in all trauma cases. May detect unsuspected underlying bony injury.

Lateral oblique
Lateral skull   specialist views for maxillofacial
Anteroposterior skull   fractures.
Occipitomental

11.4.6   Photographic examination

Good clinical photographs are useful to assess outcome of treatment and for medico-legal purposes.

●   Develop a systematic approach to history and examination.   **Key Point**

11.5   INJURIES TO THE PRIMARY DENTITION

During its early development the permanent incisor is located palatally to and in close proximity with the apex of the primary incisor. With any injury to a primary tooth there is risk of damage to the underlying permanent successor.

The most accident prone time in the primary dentition is between 2 and 4 years of age. Realistically, this means that few restorative procedures will be possible and in the majority of cases the decision is between extraction or maintenance without performing extensive treatment. A primary incisor should always be removed if its maintenance will jeopardize the developing tooth bud.

A traumatized primary tooth that is retained should be assessed regularly for clinical and radiographic signs of pulpal or periodontal complications. Radiographs may even detect damage to the permanent successor. Soft tissue injuries in children should be assessed weekly until healed. Tooth injuries should be reviewed every 3–4 months for the first year and then annually until the primary tooth exfoliates and the permanent successor is in place.

11.5.1   Uncomplicated crown fracture

Either smooth sharp edges or restore with an acid-etch restoration if co-operation is satisfactory.

11.5.2   Complicated crown fracture

Normally, extraction is the treatment of choice. However, pulp extirpation and canal obturation with zinc oxide cement, followed by an acid-etch restoration is possible with reasonable co-operation.

11.5.3   Crown–root fracture

The pulp is usually exposed and any restorative treatment is very difficult. The tooth is best extracted.

11.5.4   Root fracture

Without displacement and with only a small amount of mobility the tooth should be kept under observation. If the coronal fragment becomes non-vital and symptomatic then it should be removed. The apical portion usually remains vital and undergoes normal resorption. Similarly with marked displacement and mobility only the coronal portion should be removed.

11.5.5   Concussion, subluxation, and luxation injuries

Associated soft tissue damage should be cleaned by the parent twice daily with 0.2 per cent chlorhexidine solution using cotton buds or gauze swabs until it heals.

Concussion

Often not brought to a dentist until the tooth discolours.

Subluxation

If slight mobility then the parents are advised on a soft diet for 1–2 weeks and to keep the traumatized area as clean as possible. Marked mobility requires extraction.

Extrusive luxation

Marked mobility requires extraction.

Lateral luxation

If the crown is displaced palatally the apex moves buccally and hence away from the permanent tooth germ. If the occlusion is not gagged then conservative treatment to await some spontaneous realignment is possible. If the crown is displaced buccally then the apex will be displaced towards the permanent tooth bud and extraction is indicated in order to minimize further damage to the permanent successor.

Intrusive luxation

This is the most common type of injury. The aim of investigation is to establish the direction of displacement by thorough radiological examination. If the root is displaced palatally towards the permanent successor then the primary tooth should be extracted to minimize the possible damage to the developing permanent successor. If the root is displaced buccally then periodic review to monitor spontaneous re-eruption should be allowed (Fig. 11.7a and b). Review should be weekly for a month then monthly for a maximum of 6 months. Most re-eruption occurs between 1 and 6 months and if this doesn't occur then ankylosis is likely and extraction is necessary to prevent ectopic eruption of the permanent successor (Fig.11.8).

Exarticulation (Avulsion)

Replantation of avulsed primary incisors is not recommended due to the risk of damage to the permanent tooth germs. Space maintenance is not necessary following the loss of a primary incisor as only minor drifting of adjacent teeth occurs. The eruption of the permanent successor may be delayed for about 1 year as a result of abnormal thickening of connective tissue overlying the tooth germ.

11.6   SEQUELAE OF INJURIES TO THE PRIMARY DENTITION

11.6.1 Pulpal necrosis

Necrosis is the commonest complication of primary trauma. Evaluation is based upon colour and radiography. Teeth of a normal colour rarely develop periapical inflammation but conversely mildly discoloured teeth may be vital. A mild grey colour occurring soon after trauma may represent intrapulpal bleeding with a pulp that is still vital. This colour may recede, but if it persists then necrosis should be suspected. Radiographic examination should be 3 monthly to check for periapical inflammation (Fig. 11.9a and b). Failure of the pulp cavity to reduce in size is an indicator of pulpal death. Teeth should be extracted whenever there is evidence of periapical inflammation, to prevent possible damage to the permanent successor.

11.6.2 Pulpal obliteration

Obliteration of the pulp chamber and canal is a common reaction to trauma (Fig. 11.10). Clinically, the tooth becomes yellow/opaque. Normal exfoliation is usual but occasionally periapical inflammation may intervene and therefore annual radiography is advisable.

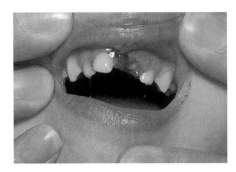

(a)

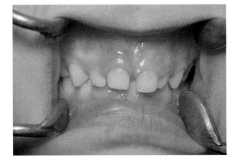

(b)

Fig. 11.7   (a) A 4 year old boy with complete intrusion of the upper right incisor.
(b) 6 months post-trauma, the tooth has spontaneously re-erupted.

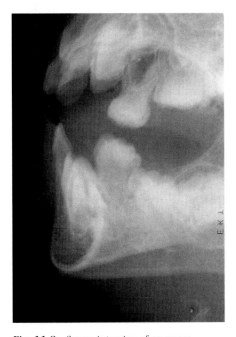

Fig. 11.8   Severe intrusion of an upper primary central incisor necessitating extraction.

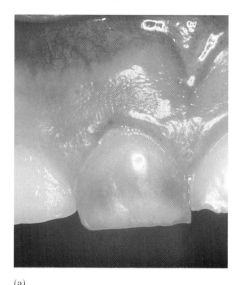

(a)

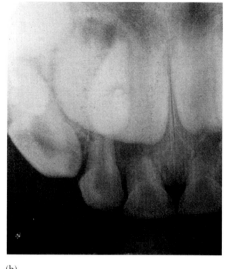

(b)

Fig. 11.9 (a) Severe discoloration of the upper right primary central incisor. (b) Radiographic evidence of periapical pathology. Extraction necessary.

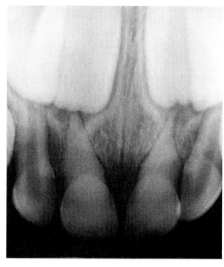

Fig. 11.10 Pulp canal obliteration and external surface resorption of upper primary central incisors after a luxation injury.

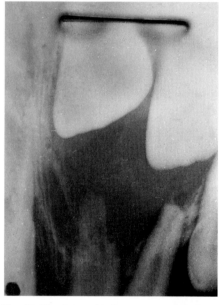

Fig. 11.11 External inflammatory resorption of previously injured primary incisors.

11.6.3 Root resorption

External inflammatory resorption is usually seen after intrusive injuries and internal resorption with subluxation and other luxation injuries. Extraction is advised for all types of root resorption (Fig. 11.11).

11.6.4 Injuries to developing permanent teeth

Injuries to the permanent successor tooth can be expected in between 12 and 69 per cent of primary tooth trauma and 19 and 68 per cent of jaw fractures. Intrusive luxation causes most disturbances and exarticulation (avulsion) of a primary incisor will also cause damage if the apex moved towards the permanent tooth bud before the avulsion. Most damage to the permanent tooth bud occurs under 3 years of age during its developmental stage. However, the type and severity of disturbance are closely related to the age at the time of injury. Changes in the morphology and mineralization of the crown of the permanent incisor are commonest but later injuries can cause radicular anomalies. Injuries to developing teeth can be classified as follows:

1. White or yellow-brown discoloration of enamel. Injury at 2–7 years (Fig. 11.12a–c).
2. White or yellow-brown discoloration of enamel with circular enamel hypoplasia. Injury at 2–7 years (Fig. 11.13).
3. Crown dilaceration. Injury at about 2 years (Fig. 11.14a–c).
4. Odontoma-like malformation. Injury at < 1–3 years.
5. Root duplication. Injury at 2–5 years.
6. Vestibular or lateral root angulation and dilaceration. Injury at 2–5 years (Fig. 11.15a and b).
7. Partial or complete arrest of root formation. Injury at 5–7 years (Fig. 11.16a and b).
8. Sequestration of permanent tooth germs.
9. Disturbance in eruption.

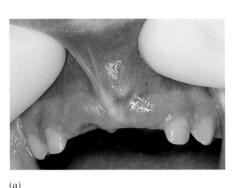

(a)

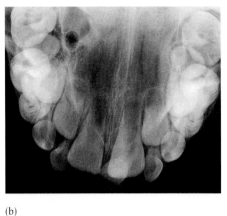

(b)

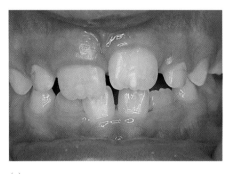

(c)

Fig. 11.12 (a)–(c) Investigation of delayed eruption of the permanent upper central incisors revealed an intruded upper left primary central incisor on radiograph. Following removal of the retained primary incisor the permanent successor erupted spontaneously with a white hypoplastic spot on the labial surface.

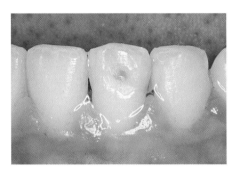

Fig. 11.13 Brown hypoplastic area on the lower left permanent central incisor resulting from trauma to the primary predecessor.

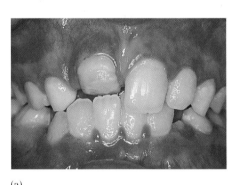

(a)

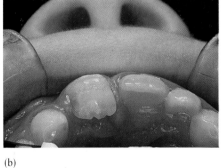

(b)

Fig. 11.14 (a)–(c) Severe crown dilaceration of the upper right permanent central incisor which erupted spontaneously.

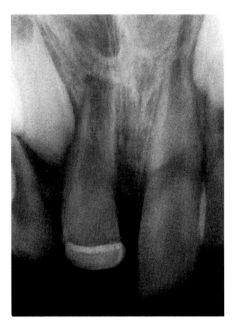

(c)

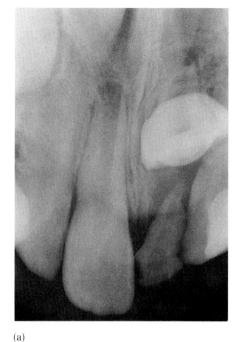

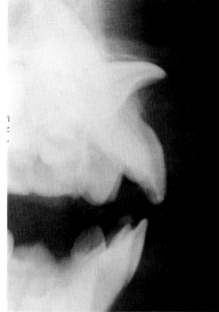

Fig. 11.15 (a) and (b) Unerupted dilacerated upper left permanent central incisor resulting from an accident at the age of 3 years.

(a)

(b)

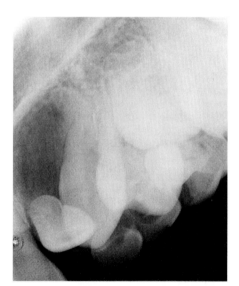

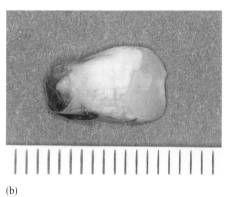

(b)

Fig. 11.16 (a) and (b) Failure of root formation of the upper left permanent lateral incisor with a history of intrusive trauma to the primary predecessor aged 5 years.

(a)

The term dilaceration describes an abrupt deviation of the long axis of the crown or root portion of the tooth. This deviation results from a traumatic non-axial displacement of already formed hard tissue in relation to developing soft tissue.

The term angulation describes a curvature of the root resulting from a gradual change in the direction of root development, without evidence of abrupt displacement of the tooth germ during odontogenesis. This may be vestibular, i.e. labiopalatal, or lateral, i.e. mesiodistal.

Evaluation of the full extent of complications following injuries must await complete eruption of all permanent teeth involved. However, most serious sequelae (disturbances in tooth morphology) can usually be diagnosed radiographically within the first year post-trauma.

Injuries that occur very early can also interfere with the development of the primary dentition e.g. intubation in premature infants.

Eruption disturbances may involve delay due to connective tissue thickening over a permanent tooth germ, ectopic eruption due to lack of eruptive guidance, and impaction in teeth with malformations of crown or root.

<table>
<tr><td>●   Risk of damage to permanent successors is high — advise parents.</td><td>**Key Point**</td></tr>
</table>

11.6.5   Treatment of injuries to the permanent dentition

Yellow-brown discoloration of enamel with or without hypoplasia

1. Acid-pumice microabrasion.
2. Composite resin restoration: localized, veneer, or crown.
3. Porcelain restoration: veneer or crown (anterior); fused to metal crown (posterior).

Crown dilaceration

1. Surgical exposure ± orthodontic realignment.
2. Removal of dilacerated part of crown.
3. Temporary crown until root formation complete.
4. Semi or permanent restoration.

Vestibular root angulation

Combined surgical and orthodontic realignment.

Other malformation

Extraction is usually the treatment of choice.

Disturbance in eruption

Surgical exposure ± orthodontic realignment.

Injuries to supporting bone

Most fractures of the alveolar socket in primary dentition do not require splinting due to rapid bony healing in small children. Jaw fractures are treated in the conventional manner, although stabilization after reduction may be difficult due to lack of sufficient teeth.

11.7   INJURIES TO THE PERMANENT DENTITION

Most traumatized teeth can be treated successfully. Prompt and appropriate treatment improves prognosis. The aims and principles of treatment can be broadly categorized into:

1. Emergency:
   (a) retain vitality of fractured or displaced tooth;
   (b) treat exposed pulp tissue;

(c) reduction and immobilization of displaced teeth;

(d) antiseptic mouthwash, antibiotics, and tetanus prophylaxis.

2. Intermediate:

(a) ± pulp therapy;

(b) minimally invasive crown restoration.

3. Permanent:

(a) apexification;

(b) root filling ± root extrusion;

(c) ± gingival and alveolar collar modification;

(d) semi or permanent coronal restoration.

Trauma cases require painstaking follow up to disclose any complications and institute the correct treatment. The intervals between examinations depends on the severity of trauma, but the following schedule is a guide: 1 week, 3 weeks, 6 weeks, 3, 6, and 12 months, and then annually for 4–5 years. At these times colour, mobility, percussion, and sensitivity are routinely noted while radiographs are examined for periradicular conditions and changes within the pulp cavity.

11.7.1 Injuries to the hard dental tissues and the pulp

Enamel infraction

These incomplete fractures without loss of tooth substance and without proper illumination are easily overlooked. Periodic recalls are necessary as the energy of the blow may have been transmitted to the periodontal tissues or the pulp.

Enamel fracture

No restoration is needed and treatment is limited to smoothing of any rough edges and splinting if there is associated mobility. Periodic review as above.

Enamel–dentine fracture

Immediate treatment is necessary due to the involvement of dentine. The pulp requires protection against thermal irritation and from bacteria via the dentinal tubules. Restoration of crown morphology also stabilizes the position of the tooth in the arch.

Emergency protection of the exposed dentine can be achieved by:

1. Fast setting calcium hydroxide over dentine then an acid-etched dressing of filled or unfilled composite resin to protect the calcium hydroxide.

2. Calcium hydroxide and glass ionomer cement within an orthodontic band or incisal end of a stainless steel crown if there is insufficient enamel available for acid-etch technique. These will serve as temporary retainers until further eruption occurs.

Intermediate restoration of most enamel–dentine fractures can be achieved by:

1. Acid-etched composite either applied freehand or utilizing a celluloid crown former. With the recent improvements in composite technology the majority of these restorations can be regarded as semi-permanent/permanent. Larger fractures can utilize more available enamel surface area for bonding by employing a complete celluloid crown former to construct a 'direct' composite crown. At a later age this could be reduced to form the core of a porcelain jacket crown preparation. The acid-etch technique is described in Chapter 7.

2. Reattachment of crown fragment. This method of restoration has become feasible since the development of dentine bonding agents. However, few long-term studies have been reported and therefore the longevity of this type of restoration is largely unknown. In addition, there is a tendency for the distal fragment to become opaque or require further restorative intervention in the form of a veneer or jacket crown (Fig. 11.17).

If the fracture line through dentine is not very close to the pulp then the fragment may be reattached immediately. If, however, it runs close to the pulp then it is advisable to place a suitably protected calcium hydroxide dressing over the exposed dentine for at least 1 month while storing the fragment in saline, which should be renewed weekly.

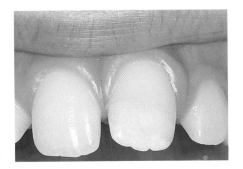

Fig. 11.17 An upper left permanent central incisor 3 years after reattachment of a fractured incisal fragment.

Technique

1. Check the fit of the fragment and the vitality of the tooth.
2. Clean fragment and tooth with pumice–water slurry.
3. Isolate the tooth with rubber dam.
4. Attach fragment to a piece of gutta percha to facilitate handling.
5. Etch enamel for 30 s on both fracture surfaces and extend for 2 mm from fracture line on tooth and fragment. Wash for 15 s and dry for 15 s.
6. Apply dentine primer to both surfaces and then dry for 15–30 s.
7. Apply enamel–dentine bonding agent to both surfaces then lightly blow away any excess. Light cure for 10 s.
8. Place appropriate shade of composite resin over both surfaces and position fragment. Remove gross excess and cure 60 s labially and palatally.
9. Remove any excess composite resin with sandpaper discs.
10. Remove a 1 mm gutter of enamel on each side of fracture line both labially and palatally to a depth of 0.5 mm using a small round or pear-shaped bur. The finishing line should be irregular in outline.
11. Etch the newly prepared enamel, wash, dry, apply composite, cure, and finish.

Complicated crown fracture

The major concern after pulpal exposures in immature teeth is the preservation of pulpal vitality in order to allow continued root growth. The injured pulp must be sealed from bacteria so that it is not infected during the period of repair. Partial pulpotomy or pulpotomy is often the treatment of choice (Chapter 8).

Uncomplicated crown–root fracture

After removal of the fractured piece of tooth these vertical fractures are commonly a few millimetres incisal to the gingival margin on the labial surface but down to the cemento-enamel junction palatally. Prior to placement of a restoration the fracture margin has to be brought supragingival either by gingivoplasty or extrusion (orthodontically or surgically) of the root portion.

Complicated crown–root fracture

As above with the addition of endodontic requirements. If extrusion is planned then the final root length must be no shorter than the final crown length otherwise the result will be unstable. Root extrusion can be successful in a motivated patient and leads to a stable periodontal condition.

Root fracture

Root fractures occur most frequently in the middle or the apical third of the root. The coronal fragment may be extruded or luxated. Luxation is usually in a lingual or palatal direction.

If displacement has occurred the coronal fragment should be repositioned as soon as possible by gentle digital manipulation and the position checked radiographically. Mobile root fractures need to be rigidly splinted to encourage repair of the fracture. Apical third fractures, in the absence of concomitant periodontal ligament (p.d.l.) injury, are often firm and do not require splinting but need to be regularly reviewed to check pulpal status and treated endodontically if necessary.

Middle third and coronal third fractures must be splinted as repair of the fracture is essential to the long-term stability and prognosis of the tooth. A rigid splint is one that includes two abutment teeth on either side of the fractured tooth and should remain in place for 2–3 months. The splint should allow colour observations and sensitivity testing and access to the root canal if endodontic treatment is required. The splint design and placement techniques are discussed in the next section on 'splinting'.

In about 80 per cent of all root fractured teeth the pulp remains viable and repair occurs in the fracture area. Three main categories of repair are recognized:

1. repair with calcified tissue: invisible or hardly discernible fracture line (Fig. 11.18a–c);
2. repair with connective tissue: narrow radiolucent fracture line with peripheral rounding of the fracture edges (Fig. 11.19);
3. repair with bone and connective tissue: a bony bridge separates the two fragments (Fig. 11.20).

In addition to these changes in the fracture area, pulp canal obliteration is commonly seen. Fractures in the cervical third of the root will repair as well as those in the middle or apical thirds as long as no communication exists between the fracture line and the gingival crevice. If such a communication exists then

Fig. 11.18 (a) An apical third root fracture of the upper right permanent central incisor with rigid splint. (b) Appearance of the fracture 15 months later. (c) Good calcified tissue repair evident 3 years post-trauma.

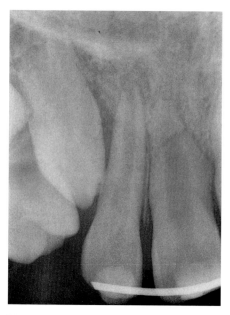

(a)

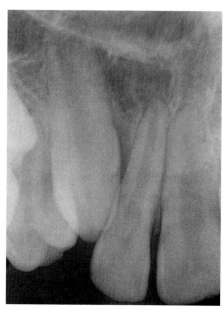

(b)

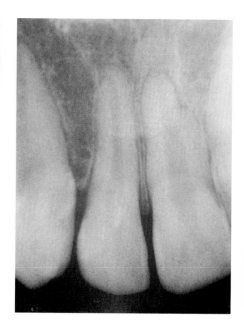

(c)

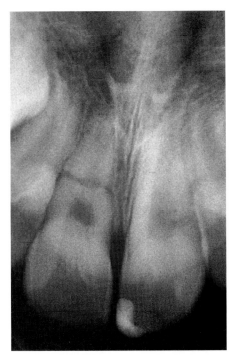

Fig. 11.19 Middle third root fracture of the upper right permanent central incisor with connective tissue repair.

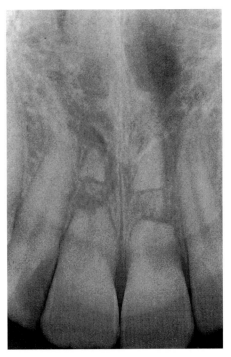

Fig. 11.20 Middle third root fracture of both upper permanent central incisors with bony repair and sclerosis of the apical fragments.

splinting is not recommended and a decision must be made either: (a) to extract the coronal fragment and retain the remaining root, or (b) extract the two fragments, or (c) internally splint the root fracture (Chapter 8).

If the root is retained then the remaining radicular pulp should be removed and the canal temporarily dressed prior to obturating with gutta percha. Three options are now available for the root treated radicular portion:

1. Post, core, and crown restoration if access is adequate.

2. Extrusion of root either surgically or orthodontically if the fracture extends too subgingivally for adequate access. Rapid orthodontic extrusion over 4–6 weeks aiming to move the root a maximum of 4 mm is the best option. This is achieved by cementing a 'J' hook made from 0.7 mm stainless steel wire into the canal and using elastic traction applied over an arch wire cemented between one abutment tooth on either side of the injured tooth. Retention for one month at the end of movement is advised to prevent relapse (Fig. 11.21). If aesthetics are a particular concern then an orthodontic bracket can be bonded to a temporary crown made over the 'J' hook. The temporary crown length will need to be reduced as extrusion occurs (Figs. 11.22a–d).

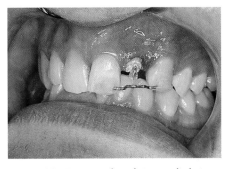

Fig. 11.21 Extrusive force being applied via a 'J' hook cemented into the root canal of the upper left permanent lateral incisor.

3. Cover the root with a mucoperiosteal flap. This will maintain the height and width of the arch and will facilitate later placement of a single tooth implant.

Pulpal necrosis occurs in about 20 per cent of root fractures and is the main obstacle to adequate repair. The amount of displacement of the coronal portion is significant in pulpal prognosis but the level of fracture and the presence of an open or a closed apex are not.

Most cases of necrosis are diagnosed within 3 months of a root fracture. A persistent negative response to electric stimulation is usually confirmed on radiography by radiolucencies adjacent to the fracture line.

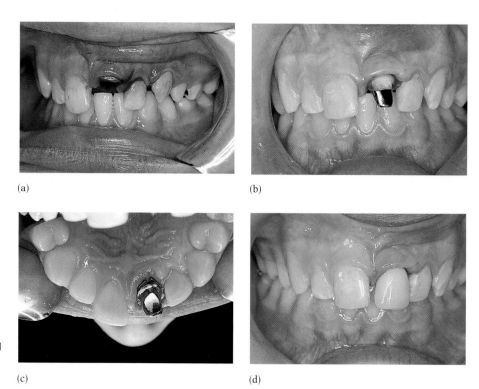

Fig. 11.22 (a) Initial presentation of high coronal root fracture which extended palatally below alveolar bone. (b) and (c) Post, core, and diaphragm after root extrusion. (d) Final coronal restoration.

The apical fragment almost always contains viable pulp tissue. In apical and middle third fractures any endodontic treatment is usually confined to the coronal fragment. (Chapter 8) After completion of endodontic treatment, repair and union between the two fragments with connective tissue is a consistent finding. In coronal third fractures that develop necrosis either the radicular portion can be retained (see above), both portions extracted, or the fracture internally splinted.

11.7.2 Splinting

Trauma may loosen a tooth either by damaging the p.d.l. or fracturing the root. Splinting immobilizes the tooth in the correct anatomical position so that further trauma is prevented and healing can occur. Different injuries require different splinting regimens.

Regimens

p.d.l. injuries

Sixty per cent of p.d.l. healing has occurred after 10 days and it is complete within a month. The splinting period should be as short as possible and the splint should allow some functional movement to prevent replacement root resorption (ankylosis). As a general rule exarticulation (avulsion) injuries require 7–10 days, luxation injuries 2–3 weeks, and dentoalveolar fractures 3–4 weeks splinting.

Root fractures

These require 2–3 months of rigid splinting to encourage a repair with calcified tissue. A connective tissue repair may be satisfactory, but with a lot of mobility the fracture site becomes filled with granulation tissue and the tooth remains mobile.

Types and methods of constructing splints

Composite resin/acrylic and wire splint

This method uses either a composite resin or a temporary crown material. The composite resin is easier to place but the acrylic resin is easier to remove. Although acrylic resin does not have the bond strength to enamel of the composite resin it is suitable for all types of splinting apart from root fractures (Fig. 11.23).

Technique for functional splint:

1. Bend a flexible orthodontic wire to fit the middle third of the labial surface of the injured tooth and one abutment tooth either side.

2. Stabilize the injured tooth in the correct position with soft red wax palatally.

3. Clean the labial surfaces. Isolate, dry, and etch middle of crown of teeth with 37 per cent phosphoric acid for 30 s, wash, and dry.

4. Apply 3 mm diameter circle either of unfilled then filled composite resin or of acrylic resin, to the centre of the crowns.

5. Position the wire into the filling material then apply more composite or acrylic resin.

6. Use a brush lubricated with unfilled composite resin to mould and smooth the composite. Acrylic resin is more difficult to handle and smoothing and excess removal can be done with a flat plastic instrument.

7. Cure the composite for 60 s. Wait for the acrylic resin to cure.

8. Smooth any sharp edges with sandpaper discs.

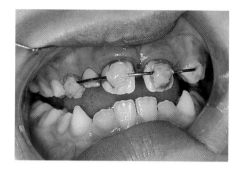

Fig. 11.23 Composite resin and wire splint for a luxation injury of both upper permanent central incisors.

Figure 11.23 shows an example of a functional splint. For a rigid splint use the same technique but incorporate *two* abutment teeth on either side of the injured tooth. These splints should not impinge on the gingiva and should allow assessment of colour change and sensitivity testing.

Orthodontic brackets and wire

For displacement injuries and exarticulations these splints have the advantage of allowing a more accurate reduction of the injury by gentle forces (Fig. 11.24a and b).

Interdental wiring

Interdental 'figure of eight' wiring on an arch wire ligated to the teeth with ligature wire are occasionally used but should only be a temporary measure. They compromise gingival health.

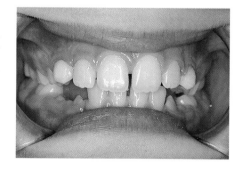

(a)

Foil/cement splint

A temporary splint made of soft metal (cooking foil or milk bottle top) and cemented with quick setting zinc oxide–eugenol cement is an effective temporary measure either during the night when it is difficult to fit a composite-wire splint as a single-handed operator or while awaiting construction of a laboratory made splint.

Technique:

1. Cut metal to size, long enough to extend over two or three teeth on each side of the injured tooth and wide enough to extend over the incisal edges and 3–4 mm over the labial and palatal gingiva.

2. Place metal over teeth and mould it over labial and palatal surfaces. Remove any excess.

3. Cement the metal to the teeth with quick setting zinc oxide–eugenol cement.

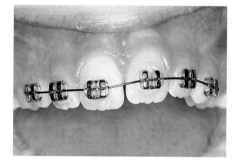

(b)

Fig. 11.24 (a) and (b) Gentle reduction and splinting of luxated upper right permanent central incisor.

Laboratory splints

(1) acrylic

(2) thermoplastic.

These are used where it is impossible to make a satisfactory splint by the direct method, e.g. a 7–8 year old with traumatized maxillary incisors, unerupted lateral incisors, and either carious or absent primary canines. Both methods require alginate impressions and very loose teeth may need to be supported by wax, metal foil, or wire ligature so they are not removed with the impression.

1. *Acrylic.* There is full palatal coverage and the acrylic is extended over the incisal edges for 2–3 mm of the labial surfaces of the anterior teeth. The occlusal surfaces of the posterior teeth should be covered to prevent any occlusal contact in the anterior region. This also aids retention and Adams Cribs may not be required. The splint should be removed for cleaning after meals and at bedtime.

2. *Thermoplastic.* The splint is constructed from polyvinylacetate–polyethylene (PVAC-PE) copolymer in the same way as a mouthguard with extension onto the mucosa. It should be removed like the acrylic splint after meals and at bedtime. However, with more severely loosened teeth it could be retained at night.

Both forms of laboratory splint allow functional movement and therefore promote normal periodontal healing. They are not suitable for root fractures as they compromise oral hygiene.

11.7.3   Injuries to the periodontal tissues

Concussion

The impact force causes oedema and haemorrhage in the p.d.l. and the tooth is tender to percussion (t.t.p.). There is no rupture of p.d.l. fibres and the tooth is firm in the socket.

Subluxation

In addition to the above there is rupture of some p.d.l. fibres and the tooth is mobile in the socket, although not displaced (Fig. 11.25). The treatment for both these injuries is:

(1) occlusal relief;

(2) soft diet for 7 days;

(3) immobilization with a splint if t.t.p. is significant;

(4) chlorhexidine 0.2 per cent mouthwash, twice daily.

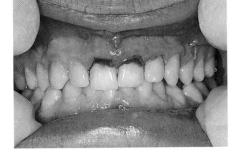

Fig. 11.25 Subluxated upper permanent central incisors.

Table 11.2   Five year pulpal survival after injuries involving the periodontal ligament

Type of injury	Open apex (%)	Closed apex (%)
Concussion	100	96
Subluxation	100	85
Extrusive luxation	95	45
Lateral luxation	95	25
Intrusive luxation	40	0
Replantation	30	0

Figures for pulpal survival 5 years after injury (Table 11.2) show that there is minimal risk of pulpal necrosis. In addition, in over 97 per cent of cases there is no evidence of any resorption.

Extrusive luxation

There is a rupture of p.d.l. and pulp.

Lateral luxation

There is a rupture of p.d.l, pulp, and the alveolar plate (Fig. 11.26a). The treatment for both these injuries is:

(1) atraumatic repositioning with gentle but firm digital pressure (Fig. 11.26b);
(2) local anaesthetic is required if there is an alveolar plate injury;
(3) non-rigid functional splint for 2–3 weeks (Fig. 11.26c);
(4) antibiotics, e.g. amoxycillin 250 mg three times daily (<6 years old 125 mg three times daily) for 5 days;
(5) chlorhexidine 0.2 per cent mouthwash twice daily while splint is in position;
(6) soft diet 2–3 weeks.

Antibiotics may have a beneficial effect in promoting repair of the p.d.l. They do not appear to affect pulpal prognosis.

After 2–3 weeks the teeth are radiographed. If there is no evidence of marginal breakdown the splint can be removed. If marginal breakdown is present then it should be retained for a further 2–3 weeks.

For both these injuries the decision whether to progress to endodontic treatment depends on the combination of clinical and radiographic signs (see later). Five year pulpal survival figures (Table 11.2) show that prognosis is significantly better for open apex teeth but nevertheless a proportion of mature closed apex teeth will retain vitality. In addition, over 4 per cent of mature teeth involved in luxation injuries will exhibit on radiographs a natural healing phenomenon known as 'transient apical breakdown' (t.a.b.) which can mimic apical infection. Ambivalent clinical and radiographic signs should be given the 'benefit of the doubt' until the next review.

With more significant damage to the p.d.l. in both extrusive and lateral luxation injuries there is an increased risk of root resorption. Thirty-five per cent of mature teeth that have undergone lateral luxation show subsequent evidence of surface resorption.

Fig. 11.26 (a) Palatally luxated upper left permanent incisor with other associated injuries. (b) Upper left permanent central incisor repositioned atraumatically. (c) Non-rigid orthodontic splint in place.

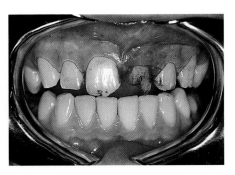

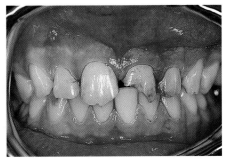

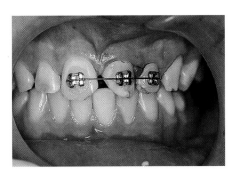

(a)   (b)   (c)

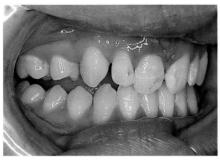

(a)

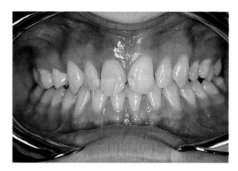

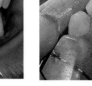

(b)   (c)

Fig. 11.27 (a) Delayed presentation of palatally luxated upper permanent central incisors in traumatic occlusion. (b) and (c) An upper removable appliance used to procline the upper incisors over 2 months.

In some cases of lateral luxation the displacement cannot be reduced with gentle finger pressure. It is not advisable to use more force as this can further damage the periodontal ligament. Orthodontic appliances, either a removable or a sectional fixed appliance can be used to reduce the displacement over a period of a few weeks (Fig. 11.27a–c).

Intrusive luxation

These injuries are the result of an axial, apical impact and there is extensive damage to PDL, pulp and alveolar plate(s).

Two distinct treatment categories exist: the open and closed apex.

Open apex:

Either

(1a) disimpact (with forceps if necessary) and allow to erupt spontaneously for 2–4 months. If there is no spontaneous movement start orthodontic extrusion;

or

(1b) disimpact and surgically reposition. Functional splint for 7–10 days;

(2) monitor pulpal status clinically and radiographically at 1, 3 and 3 weeks and start endodontics if necessary;

(3) non-setting calcium hydroxide in root canal does not preclude against orthodontic movement. Once apexification has occurred and orthodontic movement has ceased, obturate canal with gutta percha (Fig. 11.28a–c).

Closed apex:

(1) elective orthodontic/surgical extrusion immediately;

(2) functional spint 7–10 days after surgical extrrusion;

(3) elective pulp extripation at 10 days;

(3) maintain non-setting calcium hydroxide in root canal during orthodontic movement before obturation with gutta percha (Fig. 11.29 a–d).

If endodontic treatment is commenced within 2 weeks after an injury to the p.d.l. then the initial intra canal dressing should be with a polyantibiotic or antibiotic/steroid (Ledermix, Lederle) paste. (section 8.6.4 p. 168)

At the outset both categories should receive antibiotics, chlorhexidine mouthwash, and a soft diet as previously described.

The risk of pulpal necrosis in these injuries is high, especially in the closed apex (Table 11.2). The incidence of resorption and ankylosis sequelae is also high (Table 11.3).

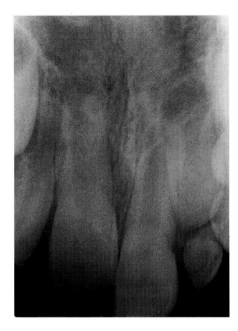

(a)

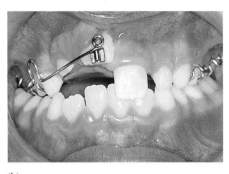

(b)

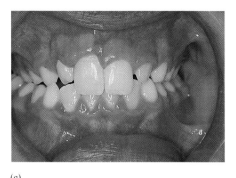

(c)

Fig. 11.28 (a) A 7 year old with intrusion of the upper right permanent central incisor which failed to re-erupt spontaneously. (b) and (c) Orthodontic extrusion of the upper right central incisor.

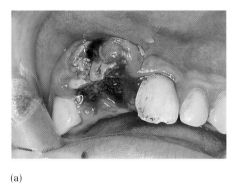

(a)

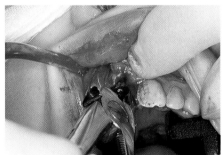

(b)

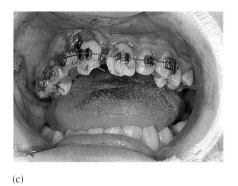

(c)

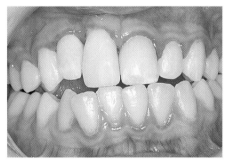

(d)

Fig. 11.29 (a) A severe intrusive injury in a 15 year old girl. (b) Surgical extrusion of the upper right permanent incisors. (c) Orthodontic splinting. (d) Completed composite restorations.

Table 11.3 Periodontal ligament healing after intrusive luxation injuries

Type of periodontal ligament	Open apex (%)	Closed apex (%)
Normal	33	0
Inflammatory resorption	41	35
Replacement resorption (ankylosis)	10	31
Surface resorption	16	34

Avulsion and replantation

Replantation should nearly always be attempted even though it may offer only a temporary solution due to the frequent occurrence of external inflammatory resorption (e.i.r.). Even when resorption occurs the tooth may be retained for years acting as a natural space maintainer and preserving the height and width of the alveolus to facilitate later implant placement.

Successful healing after replantation can only occur if there is minimal damage to the pulp and the p.d.l. The type of extra-alveolar storage medium and the extra-alveolar time (e.a.t.), i.e. the time the tooth has been out of the mouth are critical factors. The suggested protocol for replantation can be divided into: advice on phone; immediate treatment in surgery; and review.

Advice on phone (to teacher, parent, etc.)

1. Don't touch root — hold by crown.
2. Wash gently under cold tap water.
3. Replace into socket or transport in milk to surgery.
4. If replaced bite gently on a handkerchief to retain it and come to surgery.

The best transport medium is the tooth's own socket. Understandably non-dentists may be unhappy to replant the tooth and milk is an effective iso osmolar medium. Saliva, the patient's buccal sulcus, or normal saline are alternatives.

Immediate surgery treatment

1. Do not handle root. If replanted remove tooth from socket.
2. Rinse tooth with normal saline. Note state of root development. Store in saline.
3. Local analgesia.
4. Irrigate socket with saline and remove clot and any foreign material.
5. Push tooth gently but firmly into socket.
6. Non-rigid functional splint for 7–10 days.
7. Check occlusion.
8. Baseline radiographs: periapical or anterior occlusal. Any other teeth injured?
9. Antibiotics, chlorhexidine mouthwash, soft diet as previously.
10. Check tetanus immunization status.

If neighbouring teeth have root fractures then the splint will have to be a hybrid design with rigidity for the root fractures and functional movement for the replanted tooth.

Review

1. Radiograph — prior to splint removal at 7–10 days.
2. Remove splint 7–10 days.
3. Endodontics — commence prior to splint removal for categories (b) and (c):
   (a) open apex. e.a.t. < 45 min. Observe.
   (b) open apex. e.a.t. > 45 min. Endodontics.
       (i)   initial intracanal dressing — polyantibiotic or antibiotic/steroid (Ledermix, Lederle) paste.
       (ii) subsequent intracanal dressings — non-setting calcium hydroxide.
       (iii) replace calcium hydroxide 3 monthly until apical barrier (up to maximum of 2–3 years
       (iv) obturate canal with G.P.

(c) Closed apex. Endodontics.
   (i)   initial intracanal dressing polyantibiotic or antibiotic/steroid (Ledermix, Lederle) paste.
   (ii) subsequent intracanal dressing — non-setting calcium hydroxide;
   (iii) obturate with gutta percha at 6 months as long as no progressive resorption.
4. Radiographic review: 1, 3, and 6 monthly for 2 years then annually.
5. If resorption is progressing unhalted keep non-setting calcium hydroxide in the tooth until exfoliation, changing it 6 monthly.

The immature tooth with an e.a.t. of less than 45 min may undergo pulp revascularization (Table 11.2). However, these teeth require regular clinical and radiographic review because once e.i.r. occurs it progresses rapidly.

> ● splints — rigid for root fractures, functional for luxations and replantations.   **Key Points**

Replantation of teeth with a dry storage time of greater than 1 h

Mature teeth with a dry storage time of greater than 1 h will have a non-vital p.d.l. The p.d.l. and the pulp should be removed at chairside and the tooth placed in 2.4 per cent sodium fluoride solution acidulated to pH 5.5 for 20 min. The root canal is then obturated with gutta percha and the tooth replanted and splinted rigidly for 6 weeks. The aim of this treatment is to produce ankylosis allowing the tooth to be maintained as a natural space maintainer, perhaps for a limited period only. The sodium fluoride is believed to slow down resorptive processes.

Pulpal and periodontal status

Pulpal necrosis is the most common complication and is related to the severity of the periodontal injury (Table 11.2). Immature teeth have a better prognosis than mature teeth due to the wide apical opening where slight movements can occur without disruption of the apical neurovascular bundle.

Necrosis can be diagnosed in most cases within 3 months of injury but in some cases may not be evident for at least 2 years. A combination of clinical and radiological signs are often required to diagnose necrosis.

Sensitivity testing

The majority of injured teeth test negatively to e.p.t. immediately following trauma. Most pulps that recover test positively within months but responses have been reported as late as 2 years after injury. A negative test alone therefore should not be regarded as proof of necrosis. Postpone endodontics until at least one other clinical and/or radiographic sign is present.

Tooth discoloration

Initial pinkish discoloration may be due to subtotal severance of apical vessels leading to penetration of haemoglobin from such ruptures into the dentine tubules. If the vascular system repairs then most of this discoloration will disappear. If the tooth becomes progressively grey then necrosis should be suspected. A grey colour that appears for the first time several weeks or months after trauma, signifies decomposition of necrotic pulp tissue and is a decisive sign of necrosis. Colour changes are usually most apparent on the palatal surface of the injured teeth.

Tenderness to percussion

This may be the most reliable isolated indicator of pulpal necrosis.

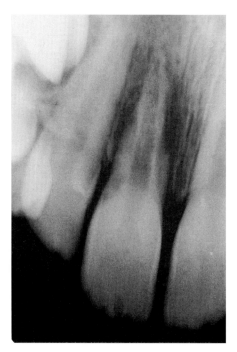

Fig. 11.30 External inflammatory resorption.

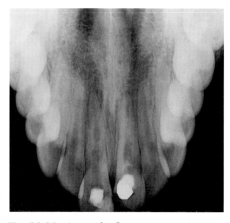

Fig. 11.31 Internal inflammatory resorption of both upper central incisors.

Periapical inflammation

Radiological periapical involvement secondary to necrosis can be seen as early as 3 weeks after trauma. In mature teeth transient apical breakdown (t.a.b.) may be mistaken for periapical inflammation.

Arrest of root development

If necrosis involves the epithelial root sheath before root development is complete, then no further root growth will occur (Fig. 11.16(a) and (b)). In an injured pulp necrosis may progress from coronal to apical portion and hence residual apical vitality may result in formation of a calcific barrier across a wide apical foramen. Failure of the pulp chamber and root canal to mature and reduce in size on successive radiographs compared with contralateral uninjured teeth is also a reliable indicator of necrosis.

Inflammatory root resorption (external)

This is a pathognomic sign of necrosis and requires immediate endodontic treatment (Fig. 11.30). Resorptive areas are usually evident within 3 weeks to 4 months after injury. E.i.r. is most frequently associated with intrusive luxation and replantation. It is initiated by p.d.l. damage resulting in resorption cavities in cementum but is propagated and potentiated by infected necrotic pulpal products stimulating an increased inflammatory response in the p.d.l. via the dentinal tubules. 'Punched out' areas of resorption on the external root surface are associated with adjacent bony radiolucencies. If e.i.r. is not present within 1 year of injury it is unlikely to occur. If untreated it will destroy the tooth completely within months and treatment consisting of extirpation, debridement, and non-setting calcium hydroxide is necessary (p. 165). The majority of cases will arrest and cemental repair occurs.

Inflammatory root resorption (internal)

This is an infrequent complication caused by chronic pulpal inflammation. It is often without clinical symptoms and is seen radiographically as a ballooning of the near parallel walls of the root canal (Fig. 11.31). It progresses rapidly and perforation of the root surface will occur. Early endodontic treatment with extirpation, mechanical and chemical debridement, and non-setting calcium hydroxide has a good chance of success (Fig. 8.32).

Pulpal canal obliteration

There is progressive hard tissue formation within the pulp cavity leading to a gradual narrowing of the pulp chamber and root canal and partial or total obliteration. There is a reduced response to vitality testing and the crown appears slightly yellow/opaque. The exact initiating factor which produces this response from the odontoblasts is unknown. It is more common in immature teeth and in luxation injuries than in concussion and subluxation injuries. Although radiographs may suggest complete calcification there is usually a minute strand of pulpal tissue remaining. Thirteen per cent of these teeth can give rise to periapical inflammation as long as 5–15 years after the initial injury. Prophylactic endodontic treatment is recommended on teeth exhibiting progressive narrowing of the pulp chamber and root canal before technical difficulties ensue.

Replacement resorption (ankylosis)

This is the most severe type of external root resorption and is significantly related to replantation of avulsed incisors with an extended extra-alveolar dry period. It is caused by extensive damage to the p.d.l. and the cementum resulting in a bony union (ankylosis) being established between the alveolar socket and the root surface. The tooth then becomes essentially part of bone and as such is constantly remodelled resulting in continuous resorption of cementum and dentine. Radiographically, the periodontal space disappears and tooth substance is gradually replaced by bone. Most resorption is evident within 2 months to 1 year of injury and can be detected clinically by a high, metallic percussion note (Fig. 11.32).

There is no effective treatment for ankylosis but as the rate of progression is relatively slow the tooth can be maintained for up to 10 years. However, such teeth can be a problem in the growing child as they may cease to 'move' or 'grow' with the rest of the jaws and cannot be moved orthodontically. Non-setting calcium hydroxide can increase replacement resorption if it is extruded through the apex of an injured tooth before p.d.l. healing has occurred. For this reason the initial intra-canal dressing should be polyantibiotic or antibiotic/steroid for the first 2 weeks after injury to the p.d.l. (section 8.6.4 p. 168).

11.7.4 Injuries to the supporting bone

The extent and position of the alveolar fracture should be verified clinically and radiographically. If there is displacement of the teeth to the extent that their apices have risen up and are now positioned over the labial or lingual/palatal alveolar plates ('apical lock') then they will require extruding first to free the apices prior to repositioning.

The segment of alveolus with teeth requires only 3–4 weeks of splintage (composite-wire type) with two abutment teeth either side of the fracture, together with antibiotics, chlorhexidine, soft diet, and tetanus prophylaxis check (Fig. 11.33a–c).

Pulpal survival is more likely if repositioning occurs within 1 h of the injury. Root resorption is rare.

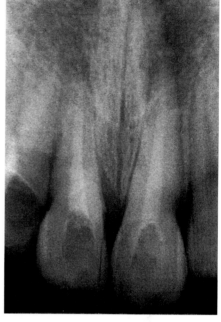

Fig. 11.32 Replacement resorption of the upper right central incisor.

● Maintain a resorbing tooth for as long as possible. It is the best space maintainer.   **Key Point**

11.8 CHILD PHYSICAL ABUSE (NON-ACCIDENTAL INJURY)

A child is considered to be abused if he or she is treated in a way that is unacceptable in a given culture at a given time (Fig. 11.4). Non-accidental injury (NAI) is now recognized as an international issue and has been reported in many countries. Each week at least four children in Britain and 80 children in the United States will die as a result of abuse or neglect. At least one child per 1000 in Britain suffers severe physical abuse; for example fractures, brain haemorrhage, severe internal injuries or mutilation and in the United States more than 95 per cent of serious intracranial injuries during the first year of life are the

Fig. 11.33 (a) Dento-alveolar fracture of the lower labial segment. (b) Fracture reduced into correct occlusion. (c) Splint *in situ* prior to removal.

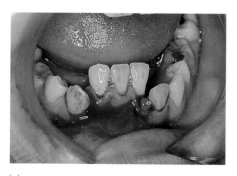

(a)

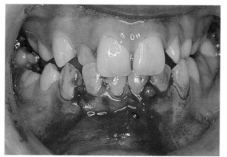

(b)

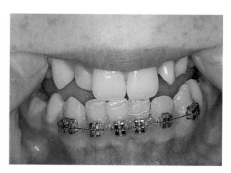

(c)

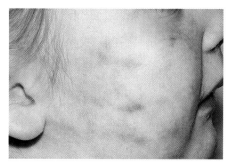

Fig. 11.34 Characteristic parallel bruising of a slap mark. (Kind permission of Munskgaard.)

Table 11.4 The incidence of common orofacial injuries in non-accidental injury

	Type of injury	Incidence (%)
Extra-oral	Contusions and ecchymoses	66
	Abrasions and lacerations	28
	Burns and bites	4
	Fractures	2
Intra-oral	Contusions and ecchymoses	43
	Abrasions and lacerations (including frenal tears)	29
	Dental trauma	29

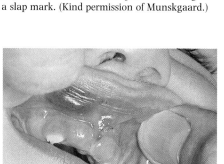

Fig. 11.35 Torn labial frenum in a young child not yet learning to walk could be an indicator of non-accidental injury. (Kind permission of Munskgaard.)

result of abuse. Although some reports will prove to be unfounded the common experience is that proved cases of child abuse are four to five times as common as they were a decade ago.

NAI is not a full diagnosis, it is merely a symptom of disordered parenting. The aim of intervention is to diagnose and cure the disordered parenting. Simply to aim at preventing death is a lowly ambition. It has been estimated in the United States that 35–50 per cent of severely abused children will receive serious re-injury and 50 per cent will die if they are returned to their home environment without intervention. In some cases the occurrence of physical abuse may provide an opportunity for intervention. If this opportunity is missed, there may be no further opportunity for many years.

Approximately 50 per cent of cases diagnosed as NAI have extra- and intra-oral facial trauma and so the dental practitioner may be the first professional to see or suspect abuse. Injuries may take the form of contusions and ecchymoses (Fig. 11.34), abrasions and lacerations, burns, bites, dental trauma (Fig. 11.35), and fractures. The incidence of common orofacial injuries are shown in Table 11.4.

The following 11 points should be considered whenever doubts and suspicions are aroused.

1. Could the injury have been caused accidentally and if so how?
2. Does the explanation for the injury fit the age and the clinical findings?
3. If the explanation of cause is consistent with the injury, is this itself within normally acceptable limits of behaviour?
4. If there has been any delay seeking advice are there good reasons for this?
5. Does the story of the accident vary?
6. The nature of the relationship between parent and child.
7. The child's reaction to other people.
8. The child's reaction to any medical/dental examinations.
9. The general demeanour of the child.
10. Any comments made by child and/or parent that give concern about the child's upbringing or life-style.
11. History of previous injury.

Dental practitioners should be aware of any established system in their locality which is designed to cope with these cases. In the United Kingdom each Local Authority Social Services Department is required to set up an 'Area Child Protection Committee'. Dental practitioners are advised how to refer and to whom, if they are concerned.

11.9 SUMMARY

1. Boys experience dental trauma almost twice as often as girls.

2. Maxillary central incisors are the most commonly involved teeth.

3. Regular clinical and radiographic review is necessary to limit unwanted sequelae, institute appropriate treatment, and improve prognosis.

4. Injuries to the developing permanent dentition occur in half of all trauma to the primary dentition.

5. Splinting for avulsion and luxation injuries should be functional to allow physiological movement and promote normal healing of the p.d.l. Splinting for root fractures should be rigid to enable a hard tissue union at the fracture line.

6. In all luxation injuries the prognosis for pulpal healing is better with an immature apex.

7. Root resorption increases with the severity of damage to the p.d.l.

8. The prognosis for replantation of avulsed teeth is best if it is undertaken within 1 h of the injury, with a hydrated p.d.l.

9. Orofacial injuries are found in 50 per cent of cases of NAI.

11.10 FURTHER READING

Andreasen, J. O. and Andreasen, F. M. (1994). *Textbook and color atlas of traumatic injuries to the teeth* (3rd edn). Munksgaard, Copenhagen. (*An excellent reference book with colour slides of each clinical procedure.*)

Andreasen, J. O., Borum, M. K., Jacobsen, H. L. and Andreasen F. M. (1995). Replantation of 400 avulsed permanent incisors. *Endodontics and Dental Traumatology* II: 51–89 (*The largest published series on avulsed permanent incisors*)

Kinirons M. J. and Sutcliffe J. (1991). Traumatically intruded permanent incisors 'a study of treatment and outcome'. *British Dental Journal* 170: 144–146 (*The largest published series on intruded permanent incisors*)

Meadow, R. (1989). *A B C of Child Abuse. British Medical Journal*, London. (*A guide to diagnosis and management of non-accident injury.*)

Welbury R. R. (1994) Child Physical Abuse (Non Accidental Injury) In *Textbook and color atlas of traumatic injuries to the teeth* (ed. J. O. and F. M. Andreasen) (3rd edn). Munksgaard, Copenhagen. (*A reference of prevalence and orofacial signs in non-accidental injury*).

12 Anomalies of tooth formation and eruption

12 Anomalies of tooth formation and eruption
G. B. WINTER

12.1 INTRODUCTION

The primary and permanent dentitions are subject to considerable variation in the number, size, and form of teeth and the structure of the dental tissues. These developmental anomalies may be genetically determined or brought about by environmentally induced systemic or local changes or possibly a combination of these factors. Similarly, abnormalities in the eruption and exfoliation of primary teeth and the eruption of permanent teeth may be subject to comparable influences which will determine the pattern of events. This chapter seeks to illustrate a number of these problems during childhood in order to give insight into the extraordinary diversity that may be encountered in clinical practice.

12.2 SUPERNUMERARY TEETH

Supernumerary teeth are common in the human community. Caucasian populations studied have indicated prevalences ranging from 0.2 to 0.8 per cent in the primary dentition to 1.5–3.5 per cent in the permanent dentition where there is a male to female ratio of approximately 2:1. Some 30–50 per cent of primary supernumeraries sited in the premaxilla are followed by permanent supernumerary units. A number of different terms have been applied to supernumerary teeth dependent on their form and location. Those resembling the normal series are called 'supplemental' while those of atypical form are named 'accessory'. Supernumeraries located in the premaxilla adjacent to the mid-line suture are known as 'mesiodens'. (Fig. 12.1). In the maxillary molar region, supernumerary teeth are known as 'paramolars' or 'distomolars' dependent on their location buccal, lingual, or distal to the arch. Primary supernumerary teeth are usually observed as single, supplemental units in the premaxilla (Fig. 12.2).

The most common region of the jaws to be affected by permanent supernumerary teeth is the premaxilla where a number of different forms have been identified. These include conical, tuberculate (multicusped), supplemental, and odontome-like types (Fig. 12.3). However, supernumeraries may be found in any region of the jaws with a maxilla to mandibular ratio of 5:1. Although permanent supernumeraries are more commonly seen unilaterally, it is not unusual to find bilateral examples and their presence in one region of the jaws warrants a full radiographic survey to rule out others elsewhere. Approximately 75 per cent of supernumerary permanent teeth never erupt and may be a chance finding on radiographs. Of the remainder, a number may lead to clinical problems such as the delayed eruption of an adjacent normal unit. Indeed the commonest cause of delayed eruption of a maxillary central incisor is the presence of a mesiodens, which is usually located palatal to the arch.

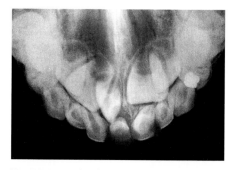

Fig. 12.1 Occlusal radiograph showing supernumerary primary incisor and unerupted 'mesiodens' to the right of the mid-line premaxillary suture.

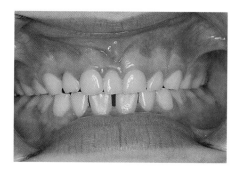

Fig. 12.2 Full eruption of a supplemental maxillary primary incisor.

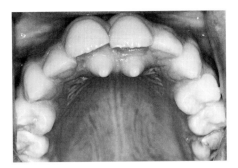

Fig. 12.3 Unusual eruption of two conical 'mesidens' palatal to maxillary permanent central incisors.

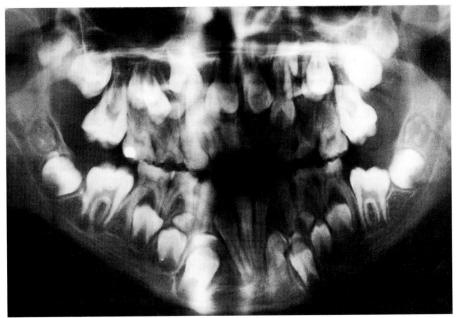

Fig. 12.4 Orthopantomogram of a 10 year old girl with cleidocranial dysplasia. There are multiple unerupted supernumerary teeth in the upper and lower labial segments and delayed eruption of permanent incisor and first molar teeth.

Key Points

Supernumerary teeth:
- 0.2–0.8 per cent in primary dentition
- 1.5–3.5 per cent in permanent dentition
- 2:1 female/male
- 5:1 maxilla/mandible

There is a significant association of supernumerary and invaginated teeth in the same dentition of some individuals. There is also a well recognized association with palatal clefts such that approximately 40 per cent present with supernumerary teeth adjacent to the alveolar deficiency.

Multiple supernumeraries are a frequent finding in cases of cleidocranial dysplasia and have been reported in association with oral–facial–digital syndrome type I and Gardner's syndrome (Fig. 12.4).

Treatment of supernumerary teeth is summarized in Chapter 13.

12.3 HYPODONTIA

Hypodontia is the generally accepted descriptive term for the absence of some teeth and anodontia for the total lack of one or both dentitions. Oligodontia is a term still used by some authors to describe the absence of many but not all the teeth.

Hypodontia in the primary dentition is more common in the maxilla and is frequently associated with the lateral incisor. (Fig. 12.5). Studies suggest this anomaly occurs in 0.1–0.9 per cent of Caucasian populations with equal frequency in males and females.

Hypodontia of permanent teeth occurs with equal frequency in the upper and lower jaws and most commonly affects the third molar. The type of permanent teeth missing and the populations prevalence for the anomaly varies with the

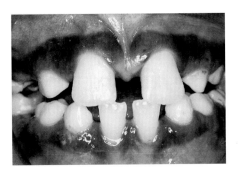

Fig. 12.5 Congenital absence of lateral incisors in both primary and permanent dentitions.

racial group and sample studied, although females are more frequently involved with a female to male ratio of 4:1. For Europeans, the mandibular second premolar is the tooth most frequently absent after the third molar, followed by the maxillary lateral incisor and second premolar. Excluding the third molar, population prevalences across the world vary between 3.5 and 6.5 per cent. The third molar is very commonly found missing in most population studies with prevalences reported of 9–37 per cent.

Key Points
Hypodontia:
● 0.1–0.9 per cent in primary dentition
● 3.5–6.5 per cent in permanent dentition
● permanent anomalies in 30–50 per cent of primary cases

The exact aetiology of isolated hypodontia in most cases is obscure but is likely to be the combined effect of a polygenic determinant with an intrauterine systemic factor. An increased frequency of hypodontia has been reported in association with multiple births, low birth weight and increased maternal age. Single gene defect has been held responsible for isolated, rare cases of hypodontia particularly of the maxillary lateral incisor.

Severe hypodontia and microdontia may be seen in a number of syndromes such as X-linked hypohidrotic ectodermal dysplasia, some autosomal dominant ectodermal dysplasias and autosomal recessive chondroectodermal dysplasia (Ellis–van Creveld syndrome) (Fig. 12.6). Hypodontia and microdontia affecting the maxillary lateral incisor is a frequent finding in clefts of the lip and palate. Down syndrome (trisomy 21) has a high correlation with hypodontia and cases have also been reported in association with rubella and thalidomide embryopathy.

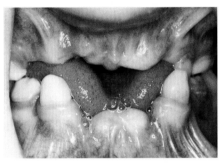

Fig. 12.6 Four year old chondro-ectodermal dysplastic boy with congenital absence of primary and permanent teeth most marked in the labial segments of the jaws. Note the virtual obliteration of the labial sulci by frenal tethering of the lip mucosa to the gingiva.

Treatment

The treatment of anodontia or severe hypodontia in children can be complex and is best undertaken in specialist centres with access to paediatric dentistry, orthodontics, and prosthodontics. In these circumstances anodontia affecting both dentitions can be corrected in childhood by the appropriate use of full dentures. Children as young as 3 years can manage full dentures successfully. Similarly severe hypodontia can be remedied by the use of partial dentures with the added advantage of retention from adjacent teeth. In later childhood a progressive increase in the 'freeway space' and true over-closure may indicate the need for overdentures when severe hypodontia affects the permanent dentition.

More mild cases of hypodontia require careful planning with particular reference to the orthodontic considerations (Chapter 13).

12.4 ABNORMALITY OF TOOTH SIZE

12.4.1 Crown size

Tooth size is diagnosed as anomalous when the norms for the sex and racial group concerned are exceeded. These abnormalities may affect the whole tooth or be limited to the crown or root portion. Such changes may be restricted to isolated teeth or affect multiple teeth unilaterally or bilaterally. Teeth which exceed the range of normal variation for a given population are described as 'megadont' or 'macrodont', whereas teeth smaller than the norm are known as 'microdont'. The size and shape of tooth crowns are not easily separated and are often interdependent.

Megadontia

Megadont maxillary incisors may be distinguished from double teeth by the absence of incisal notching and a normal morphology (albeit enlarged) in radiographs of the pulp chamber and root canal (Fig. 12.7). Bilateral symmetry frequently exists and the teeth most often affected are permanent maxillary incisors and mandibular second premolars with an overall prevalence for British school children of 1.1 per cent in the permanent dentition.

Generalized megadontia has been reported in association with pituitary gigantism and patients with unilateral facial hyperplasia may exhibit megadont teeth on the affected side. Children with hereditary gingival hyperplasia and hypertrichosis may also have isolated megadont permanent teeth.

Microdontia

Microdont primary teeth are uncommon with a reported prevalence of 0.2–0.5 per cent. For permanent teeth, the overall occurrence in British school children is 2.5 per cent, with generalized microdontia affecting 0.2 per cent. Females are more frequently affected by the anomaly than males. Microdont teeth may be either of usual form or with tapering (peg or conical) crowns (Fig. 12.8).

The association of microdontia and hypodontia is well established and in population studies the relationship has been shown to be statistically significant. The majority of affected cases are probably determined multifactorially by a combination of polygenic and environmental factors. Single gene inheritance has been described in family studies and the anomalies are frequently seen in association with Down syndrome and various types of ectodermal dysplasia.

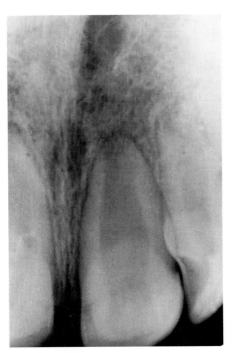

Fig. 12.7 Megadont maxillary permanent central incisor in periapical radiograph showing enlarged single pulp chamber and root canal. The antemere was of similar size and morphology.

12.4.2 Root size

Root length appears to be subject to racial variation, with shorter roots generally being observed in people of Mongoloid origin.

Large root size

Isolated teeth with increased root size is most common in canines — especially permanent maxillary canines. Increased root length affecting permanent maxillary central incisors tends to occur in individuals with generalized increase in root length. A Swedish study estimated a population prevalence for long-rooted central incisors at 2.3 per cent. Males are five times more frequently affected than females.

Small root size

Short-rooted teeth in the primary dentition have been described, usually in association with a gross dental disturbance. Similarly, generalized reduction in the root length of permanent teeth may be seen in association with dentine and pulp dysplasias, frequently with disturbance of root form. Such dysplasias include dentinogenesis imperfecta types I and II, dentine dysplasias types I and II, and pulpal dysplasia. Teeth in odontodysplasia may show little evidence of root formation in the affected region of the jaws. Irradiation of the jaws during the later stages of odontogenesis may also lead to a shortened root form.

Short root anomaly is the descriptive term which, by definition, is confined to the abnormality observed in permanent maxillary central incisors. The anomaly

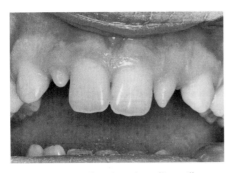

Fig. 12.8 Microdont 'peg shaped' maxillary permanent lateral incisors.

is common affecting approximately 2.5 per cent of children and of these some 15 per cent have other shortened teeth, usually premolars and/or canines.

Treatment

Isolated megadont permanent maxillary central incisors may present a considerable cosmetic disability and a decision will have to be made soon after eruption on their retention or extraction. This decision will be based on a full orthodontic assessment including the amount of available space in the upper labial segment for the eruption of the maxillary lateral incisors. Should extraction be considered the best option, further consideration will have to be given to either orthodontic space closure with coronal conversion of the lateral incisors to simulate the missing centrals or appropriate and controlled space retention with the subsequent provision of an etch retained bridge or partial denture.

Modification of the crown of a 'peg-shaped' tooth may be undertaken during childhood on full eruption of these teeth by means of etch retained composite restorations or porcelain veneers (Chapter 9).

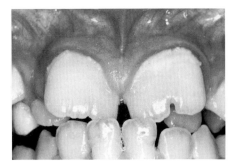

Fig. 12.9 Double maxillary permanent central incisors, the incisal notching of which is more evident in the left incisor.

12.5 ABNORMALITY OF TOOTH FORM

Considerable variety may be seen in *Homo sapiens* in relation to anomaly of tooth form and the examples discussed below are selective.

12.5.1 Abnormality of crown form

Double teeth

A variety of different terms have been used to describe the process of formation of double teeth in either the primary or permanent dentitions. Included in this list of terms are fusion, gemination, dichotomy, synodontia, schizodontia, and connation. However, the mode of development in humans remains unclear and the neutral term double teeth is at least uncontentious.

The anomaly has been observed since the Neolithic period and recent studies have suggested a prevalence in the primary dentition of 0.5–1.6 per cent for Caucasians. The permanent dentition is less commonly involved with a prevalence of 0.1–0.2 per cent. Both sexes are affected with equal frequency. Studies in the Lakeland terrier have suggested a genetic basis for the anomaly but in humans no clear Mendelian pattern has been established.

The clinical manifestation of the anomaly may vary considerably from a minor notch in the incisal edge of an abnormally wide incisor crown to the appearance of almost two separate crown (Fig. 12.9). There may be continuity of hard tissue either between the crowns or roots of the two elements or between both crowns and roots. Similarly, the pulp chamber and root canal may be common to both elements or separate for each component (Fig. 12.10). Double teeth are distinct from concrescences which are teeth united by cementum after completion of development. In the primary dentition double teeth are mainly confined to the labial segments of the arch and more frequently seen in the mandible (Fig. 12.11). A double tooth involving the mandibular lateral incisor and canine is common whereas in the maxilla it is comparatively rare. Double permanent teeth may occur in any region of the arch but incisors are probably more frequently observed. Counting a double tooth as one unit means that there may either be a full complement of teeth present or hypodontia. This is of particular diagnostic importance in the primary dentition as observation of which state

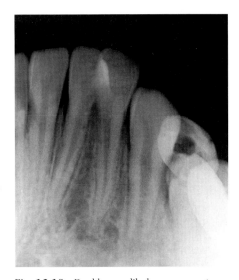

Fig. 12.10 Double mandibular permanent lateral incisor showing hard tissue continuity of the coronal portions in which there is evidence of a common pulp space.

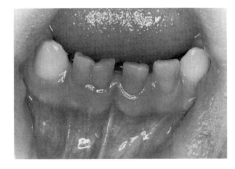

Fig. 12.11 Double mandibular primary central incisor associated with a missing permanent lateral incisor.

exists may be prognostically important for planning treatment in the permanent dentition. Double primary teeth with hypodontia are usually followed by missing permanent teeth, whereas double primary teeth without hypodontia are often associated with permanent supernumeraries. This rule is not invariable and the permanent dentition may be normal. The overall frequency of permanent anomalies following double primary teeth is 30–50 per cent in Caucasians and 75 per cent in the Japanese. Physiological root resorption of double primary teeth is sometimes retarded leading to delayed eruption of the permanent successors.

Treatment

Double primary teeth do not require treatment *per se* but as stated above are good prognostic indicators of possible problems in the underlying permanent dentition. Radiographic examination of the affected segment of the jaw prior to the expected date of permanent tooth eruption is a wise precaution. Should a permanent anomaly appear evident the parent can be advised and appropriate treatment plan can be advanced. Extraction may be required for double primary teeth that are retained unduly beyond the date of normal exfoliation and the surgical removal of supernumerary permanent units may be necessary to facilitate the eruption of adjacent normal permanent teeth.

The decision of whether to retain, extract, or otherwise treat double permanent teeth will depend on a number of factors including space in the arch, type of pulp chambers, and/or root canals present and whether hard tissue conjunction exists between coronal or root elements or both.

Key Points	Double teeth:
	• 0.5–1.6 per cent in primary
	• 0.1–0.2 per cent in permanent
	• 1:1 female/male
	• permanent anomalies in 30–50 per cent of primary cases

12.5.2   Accessory cusps

Additional cusps are common in the human dentition both in primary and permanent teeth, larger teeth tending to have more cusps.

In the primary dentition the most common accessory cusps are seen on the mesiobuccal aspects of the maxillary first molar and the mesiopalatal aspect of the maxillary second molar where they are comparable with the tubercle of Carabelli seen on the first permanent molar.

Permanent incisor teeth may show an additional cusp arising from the lingual cingulum, more often in the maxilla than the mandible. This accessory cusp is often referred to as a talon cusp, as it is said to resemble an eagle's claw (Fig. 12.12). The cusp is composed of enamel, dentine, and a horn of pulp tissue. Maxillary talon cusps may present problems because of their unsightly appearance, interference with the occlusion or the development of caries in the deep grooves found between the cusp and the sloping palatal surface of the incisor.

The lingual tuberculum in permanent canines may be accentuated to form an accessory cusp and the tooth may resemble a premolar.

While premolars may occasionally show an additional buccal cusp in the maxilla the commonest accessory cusp in the permanent dentition is the mesiopalatally sited tubercle of Carabelli on the maxillary first molar. The tubercle is frequently bilateral and its prevalence ranges from 10–60 per cent in different population groups.

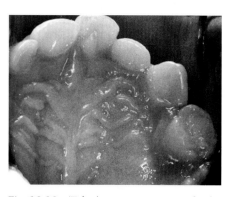

Fig. 12.12 'Talon' accessory cusp on palatal aspect of maxillary permanent central incisor.

Treatment

The talon cusp affecting the maxillary incisor teeth is the only accessory cusp likely to require treatment. Two methods of treatment have been advocated: a) selective grinding of the cusp over a period of time to encourage obliteration of the pulp horn by secondary dentine; and b) aseptic removal of the cusp under rubber dam with ultra-speed diamond burs and to undertake a limited pulpotomy procedure.

12.5.3 Invaginated teeth

A number of different terms have been used to describe teeth which are the result of invagination of the enamel epithelium into the dental papilla of the underlying tooth germ. Some of these terms are based on misconceptions, these include dens in dente, gestant composite odontome, and dilated composite odontome. However, the correct descriptive term is dens invaginatus or invaginated tooth.

The anomaly may vary clinically from a deep cingulum pit in a tooth of normal form, to a tooth with a grossly distorted crown and root. The simplest type may be seen involving the upper permanent incisors, particularly the lateral, where the small palatal invagination commences in the cingulum pit (Fig. 12.13). Invaginations of this type are commonly seen in incisors where the coronal form is 'shovel' shaped. In more severe types involving incisors or canines the crown tends to a conical or barrel form with the orifice of the invagination near the incisal edge. In such cases the root morphology may be similarly deformed by the extensive invagination, with the pulp space seen in radiographs as slits in the dentine on either side of the invagination cavity.

Invaginated primary teeth are rare but in the permanent dentition the anomaly is common affecting 1–5 per cent of population groups. There may be true racial variation as there has been reported a significantly higher proportion of Singaporian children of Chinese origin with the anomaly than those of Malay stock. Males are more commonly affected by the anomaly than females in the ratio of 2:1.

Invaginated teeth frequently cause problems during childhood. The most acute problems occur in the more severe cases where the enamel lining of the invagination may be incomplete. In some areas the dentine may be missing and bacterial ingress into the underlying pulp causes a rapidly spreading infection. Such patients may present with acute facial cellulitis or acute dento-alveolar abscess formation soon after tooth eruption. In the more minor invagination where the enamel lining is complete, plaque collection in the cingulum pit may lead to caries with subsequent pulp death and periapical infection. Bilateral symmetry is frequent in invaginations of the more simple type and the clinical detection of an invagination in one tooth should lead to clinical and radiographic examination of its antemere. A further complication of grossly invaginated teeth with massive root dilatation is impaction of adjacent teeth preventing their eruption (Fig. 12.14). There is also an association between invaginated and supernumerary teeth, and a full radiographic examination is justified when invaginated teeth are identified and vice versa.

Treatment

Acute infective episodes with associated facial cellulitis must be treated initially with appropriate antibiotic therapy. Subsequently, a conservative approach should be adopted with appropriate endodontic treatment if the root form of the invaginated tooth is amenable. With gross anomaly and distortion, particularly when this involves impaction of adjacent teeth, surgical removal is required.

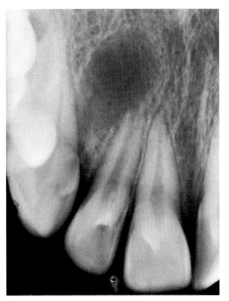

Fig. 12.13 Palatal invagination of maxillary permanent lateral incisor seen in periapical radiograph. The pear-shaped invagination is superimposed on the pulpal shadow. Note the incomplete root formation and area of periapical radiolucency associated with this tooth — suggesting a non-vital and infected pulp space. Also of interest is the uncommon minor palatal invagination in the adjacent permanent canine.

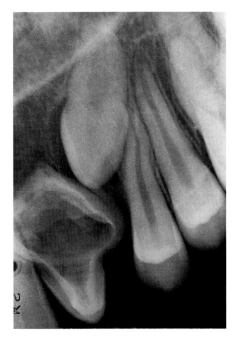

Fig. 12.14 Periapical radiograph of grossly invaginated maxillary permanent lateral incisor preventing the eruption of the adjacent canine. This type of dens invaginatus has been described as a dilated odontome.

Simple invaginations should be sealed with etch retained resin sealants soon after eruption to prevent ingress of plaque and carious tooth destruction.

12.5.4   Evaginated teeth

The abnormality known as evaginated tooth, dens evaginatus, or tuberculated tooth is principally seen in premolar teeth as a conical tuberculated projection arising from the occlusal surface in the region of the central fissure or lingual plane of the buccal cusp. Occasionally, permanent molar or canine teeth may be affected. The condition is said to arise as the result of either an outflow of enamel epithelium or a focal hyperplasia of the ectomesenchyme of the primitive dental papilla. The condition is mainly seen in people of Mongoloid stock with an estimated prevalence of 1–4 per cent. Rare cases have been reported in Caucasians.

The size of the evagination may be comparable with an accessory cusp or a long slender spicule. Evaginations are composed of enamel, dentine and pulp, and pulpal extension into the evagination may vary considerably but is a potential source of complications. The more slender variety of anomaly are liable to fracture during mastication. This in turn may lead to pulpal exposure, infection, necrosis, and subsequent periapical infection (Fig. 12.15).

Treatment

The treatment of evaginations is comparable with that suggested for talon cusps but is only required when there is occlusal interference. Selective grinding of the tubercle as a method of therapy must be undertaken with considerable care as secondary dentine obliteration of the pulp space is reported to occur only in evaginations with a wide base. The preferred approach is the aseptic excision of the tubercle under rubber dam. This involves removal of the tubercle with ultra-speed diamonds, a limited pulpotomy procedure and restoration of the tooth to a normal coronal form.

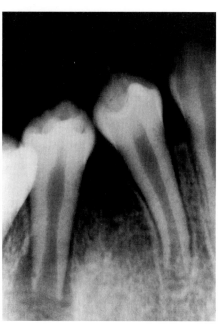

Fig. 12.15 Both lower premolars seen in this periapical radiograph have occlusal evaginations. The evagination in the second premolar has fractured with subsequent pulpal exposure and infection. The area of periapical bony rarefaction is evidence of pulpal necrosis.

12.6   ABNORMALITY OF ROOT FORM

12.6.1   Taurodontism

The descriptive term taurodontism (bull-like teeth) applies to multirooted teeth in which the body is enlarged corono-apically at the expense of the roots. Three degrees of severity have been suggested under the titles of hypo-, meso-, and hypertaurodont teeth, in the latter the pulp chamber extends nearly to the apex with little division of the root. Clinically, the diagnosis is most appropriately established by means of extra-oral radiographs which show apparent enlargement of the coronal pulp chamber, usually extending below the level of the alveolar crest before root division. The normal constriction at the level of the amelocemental junction is frequently absent in affected teeth.

Taurodontism is uncommon in the primary dentition where it may be seen affecting molars and rarely multirooted canines. In the permanent dentition molars are most often affected but occasionally multirooted premolars may show a similar anomalous form.

Precise prevalence data for the anomaly are difficult to ascertain due to wide variations in diagnostic criteria and sampling methods. However, one study of British school children showed a prevalence of 6.3 per cent for mandibular first permanent molars which is probably an underestimate for all permanent molars. The prevalence for permanent molars is probably higher in other racial groups for example, the Bantu in Southern Africa.

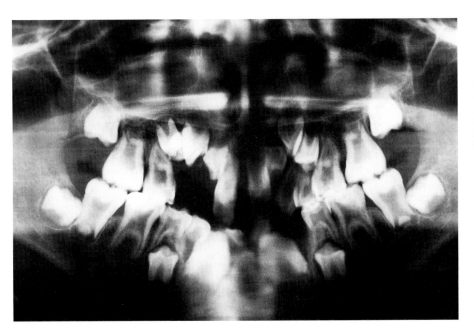

Fig. 12.16 Orthopantomogram of 8 year old boy with mild ectodermal dysplasia showing marked taurodontism of both primary and permanent molar teeth together with congenital absence of mandibular permanent incisors and second premolars (except in right maxilla).

Taurodontism is found in association with amelogenesis imperfecta, trichodento-osseous syndrome, ectodermal dysplasia with hypodontia, Ellis–van Creveld syndrome, achondroplasia, and Klinefelter's syndrome (Fig. 12.16). In all these cases the pattern of inheritance is well established but in the general population the trait is most likely determined polygenically. The defect is thought to originate from a defect in the epithelium of Hertwig's root sheath, which either fails to invaginate at the normal horizontal level or fails to achieve union of the flaps which determine root morphodifferentiation.

12.6.2 Accessory roots

Accessory roots in excess of the normal number may occur in almost any tooth. Branched roots have been described in primary canines and accessory roots reported in maxillary primary incisors and molars in both jaws. In permanent teeth, accessory roots may occasionally affect upper incisors but are rare on lower incisors or upper canines. Extra roots are more commonly seen in lower canines, premolars, and molars, particularly the lower first molar. Accessory roots on these teeth are usually distolingually placed but on occasions may arise lingual to the bifurcation. Such accessory roots are usually fine, rounded, tapering, and curved.

The prevalence of accessory roots in the primary dentition has variously been reported as 1–9 per cent whereas in the permanent dentition prevalence figures range from 1 to 45 per cent.

Accessory roots in the permanent dentition have been found associated with an increased size in the tubercle of Carabelli on the upper first molar, with paramolar tubercles on upper second and third molars and a pulp containing type of enamel pearl. There is a tendency for the crowns of teeth with accessory roots to be abnormally large and there is also a possible association with supernumerary teeth.

Apart from rare examples of an accessory root which is the direct consequence of early trauma to a forming root, the majority are likely to be due to genetic factors which remain to be clarified.

12.6.3   Pyramidal roots

Reduction of root number in teeth which are normally multirooted is variously described under the terms pyramidal, cuneiform, or fused roots. Cuneiform roots show a single root canal whereas other more complex variations of pyramidal root may have two or more root canals. Any molar tooth may be affected but anomalous second and third permanent molars are the most frequently seen in radiographs. Prevalence figures for the first permanent molars are 1 per cent or less whereas figures range from 15 to 40 per cent for second and third permanent molars. Females are more frequently affected than males.

Treatment

The only treatment considerations affected by these anomalies of root form are the increased complexity of endodontic treatment and the increased fragility of some types on extraction.

12.7   ABNORMALITY OF TOOTH STRUCTURE

12.7.1   All tissues

Arrested development of tooth germs

Arrested development of one or more tooth germs may occur as a sequela to irradiation, severe trauma, or osteomyelitis of the jaws during childhood. Similarly, systemic chemotherapy for malignant disease in childhood may lead to failure or arrested development of tooth germs (Fig. 12.17). Rarely, developmental arrest of a single permanent tooth germ may result from acute infection spreading from a cariously exposed pulp of a primary predecessor.

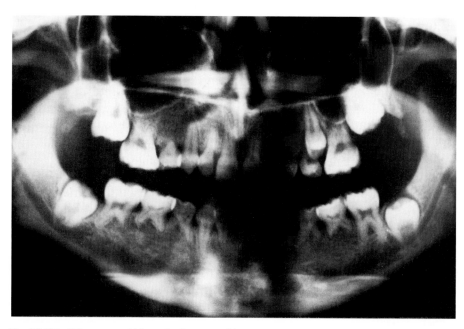

Fig. 12.17 Fifteen year old boy who has treated for 4 years with chemotherapy for a stage IV neuroblastoma of the adrenal in early life. This orthopantomogram shows the arrested development of permanent molar tooth roots and the apparent complete arrest of all mandibular and right maxillary premolar tooth germs.

Odontodysplasia

Odontodysplasia is a rare developmental anomaly occurring with equal frequency in both sexes and affecting teeth in both primary and permanent dentitions. Although accepted as a clinicopathological entity its precise aetiology remains obscure. A few cases have been described as a component of the epidermal naevus syndrome. A number of different terms have been used to describe the condition among which are ghost teeth, odontogenic dysplasia, and regional odontodysplasia. The most common presenting symptoms are pain on eruption or delayed eruption of teeth. The abnormal teeth, particularly in the primary dentition, may be mistakenly diagnosed as grossly carious. The crowns of affected teeth are reduced in size and have a rough, brown-stained surface which is soft to the probe, and may show globular masses. Teeth are affected in a segmental or regional pattern, although especially in the maxilla, which is twice as commonly affected as the mandible, the abnormality may cross the mid-line. The 'ghost like' radiographic appearance often described as characteristic for the anomaly is only seen in severely affected or developing teeth (Fig. 12.18). Roots are usually short, with very wide pulp canals and open apices, although occasionally late development of more normal looking root form may occur on affected permanent teeth which have failed to erupt.

Histopathologically, the enamel is markedly irregular with areas of prismatic enamel covered by a mineralized tissue made up of mixed calcified enamel organ and cementum-like material. The pathognomonic feature is basophilic amorphous areas in the coronal dentine.

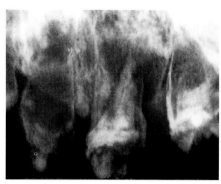

Fig. 12.18 'Ghost-like' appearance of odontodysplastic maxillary primary canine and molar teeth seen in periapical radiograph. Note the periapical bony rarefaction distal to the first molar indicative of pulpal necrosis and infection.

Treatment

Surgical removal of an infected and arrested tooth germ is required to avoid recurrent suppurative episodes. Severely affected teeth are rarely suitable for restorative treatment and require extraction to avoid further symptoms. However, asymptomatic teeth which have failed to erupt may be retained during childhood when multiple teeth are involved and orthodontic space closure is thought to be impossible. In these circumstances a prosthetic replacement will be required.

12.7.2 Enamel defects

Defective enamel formation may be caused by genetic or environmental factors. The extent to which these factors act independently or in combination to produce the end result is presently unknown. The defective enamel will exhibit either hypoplasia due to deficient matrix production or hypomineralization from imperfect mineralization of the matrix proteins. The clinical features depend on the principal changes that have occurred. In hypoplasia the enamel may be thin, grooved, or pitted, whereas in hypomineralization it may appear mottled. The main clinical characteristics will govern classification of the anomaly (Table 12.1); however, combinations of hypoplasia and hypomineralization usually coexist, particularly at the histological level.

Enamel defects:
- hypoplasia — deficient matrix
- hypomineralization — poor mineralization

Key Points

Genetically determined enamel defects

Enamel defects of genetic origin may occur either as a phenomenon primarily involving the enamel with possible secondary defects in other dental tissues and

Table 12.1 Developmental abnormalities of enamel

General factors
1.   Genetic influences:
(i)   primarily involving enamel — amelogenesis imperfecta
(ii) associated with generalized defects
2.   Systemic influences (chronological):
(i)   nutritional deficiencies
(ii) metabolic or biochemical disorder
(iii) toxic substances
(iv) infectious illnesses: prenatal; perinatal; neonatal; infancy; early childhood
3.   Idiopathic
Local factors
(i)   trauma
(ii) infection

craniofacial structures, or as a component of a more complex syndrome in which defective enamel is only one of a number of more generalized abnormalities.

Genetic defects primarily involving enamel — amelogenesis imperfecta

Hereditary enamel defects unassociated with systemic abnormality or disease are collectively known as amelogenesis imperfecta (AI). These changes are the result of single gene mutations which follow autosomal dominant, autosomal recessive, or X-linked patterns of inheritance. Prevalence of AI varies considerably around the world with reported rates of one in 718 in northern Sweden and one in 14 000 in Michigan, USA. Both hypoplastic and hypomineralized variants have been observed, the latter being subdivided by clinical expression or phenotype into two types. The more severe form is described as hypocalcification and the relatively mild variant as hypomaturation of the enamel. However, a number of 'mixed' types exist exhibiting both hypoplasia and hypomineralization at the clinical level. To date 14 different types of AI have been delineated on the basis of genetic pattern, clinical and radiological features, and histological changes (Table 12.2). In most, but not all, types of AI, teeth in both the primary and permanent dentitions are affected by the defect.

A significant association has been established between AI and anterior open bite of skeletal origin. Indeed, AI is frequently associated with an underlying craniofacial anomaly the cause of which remains obscure.

Taurodontism appears to be another feature associated with AI. This is most marked in type IV but appears to affect permanent molars, particularly in the maxilla, in other types of AI more frequently than is the norm for the Caucasian population. Genetic linkage studies of families with X-linked AI have assigned the locus of the defect to the short arm of the X chromosome at Xp22.1–22.3, the region of the amelogenin gene. More recent molecular genetic research has demonstrated a number of different mutations in the amelogenin gene, which is thought responsible for the different types of X-linked AI. Further linkage of AI to the long arm of the X chromosome at Xq22–28 has been reported, although the significance of this finding has yet to be established.

Key Points

Amelogenesis imperfecta — inheritance:
- autosomal dominant
- autosomal recessive
- X-linked

The general features of a number of specific types of AI will be described in detail.

Table 12.2 Types of amelogenesis imperfecta

Type I	Hypoplasia	
1A	Autosomal dominant thin and smooth hypoplasia with eruption defect, coronal resorption and pulpal calcification	
1B	Autosomal dominant thin and rough hypoplasia	
1C	Autosomal dominant randomly pitted hypoplasia	
1D	Autosomal dominant localized hypoplasia	
1E	Autosomal recessive localized hypoplasia	
1F	X-linked hypoplasia	
1G	Autosomal recessive thin and rough hypoplasia (agenesis)	
Type II	Hypocalcification	
IIA	Autosomal dominant hypocalcification	
IIB	Autosomal recessive hypocalcification	
Type III	Hypomaturation	
IIIA	X-linked hypomaturation	
IIIB	Autosomal recessive pigmented hypomaturation	
IIIC	Autosomal dominant snow-capped teeth	
Type IV	Hypomaturation–Hypoplasia with taurodontism	
IVA	Autosomal dominant hypomaturation with pitted hypoplasia and taurodontism	
IVB	Autosomal dominant hypomaturation with thin hypoplasia and taurodontism	

Hypoplasia type IA

The autosomal dominant thin and smooth hypoplasia type of AI exhibits one of the most severe forms of hereditary hypoplasia. The grossly thin enamel is hard, shiny, and discoloured yellow to yellow-brown (Fig. 12.19). Many permanent teeth are delayed in their eruption or fail to erupt completely and may exhibit coronal resorption. These features have been attributed to a premature degeneration of the reduced enamel epithelium covering the crowns of the unerupted teeth. Radiographs may fail to demonstrate the extremly thin enamel but may show dystrophic pulpal calcification. Histologically, the enamel demonstrates little evidence of prism formation and presents a largely homogeneous glass-like appearance with occasional incremental lines running parallel to the outer surface.

Hypoplasia type IF

The X-linked dominant type of hypoplasia shows a significant variation between the sexes. In the affected male, the enamel is extremely thin, hard, and the surface either smooth or finely pitted and granular. The heterozygotic female, however, exhibits alternating vertical bands of near normal enamel with bands of vertically pitted, grooved, or wrinkled enamel (Fig. 12.20). The female may also show areas of whitish or yellowish-white enamel mottling some of which may have a vertically banded distribution. The curious banded distribution of normal and abnormal enamel in the female is attributed to the Lyon effect whereby alternate clones of pre-ameloblasts are randomly governed by either normal or abnormal genes on the X-chromosome. Recent research has shown mutations on exons 5 and 6 of the amelogenin gene to account for some families with this type of AI. Histologically, the defective enamel lacks a normal prismatic structure.

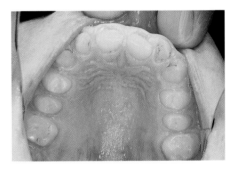

Fig. 12.19 Maxillary permanent teeth showing a thin and smooth enamel surface. Note the almost total absence of cusps on the first molars due to the extremely thin enamel covering.

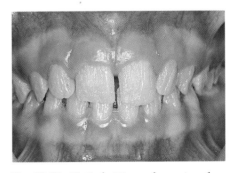

Fig. 12.20 Vertical pitting and grooving of the enamel affects the entire permanent dentition in this adolescent heterozygote female with X-linked hereditary hypoplasia.

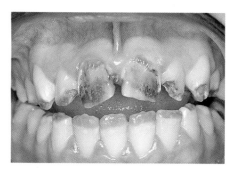

Fig. 12.21 Fragmentation of the severely hypomineralized enamel is most evident in the maxillary permanent incisors and canines in this patient and caused considerable sensitivity to external stimuli.

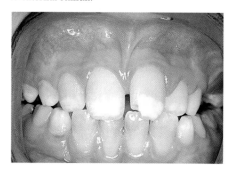

Fig. 12.22 Whitish mottling of the hypomature enamel in this child was limited mainly to the incisal portions of the crowns of the maxillary permanent teeth.

Hypocalcification type IIA

In this type of AI both primary and permanent teeth erupt with enamel which has a dull, lustreless, opaque white, honey coloured, or light brown surface. The degree to which teeth are affected is not usually evenly distributed around the arch, although there is frequent bilateral symmetry. In severely affected teeth, the soft enamel wears away rapidly leaving rough, discoloured, highly sensitive dentine exposed to the oral environment (Fig. 12.21). In the same teeth portions of the enamel, especially towards the cervical region of the crown, may be more highly mineralized and may resist wear. A few reported cases have shown delayed or failed eruption of teeth, the latter exhibiting evidence of coronal resorption. Radiographic contrast between enamel and dentine is lacking and the crowns may appear moth-eaten from irregular loss of enamel. Supragingival calculus is curiously often abundant in affected individuals with associated severe gingivitis or periodontitis. The organic matrix of the enamel appears relatively normal on histological examination.

Hypomaturation type IIIC

The descriptive term snow-capped teeth has been given to this type of hypomaturation defect. The hypomineralized defects are limited to the incisal portions of crowns in anterior teeth and to the occlusal portions in posterior teeth. The affected areas of the crown are mottled with either flecks of opaque white enamel or larger demarcated lesions resembling opaque white ground glass. Maxillary teeth are always involved to a greater extent than mandibular teeth. In the maxilla incisors and canines are commonly affected but the lesions may extend backwards to involve premolars and even molars (Fig. 12.22). The defect appears to be conveyed by an autosomal dominant gene of variable expressivity and occasional lack of penetrance.

Key Points

Amelogenesis imperfecta — main types:
- hypoplastic
- hypomineralized — hypocalcified
             — hypomature
- 'mixed'

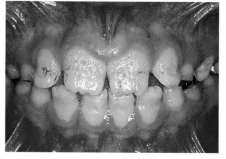

Fig. 12.23 Marked hypoplastic pitting of the enamel was evident in the primary and permanent teeth of this child with epidermolysis bullosa.

Genetic enamel defects associated with generalized disorders

A number of uncommon or rare genetically determined diseases and clinical syndromes have been described in which anomalous enamel development appears to be a significant component of the condition. These diseases and complex syndromes include epidermolysis bullosa (Fig. 12.23), tuberous sclerosis, pseudohypoparathyroidism, trichodento-osseous syndrome, oculodento-osseous dysplasia, vitamin D-dependent rickets, amelocerebrohypohidrotic syndrome, ameloonychohypohidrotic syndrome, and some types of mucopolysaccharidosis.

Environmentally determined enamel defects

Enamel defects of environmental origin may either be associated with a systemic upset or result from a local factor involving the developing tooth. The defect resulting from systemic upset will be related to the timing of the event which may have occurred prenatally, perinatally, neonatally, during infancy, or early childhood (or later in the case of the third permanent molar); that is, during the period of enamel development in the primary and permanent dentitions. Furthermore, the portion of enamel affected will vary with tooth type dependent on its stage of development. In other words the defect will be chronologically arranged around the dental arch. The terms systemic or chronological enamel defects have been used to describe these changes.

Systemic (chronological) enamel defects

A wide range of maternal and fetal conditions may adversely influence enamel development *in utero*. Examples include endocrine disturbances (e.g. hypoparathyroidism), infections (e.g. rubella), drugs (e.g. thalidomide), nutritional deficiencies (e.g. maternal vitamin D), and haematological and metabolic disorders (e.g. rhesus incompatibility followed by hyperbilirubinaemia and kernicterus). In these circumstances hypoplasia or hypomineralization of the enamel may effect the incisal portions of the crowns of the primary incisors. Similar changes have been reported for pre-term, low-birth-weight children particularly affecting the maxillary incisors. Recent evidence suggests the latter phenomenon may be associated with the use of orotracheal intubation in these children. Neonatal disorders in children born at term may lead to enamel defects in the primary dentition and first permanent molars which follow the position of the neonatal line (Fig. 12.24). This has been reported in cases of maternal vitamin D deficiency followed by neonatal tetany. Similarly, systemic upset following the neonatal period may have effects on the later forming enamel in the primary and permanent dentitions. Enamel defects of these types will be seen as chronologically arranged changes varying from hypomineralized enamel mottling to more severe hypoplastic pitting or grooving (Fig. 12.25). The degree of disturbance to amelogenesis is generally determined by the severity of the systemic upset. For instance, exanthematous fevers, e.g. measles, rarely cause significant enamel changes unless complicated by pneumonia or encephalitis.

Amelogenesis may also be disturbed by the excessive chronic ingestion of fluoride. This may come from the excessive intake of fluoride from naturally occurring sources in drinking water as in endemic fluorosis, or from overdosage by fluoride supplements and fluoride toothpastes. Endemic fluorosis is common in parts of East Africa and India. Recent observations suggest that fluorosis may also occur in children continuously resident in areas of artificial fluoridation who also use (and consume) fluoride toothpaste. Enamel fluorosis is dose dependent and varies with the level and period of consumption and the age of the child. In areas of endemic fluorosis such as Ethiopia, teeth in both the primary and permanent dentitions may be affected (Fig. 12.26). In most other cases the enamel changes are largely confined to the permanent dentition. The third year of life is thought to be a particularly vulnerable time for ingested fluoride as far as the permanent incisors are concerned. Fluorosis commonly effects the outer enamel

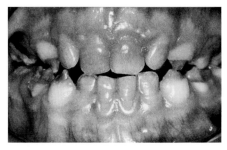

Fig. 12.24 The chronological enamel hypoplasia in this child's primary dentition marks the position of the neonatal line. A history of postmature birth and neonatal asphyxia could account for the changes.

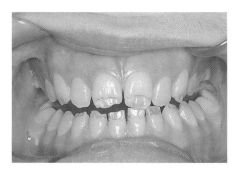

Fig. 12.25 Infantile rickets probably was responsible for the chronological enamel hypoplasia affecting the early mineralizing permanent teeth in this child.

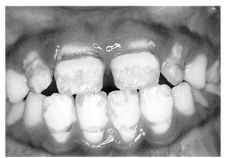

Fig. 12.26 Endemic enamel fluorosis in a child born and raised for the first few years of life in Ethiopia. The horizontal linear enamel defect seen in the permanent incisors was probably caused by a severe attack of measles.

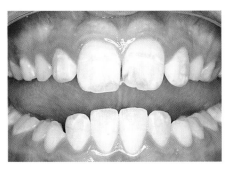

Fig. 12.27 Girl of 11 years with brownish white enamel mottling of her permanent incisors from the combined ingestion of fluoride supplements and toothpaste from early infancy. The horizontal linear enamel defect in the central incisors was probably caused by an attack of rubella.

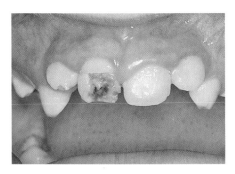

Fig. 12.28 Localized enamel hypoplasia affecting the maxillary permanent right central and lateral incisors. A history of early trauma to the primary incisors was given. Note also the line of dilaceration in the central incisor which assists in timing the event.

layers and may vary from white, opaque lines which follow the perikymata, to scattered white flecking, and to more diffuse areas of opaque mottling which may be chalky white or brownish in appearance (Fig. 12.27). Fragmentation of the outer surface layers of fluorosed enamel leads to pitting or more extensive areas of loss which may resemble hypoplastic changes and which frequently stain brown. Many of these changes have been described as pathognomonic for fluorosis but caution should be exercised in making this diagnosis as some hypomaturation types of AI may be indistinguishable at the clinical level. The changes in the permanent dentition are usually symmetrically distributed around the arch but vary in intensity with tooth type. The most severely affected teeth are often the maxillary incisors, premolars, and second permanent molars.

A number of severe or chronic childhood illnesses have been associated with a high level of enamel defect. Among these are endocrine disorders such as hypothyroidism and hypoparathyroidism, chronic renal disease associated with the nephrotic syndrome, and gastrointestinal disorders such as coeliac disease. The prolonged or recurrent use of tetracycline antibiotics has been associated with tooth discoloration in childhood. Whether at therapeutic levels these drugs have been responsible for enamel hypoplasia is uncertain.

Localized enamel defects

Local infection or trauma may result in enamel defects. Attention has already been drawn above to the apparent local effect of the orotracheal tube imposing pressure on the premaxilla and leading to enamel defects in the unerupted primary incisor teeth.

Trauma to the primary dentition particularly where it involves intrusion or avulsion of teeth is likely to inflict damage to an underlying permanent successor (Chapter 11). Similarly, long-standing periapical or periradicular infection of primary teeth whether the result of trauma or caries may lead to changes in the underlying permanent tooth germ.

Enamel defects arising in these circumstances are mainly confined to areas of hypomineralization which present clinically as patches of opaque white or yellow-brown discoloration. More severe changes are much less common but may be seen as isolated hypoplastic areas in the enamel. In the case of early trauma to primary incisor teeth, hypoplastic or hypomineralized enamel defects may be associated with coronal dilaceration. The teeth most commonly involved are the maxillary central incisors (Fig. 12.28). Children with cleft lip and palate have a high prevalence of enamel defects in maxillary incisors which may be attributable in part to the effects of surgical repair.

Idiopathic enamel defects

The type of enamel defect for which it is difficult to establish a cause is seen in children with one or more hypomineralized and/or hypoplastic first permanent molars without changes in other primary or permanent teeth. In these circumstances there may not be a familial history nor a history of systemic or local upset to account for the abnormality. It is possible that an autosomal recessive genetic defect may account for the changes observed but this remains to be established.

Treatment

The treatment of children and adolescents with enamel defects has three principal requirements. First, to alleviate symptoms; secondly, to maintain or restore occlusion and masticatory efficiency; and thirdly, to improve appearance when the defect(s) has an adverse cosmetic effect. These treatments are discussed in Chapter 9.

12.7.3 Dentine defects

Dentine defects may be subdivided by cause into two main groups, which are of genetic or environmental origin.

Genetically determined dentine defects

Dentine anomaly which is genetically determined may appear to be limited to the dentition or form part of a more complex generalized disorder (Table 12.3). Recent research has suggested that in some cases this distinction may be difficult to sustain.

Genetic defects primarily involving dentine

A number of different genetic variants of anomalous dentine formation have been classified under this heading.

Dentinogenesis imperfecta type II (hereditary opalescent dentine)
In this genetic variant all teeth in both dentitions are usually affected. The teeth are opalescent on transillumination and bluish or brownish in colour. Severity of the defect varies considerably between families and within families. Primary teeth tend to be more severely affected than permanent teeth and the later forming permanent teeth may be the least affected. This variability of effect in the permanent dentition is not as marked as that seen in dentinogenesis imperfecta type I in association with osteogenesis imperfecta (*vide infra*). Enamel tends to chip away from the underlying amelodentinal junction exposing the abnormally soft dentine which undergoes rapid wear. This is most marked in the primary dentition where, within 2 years, the crowns may be worn to the gingival margin and appear as smooth amber-coloured remnants, which are frequently infected and abscessed. In the permanent dentition following eruption the enamel may look reasonably normal but histological studies have shown hypomineralized areas in approximately one-third of cases. A few families exhibit more severely defective enamel which is thin and has a greyish, friable surface layer (Fig. 12.29). Radiographically, the crowns appear bulbous and the roots may be short and thin. The pulp chambers obliterate soon after eruption and the root canals are

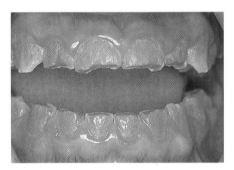

Fig. 12.29 Fragmentation of the thin and dysplastic enamel is evident in the permanent incisor teeth of this child with dentinogenesis imperfecta type II. Generalized discoloration of both primary and permanent teeth is present.

Table 12.3 Hereditary dentine defects

1. Limited to the dentine
    (a) dentinogenesis imperfecta type II (hereditary opalescent dentine)
    (b) dentine dysplasia type I (radicular dentine dysplasia)
    (c) dentine dysplasia type II (coronal dentine dysplasia)
    (d) fibrous dysplasia of dentine

2. Associated with generalized disorder:
    (a) osteogenesis imperfecta (dentinogenesis imperfecta type I)
    (b) Ehlers–Danlos syndrome
    (c) brachio-skeleto-genital syndrome
    (d) vitamin D resistant rickets
    (e) vitamin D dependent rickets
    (f) hypophosphatasia

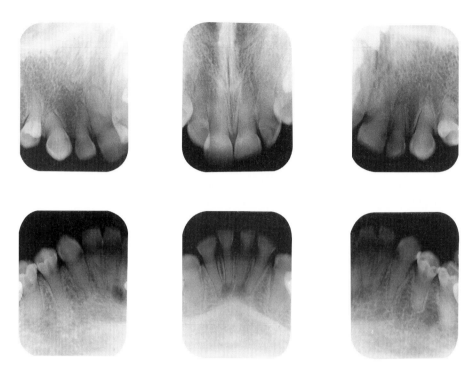

Fig. 12.30 Periapical radiographs of adolescent with dentinogenesis imperfecta type II showing almost total calcific obliteration of the pulp chambers and root canals in incisors and canines.

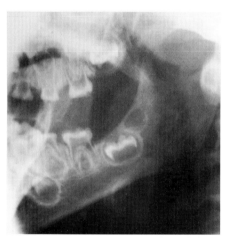

Fig. 12.31 A severe form of dentinogenesis imperfecta type II in the primary dentition of a 2 year old child is seen in this oblique lateral jaw radiograph. The descriptive term 'shell teeth' has been used for this condition.

progressively narrowed by the rapid deposition of abnormal dentine (Fig. 12.30). Histologically, the amelodentinal junction may appear flattened and while the subadjacent peripheral dentine may approach normality, the remainder is grossly disordered. This anomalous tissue has an amorphous matrix with areas of interglobular calcification, abnormally shaped and sized tubules and a highly disorganized pattern with cellular inclusions.

Prevalence of the defect has been estimated at about one in 8000 of the population. The inheritance pattern is invariably autosomal dominant with marked expressivity and good penetrance. Very long family pedigrees have been described extending over many generations. The defect has been linked to the Gc locus on chromosome 4q. Two clinical variants of this condition have been described under the titles of 'shell teeth' and dentinogenesis imperfecta type III or the brandywine type. The former type is rare and may be seen in the primary dentition of severely affected cases where the pulp chambers remain enlarged, the thin enamel and dentine fragments rapidly, and the pulps become infected at an early age (Fig. 12.31). The latter was first described in a triracial isolate in Maryland, USA and has more recently been linked to the same locus on chromosome 4q as dentinogenesis imperfecta type II.

Key Points	Dentinogenesis imperfecta — main types:
	● I — associated with osteogenesis imperfecta
	● II — teeth only

Dentine dysplasia type I (radicular dentine dysplasia, rootless teeth)
In this anomaly teeth in both dentitions are affected, their colour varying from normal to a slight bluish or brownish tinge. Radiographs show the crowns to have a normal morphology but the roots are seen as excessively short and blunt. The pulp chambers appear as small demilunes or are completely obliterated and the root canals absent. Histologically, the coronal enamel and dentine may appear to be within normal limits but the pulp chamber is part or fully obliter-

ated with large masses of dysplastic dentine with a distinctive 'waterfall' appearance.

Teeth in this condition are usually lost early due to their extreme mobility and ease of avulsion with minor trauma. The condition is rare and is probably inherited as an autosomal dominant.

Dentine dysplasia type II (coronal dentine dysplasia)
The remarkable feature in this anomalous condition is the disparity of effect in the primary and permanent conditions. The defect in the primary dentition is difficult to distinguish clinically and radiologically from dentinogenesis imperfecta type II. Histologically, beneath a thin layer of normal dentine lies a largely amorphous calcified tissue with only a few haphazard tubules.

Permanent teeth are clinically of normal colour but radiographically show thistle or flame-shaped pulp chambers partially occluded by pulp stones. The root canals gradually become narrowed to the point of almost total obliteration (Fig. 12.32). Histologically, the coronal dentine approaches a near normal appearance, whereas the radicular dentine is largely amorphous without a tubular structure. Reticulum staining of this abnormal tissue suggests a large content of type III collagen in distinction to the type I collagen found in normal dentine. The condition is rare and the inheritance pattern autosomal dominant.

Fibrous dysplasia of dentine
In this very rare anomaly the permanent teeth have a normal colour and form. Radiographs show the pulp chambers and root canals to be represented by only a few radiolucent areas. This histological appearance of the dentine varies from area to area, some showing numerous lacunae and cellular inclusions whereas other areas are taken up by predentine-like collagen. The nature of the defect in the primary dention has not been recorded.

Genetic dentine defects associated with generalized disorders
A number of genetically determined disorders have been reported in which anomalous dentine forms a significant clinical feature. Listed under these conditions are osteogenesis imperfecta, Ehlers–Danlos syndrome, vitamin D resistant rickets and vitamin D dependent rickets.

Osteogenesis imperfecta with dentinogenesis imperfecta type I
Osteogenesis imperfecta is a heterogeneous group of connective tissue disorders involving inherited abnormalities of type I collagen. Increased bone fragility is only one aspect of the condition which may include lax joints, blue sclerae, opalescent teeth, hearing loss, and a variable degree of bone deformity. The inheritance pattern is either autosomal recessive or dominant; of these the recessive varieties are the most severely affected and are frequently lethal at or shortly after birth.

Opalescent teeth are only rarely seen in the surviving recessive types, more commonly this feature is observed in the dominantly inherited varieties accompanying a variable degree of bone deformity, mild to moderately severe bone fragility, and blue sclerae in childhood.

The primary teeth resemble in every feature those seen in dentinogenesis type II. In the permanent dentition the defect is extremely variable. In many cases the upper anterior teeth in children may have a normal colour and appearance whereas the lower incisors and canines are opalescent, discoloured bluish-brown and wear at the incisal edges. In most cases the enamel appears clinically well formed and does not chip as readily from the underlying dentine as seen in the genetic isolate. Indeed the prognosis for the permanent dentition

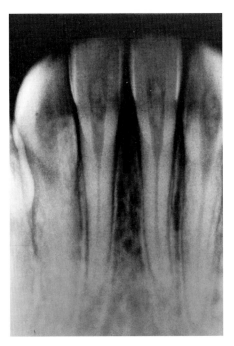

Fig. 12.32 The characteristic thistle-shaped pulp chambers and narrowed root canals are seen in this periapical radiograph of dentine dysplasia type II. Note the multiple pulp stones in the pulp chambers.

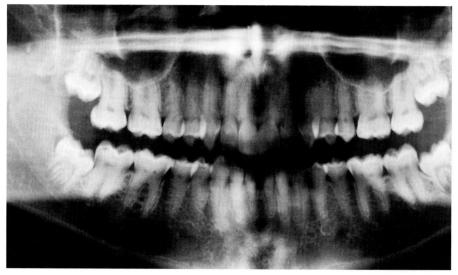

Fig. 12.33 Adolescent patient with osteogenesis imperfecta and dentinogenesis imperfecta type I. Note the patency of many pulp chambers and root canals and the absence of significant coronal attrition on the posterior teeth.

during childhood, adolescence, and early adult life is much better than in hereditary opalescent dentine. However, this feature is not observed in all cases. Radiographically, the permanent teeth show a variable calcific occlusion of the pulp chambers and root canals during childhood which does not follow any strict pattern, although the upper anterior teeth may retain their pulp spaces long after those in the lower jaw (Fig. 12.33). This feature differentiates the condition from dentinogenesis imperfecta type II. But histological appearances of affected portions of the dentine are indistinguishable.

A number of families have been observed with teeth similar to those found in osteogenesis imperfecta, with mildly blue sclerae and lax joints but without a history of bone fragility. The exact nature of this inherited abnormality of collagen remains to be resolved.

Environmentally determined dentine defects

Although these abnormalities exist they have been much less well documented than corresponding anomalies of enamel, principally because dentine is less available to inspection. Local trauma may interfere with the process of dentine formation as may a number of systemic influences such as nutritional deficiencies of minerals, proteins and vitamins, drugs such as tetracycline, and chemotherapeutic agents such as cyclophosphamide. The likely effects are the increased formation of interglobular dentine, predentine, and osteoid.

Treatment

Early intervention is required in cases of dentinogenesis imperfecta types I and II due to the rapid wear. The principles of treatment are covered in Chapter 9.

12.7.4 Cementum defects

During childhood and adolescence defective cementum of clinical relevance is associated with a number of genetically determined disorders. Two rare conditions are important in this respect, cleidocranial dysplasia and hypophosphatasia.

Cleidocranial dysplasia is an autosomal dominant defect characterized by aplasia or hypoplasia of the clavicles, a brachycephalic skull, with pronounced frontal and parietal bossing, hypoplasia of the maxilla and zygomas, hypertelorism, and delayed closure of the anterior frontanelle, frontal and metopic sutures. Numerous wormian bones are formed in the line of the cranial sutures, especially the lambdoidal suture. The most significant dental feature is the presence of multiple supernumerary teeth in the permanent series, especially in the anterior segments of the jaws (see Fig. 12.4). While primary tooth eruption is within normal limits, permanent teeth are frequently delayed in their eruption or fail to erupt at all. Primary tooth resorption is similarly delayed or arrested. The disorder of permanent tooth eruption has been attributed to a primary failure of bone resorption mechanisms. Histologically, hypoplasia of root cementum has been observed, particularly affecting the cellular component.

Hypophosphatasia is a rare genetically determined disorder of bone mineralization conveyed by both autosomal recessive and dominant genes. The homozygote for the recessive defect may present in the neonatal and infantile periods with severe metabolic disturbances, which may prove fatal. Later in childhood the condition may present in a milder form with a ricketic form of bony abnormality and premature loss of primary teeth and spontaneous loss of permanent teeth. Serum alkaline phosphatase levels are extremely low and phosphoethanolamine is excreted in excess in the urine (Fig. 12.34). Early and spontaneous loss of teeth may on occasions be the only manifestation of the disease. In these cases histological investigation of the shed teeth may be crucial to the diagnosis. Aplasia or marked hypoplasia of cementum is characteristic of the condition. Significant changes may also be observed in the pattern of dentine formation with a wide predentine zone and considerable amounts of interglobular dentine.

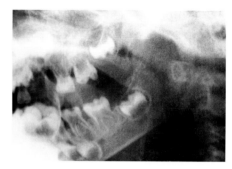

Fig. 12.34 Radiograph of 2 year old child with the autosomal recessive form of hypophosphatasia. Primary incisor and canine teeth have been already shed prematurely. Note the bony rarefaction associated with the first primary molars and the large size of the pulp chambers in all the primary teeth.

Treatment

Extraction of retained primary teeth and surgical removal of unerupted supernumerary teeth should be performed with caution in cases of cleidocranial dysplasia as this will not necessarily guarantee the subsequent successful eruption of the permanent dentition. Parents and children should be warned of the possible outcome prior to a decision on surgical approach.

Prosthetic replacement of teeth in the primary and permanent dentitions may be required in cases of hypophosphatasia.

12.8 DISTURBANCES OF ERUPTION

In discussing disturbances of eruption it is important to take into account the considerable racial variations that exist in the eruption of the permanent dentition. As a generalization, Negroids tend to erupt their permanent teeth earlier than Mongoloids, who in turn are in advance of Caucasians. However, there is little doubt that other factors such as nutrition and chronic illnesses in population groups of children may modify the basic racial chronology for the eruption of teeth. Eruption times of primary teeth do not appear to vary with racial group but the eruption pattern in the primary dentition is extremely variable in contrast to the later erupting permanent teeth. Sexual differences exist in the eruption times of permanent teeth with females several months ahead of males, this difference tends to be greater for later erupting teeth.

12.8.1 Premature eruption

Premature tooth eruption may be a familial feature and children with high birth weights tend to erupt their primary teeth early. Excessively early eruption of the permanent dentition is seen in children with precocious puberty and those with endocrinological abnormalities associated with excessive secretion of growth or thyroid hormones.

Natal and neonatal teeth

Teeth present in the mouth at birth are known as natal teeth and those which erupt within the subsequent 30 days as neonatal teeth. Prevalence rates for both natal and neonatal teeth are reported as approximately one in 2000–3000 live births. The tooth most commonly presenting in this way is the lower central incisor, although rarely maxillary incisors or first molars have been observed. This precocious eruption is thought to be caused by the ectopic position of the tooth germ during fetal life. Apart from these sporadic cases in the general population, which may show a familial pattern, natal/neonatal teeth may be seen associated with pachyonychia congenita or as a feature of the Ellis–van Creveld and Hallermann–Streiff syndromes.

Natal/neonatal teeth are often very mobile from lack of root development, the crowns occasionally dilacerated and the enamel hypoplastic or hypomineralized. The surrounding gingival tissue is frequently inflamed and the ventral surface of the tongue may be ulcerated. These complications may interfere with the normal suckling of the baby at the breast. Teeth left *in situ* will continue root development and will eventually attain normal mobility.

Treatment

Extraction of these precocious teeth is required when there is a danger of detachment and inhalation or there is significant disturbance of feeding. Occasionally, the lingual ulceration may respond to treatment with Carmellose sodium oral paste applied with a cotton bud prior to feeds without the need for extraction.

12.8.2 Retarded eruption

Delayed eruption of primary teeth tends to occur in children born pre-term or with very low birth weights.

There are a number of conditions associated with generalized retarded eruption of teeth in both dentitions. Examples of this phenomenon may be seen in some children with the chromosomal abnormalities of Down and Turner syndromes. Significantly delayed eruption may also be associated with gross nutritional deficiency, hypothydroidism, or hypopituitarism in childhood (Fig. 12.35). Cleidocranial dysplasia is associated with grossly delayed or failed eruption of teeth in the permanent dentition. Hereditary gingival hyperplasia associated with hypertrichosis is similarly associated with gross delay in the eruption of both primary and permanent teeth.

Fig. 12.35 Orthopantomogram of a teenage child with failure of eruption of mandibular second primary molars, premolars and permanent molars. In the maxilla teeth distal to the first premolars have also failed to erupt. The cause is unknown.

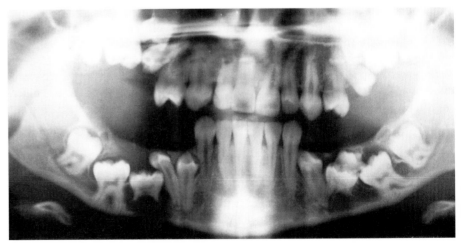

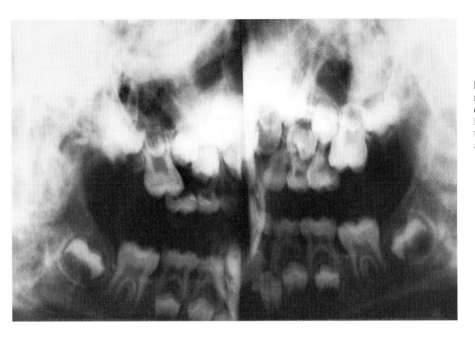

Fig. 12.36 Both maxillary first permanent molars have failed to erupt in this 6 year old child. Oblique lateral jaw radiographs show impaction of these teeth on the distal aspect of the maxillary second primary molars which are affected by gross root resorption.

Localized causes within the oral cavity for delayed eruption of teeth include ectopic crypt positions, e.g. maxillary permanent canines, impaction of maxillary permanent first molars on distal aspect of maxillary primary second molars (Fig. 12.36), and the presence of supernumeraries or odontomes impeding the eruptive pathway of adjacent permanent teeth. The very early extraction of primary molar teeth may often be associated with the delayed eruption of the permanent successors.

Treatment

Apart from management of any systemic factor, e.g. hormone replacement therapy, treatment relates to removal of obstructions such as supernumeraries and odontomes, surgical exposure and orthodontic traction for ectopic maxillary canines, and gingivectomy in hereditary gingival hyperplasia. Surgical treatment in cleidocranial dysplasia with the removal of supernumeraries and possible exposure of unerupted teeth has an uncertain prognosis for the successful eruption of permanent teeth.

12.9   DISTURBANCES OF EXFOLIATION

12.9.1   Premature exfoliation

Apart from the common early loss of primary teeth from accidental trauma or extraction there are a number of comparatively uncommon or rare conditions which may result in the premature loss of teeth in the primary dentition. Occasionally, these pathological processes may proceed to involve the permanent dentition with consequent loss of teeth. Examples of such diseases are hereditary hypophosphasia where aplasia or hypoplasia of cementum may result in premature loss of both primary and permanent teeth, immunological deficiencies such as severe congenital neutropenia (Kostmann's disease), cyclic neutropenia, and the Chediak-Higashi syndrome which may lead to gross periodontal destruction and finally the invasion of histiocytic tissue in histiocytoses X which may destroy the supporting alveolar bone.

12.9.2 Delayed exfoliation

Infra-occlusion

Infra-occlusion is the preferred term to 'submerged teeth' or 'ankylosis' when describing teeth which have failed to achieve or maintain their occlusal relationships to adjacent and opposing teeth. The majority of infra-occluded teeth in the primary dentition have reached the normal occlusal level but have then been subject to secondary changes which result in them falling below the level of the occlusion. Rarely primary molar teeth may fail to erupt completely and this may be seen in association with infra-occlusion of primary and permanent molar teeth in the same individual (Fig. 12.37). Different diagnostic criteria between studies make it difficult to give precise prevalence figures for infra-occlusion but the range is from 1 to 9 per cent with no difference between the sexes. The primary dentition is far more often affected than the permanent dentition and primary molars are the most frequently involved. The mandibular first primary molar is the most commonly affected tooth. Not infrequently more than one primary molar is infra-occluded in the same patient and the condition may be bilaterally symmetrical. Congenital absence of premolars is more common in children with infra-occluded primary molars than in the general population. Varying degrees of infra-occlusion have been described as minimal, moderate, or severe depending on the relationship to adjacent teeth and the gingival margin (Fig. 12.38). Severely infra-occluded primary molars may rarely become totally reincluded by the surrounding tissues, the only visible evidence sometimes being a portion of the occlusal surface. Radiographs may show some blurring of the periodontal space but this cannot be relied upon to show the degree of ankylosis. Histological evidence of ankylosis has frequently been reported for infra-occluded teeth.

The aetiology of the condition is not clear. Ankylosis is thought to be due to an imbalance in the normal pattern of resorption and repair in primary teeth. Trauma and infection have been suggested as precursors to ankylosis but evidence for this is scanty. Protagonists for the view that ankylosis is a primary pathological process suggest that this may cause growth to cease in the affected portion of the alveolus while adjacent teeth continue to move occlusally. An alternative view suggests that ankylosis is secondary to a failure in the continued

Fig. 12.37 Failure of eruption of the right mandibular second primary molar associated with varying degrees of infra-occlusion in other primary molar teeth are seen in the orthopantomogram of this unusual case. The first permanent molars on the right are also infraoccluded, and the right second premolars are absent.

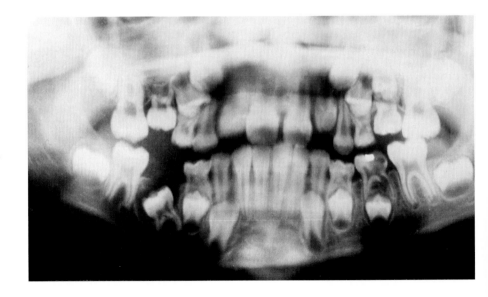

eruption of the affected tooth associated with a localized failure in vertical growth of the alveolus. Familial examples of infra-occlusion have been reported and genetic factors are likely to be of importance. Studies of infra-occluded primary molars have shown that apart from those with missing permanent successors the teeth are not generally delayed in their exfoliation. Furthermore, leaving aside rare examples of severely infra-occluded primary molars which become impacted between adjacent primary or permanent teeth the majority exfoliate naturally within the normal age range.

Other causes of delayed exfoliation

Delay in the normal exfoliation of primary teeth may be seen in association with double primary teeth, hypodontia affecting permanent successors, ectopically placed permanent successors, and subsequent to trauma or severe periradicular infection of primary teeth.

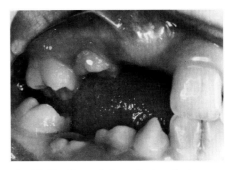

Fig. 12.38 Severe infra-occlusion of primary second molars in the right mandible and maxilla, the lower tooth is almost reincluded in the tissues. The first permanent molars on this side of the jaws are also infra-occluded.

Key Points

Infraocclusion:
- 1–9 per cent prevalence
- 1:1 female/male
- primary > permanent
- higher incidence of absent permanent successors

Treatment

While many infra-occluded primary molar teeth with permanent successors respond to a conservative approach and exfoliate normally this is not true for all. Particular care should be taken with infra-occluded second primary molars which show signs of becoming severely infra-occluded under the age of 5–6 years. In these circumstances extraction or surgical removal, dependent on the degree of ankylosis, may be required prior to the eruption of the first permanent molar and the possible complication of impaction.

Retained primary teeth without permanent successors may in some circumstances be kept for many years and provide a useful functional unit with or without the addition of resin-bonded ceramic or composite resin onlays. Minimal enamel preparation of less than 0.5 mm buccally, lingually, and occlusally, and rounding of cusp tips is recommended. Onlays are constructed on dies produced from elastomeric impressions and under effective isolation are cemented after prior etching of the infra-occluded surface. Ceramic onlays require addition of a silane coupling agent prior to application of the bonding resin. The prospective longevity of these bonded onlays is unknown. Although growth influences and associated occlusal changes may be minimal the primary molar roots could eventually resorb and the tooth require removal. Other prosthodontic options will then need to be considered, e.g. osteo-integrated implants, resin bonded or fixed-fixed bridgework.

12.10 SUMMARY

1. Presence of one dental anomaly may be associated with others; thorough clinical and radiographic examination is essential.
2. An anomaly in the primary dentition is often associated with an increased risk of an anomaly in the permanent dentition.
3. All cases of hypodontia require careful treatment planning with multi-specialist input.

4. Developmental enamel defects may be genetic or environmental in aetiology.

5. The distribution of an environmental enamel defect will depend on the stage of tooth development at the time of the upset.

6. Excessive fluoride ingestion can cause enamel defects.

7. Hereditary dentine defects may be limited to the teeth or may form part of a more general condition.

8. Dentinogenesis imperfecta type II may be associated with enamel defects.

12.11 FURTHER READING

Backman, B. (1989). Amelogenesis imperfecta. An epidemiologic, genetic morphologic and clinical study. Umea University odontological dissertations. (*A good example of carefully conducted population study of enamel defects.*)

Crawford, P. J. M. and Aldred, M. J. (1992). X-linked amelogenesis imperfecta — presentation of two kindreds and a review of the literature. *Oral Surgery, Oral Medicine, Oral Pathology*, **73**, 449–55. (*A good review of the literature on the subject of amelogenesis imperfecta.*)

Gorlin, R. J., Cohen, M. M. and Levin, L. S. (1990). *Syndromes of the head and neck* (3rd edn). Oxford University Press, New York. (*Excellent account of osteogenesis imperfecta.*)

Lagerstrom, M., Dahl, N., Nakahori, Y., *et al.* (1991). A deletion in the Amelogenin Gene (AMG) causes X-linked amelogenesis imperfecta (AIHI). *Genomics*, **10**, 971–5. (*Landmark research in this field. The first workers to identify a mutant gene for an enamel defect.*)

Rowe, A. H. R., Alexander, A. G., and Johns, R. B. (1989). *A comprehensive guide to clinical dentistry*. Class Publishing, London. (*More comprehensive and detailed account in chapter devoted to tooth abnormalities.*)

Stewart, R. E. and Prescott, G. H. (1976). *Oral facial genetics*. Mosby, St Louis. (*Good chapter on enamel dysplasias.*)

Witkop, C. J. Jr. (1988). Amelogenesis imperfecta, dentinogenesis imperfecta and dentine dysplasia revisited: problems in classification. *Journal of Oral Pathology*, **17**, 547–53. (*Thoughtful account of the difficulties of classification in this field of study.*)

13 The paedodontic/orthodontic interface

13 The paedodontic/orthodontic interface

N. E. CARTER

13.1 INTRODUCTION

The long-term management of a child's developing occlusion often benefits greatly from a good working relationship between the paediatric dentist and the orthodontist. Typical problems range from minimizing damage to the occlusion caused by enforced extraction of poor quality teeth, through the management of specific local abnormalities such as impacted teeth, to referral for comprehensive treatment of all aspects of the malocclusion. This chapter discusses the principles of when to refer to a specialist colleague, and looks at some common clinical situations where collaboration is often needed.

13.2 RECOGNITION OF MALOCCLUSION

13.2.1 Orthodontic assessment

All children from the age of 8 years should be screened for the presence of malocclusion when they attend for a routine dental examination. Although orthodontic treatment is usually carried out in the late mixed and early permanent dentition, some conditions do benefit from treatment at an earlier stage. The screening need only be a brief clinical assessment but it should be carried out systematically to ensure that no important findings are overlooked.

An outline of a basic orthodontic assessment is given in Table 13.1. With practice this can be carried out quite quickly to give an overall impression of the nature and severity of a malocclusion. In essence, it comprises assessments of the following elements:

(1) the patient's awareness of their malocclusion (the complaint, if any);
(2) their general level of dental awareness;
(3) an extra-oral examination of facial form (skeletal pattern and soft tissues);
(4) general oral condition — oral hygiene and tooth quality;
(5) the presence or absence of all teeth;
(6) the alignment and form of each arch;
(7) the teeth in occlusion.

Radiographs are not necessary routinely when screening for the presence of malocclusion, and should only be taken when there is a clinical indication for them. A panoramic radiograph gives a useful general scan of the dentition and indicates the presence or absence of teeth, but some authorities advise that it should be supplemented with a naso-occlusal view as the premaxillary region is often poorly shown on panoramic views and is commonly the site of dental

Table 13.1 Orthodontic assessment

Complaint	
Medical history:	May affect decisions about extractions, or where appliances may compromise gingival health
Dental history:	Caries experience, previous extractions, dental awareness
Attitude to treatment:	Of patient and parents. Likely level of co-operation: with dentistry generally, with orthodontic appliances, monthly adjustment visits (time off school, travelling), etc
Extra-oral examination	
General	Height, developmental stage
Facial skeletal pattern	
Anteroposterior:	Facial profile – skeletal I, II, or III. Mild, moderate, severe
Vertical:	Steepness of mandibular plane. Facial proportions – increased, normal, reduced
Transverse:	Facial asymmetry. Discrepancies in widths of upper and lower arches
Soft tissues	
Lips:	Competent or incompetent. Relationship of lower lip to upper incisors
Tongue:	Tongue thrust (rare); tongue to lower lip seal
Habits:	Digit sucking or other habit
TMJ	Pain, clicks, limitation of opening, mandibular deviation
Intra-oral examination	
Dentition:	Teeth present in the mouth. Delayed eruption of teeth. Oral hygiene. Teeth of poor prognosis: caries, extensive restorations, trauma
Lower arch:	Crowding, misplaced teeth. Angulation of incisors and canines
Upper arch:	Crowding, misplaced teeth. Palpate for unerupted canines. Angulation of incisors and canines
Incisor relationship:	Overjet (mm). Overbite — increased or reduced, complete or incomplete. Centrelines — coincident, correct within face? Anterior cross-bites. Check for premature occlusal contact and associated displacement of mandible on closure — forward and/or lateral
Posterior occlusion:	Both sides: class I, II, or III. Check first molars and canines. Posterior cross-bites – local, unilateral, bilateral. Mandibular displacement?
Radiographs	Presence of permanent teeth: absent teeth, supernumerary teeth, ectopic teeth. Pathology. (Skeletal assessment using cephalometric radiographs is not needed for routine screening for malocclusion)

anomalies. A radiographic assessment must always be made when considering any extractions.

Good quality study models are often helpful when planning orthodontic treatment, and full orthodontic records comprising study models, relevant radiographs and photographs should be obtained before any active treatment is started. Full face and profile photographs are a record of facial form, including lip morphology. Intra-oral photographs are a further record of the malocclusion, give some indication of the standard of oral hygiene, and are valuable where enamel defects are present before treatment.

13.2.2   Need and demand for orthodontic treatment

The Index of Orthodontic Treatment Need (IOTN) is based upon the severity of the malocclusion and has been developed to try to establish a consensus within the profession as to which malocclusions will gain a worthwhile benefit from orthodontic treatment. The complexity and difficulty of treatment do not necessarily depend upon the severity of the malocclusion, and mild malocclusions often need extensive and sophisticated treatment if any improvement is to be made at all. The IOTN has two components:

1. *The Dental Health Component* categorizes malocclusion into five grades (Table 13.2) according to severity, based upon current evidence for the detrimental effects of various occlusal features. A malocclusion is graded according to its worst feature. Patients in grades 1 and 2 have little or no indication for

Table 13.2 Dental health component of the Index of Orthodontic Treatment Need

Grade 5 (need treatment)
- 5.i Impeded eruption of teeth (except for third molars) due to crowding, displacement, the presence of supernumerary teeth, retained primary teeth and any pathological cause
- 5.h Extensive hypodontia with restorative implications (more than one tooth missing in any quadrant) requiring pre-restorative orthodontics
- 5.a Increased overjet greater than 9 mm
- 5.m Reversed overjet greater than 3.5 mm with reported masticatory and speech difficulties
- 5.p Defects of cleft lip and palate and other craniofacial anomalies
- 5.s Submerged primary teeth

Grade 4 (need treatment)
- 4.h Less extensive hypodontia requiring pre-restorative orthodontics or orthodontic space closure to obviate the need for a prosthesis
- 4.a Increased overjet greater than 6 mm but less than or equal to 9 mm
- 4.b Reverse overjet greater than 3.5 mm with no masticatory or speech difficulties
- 4.m Reverse overjet greater than 1 mm but less than 3.5 mm with recorded masticatory and speech difficulties
- 4.c Anterior or posterior cross-bites with greater than 2 mm discrepancy between retruded contact position and intercuspal position
- 4.l Posterior lingual cross-bite with no functional occlusal contact in one or both buccal segments
- 4.d Severe contact point displacements greater than 4 mm
- 4.e Extreme lateral or anterior open bites greater than 4 mm
- 4.f Increased and complete overbite with gingival or palatal trauma
- 4.t Partially erupted teeth, tipped and impacted against adjacent teeth
- 4.x Presence of supernumerary teeth

Grade 3 (borderline need)
- 3.a Increased overjet greater than 3.5 mm but less than or equal to 6 mm with incompetent lips
- 3.b Reverse overjet greater than 1 mm but less than or equal to 3.5 mm
- 3.c Anterior or posterior cross-bites with greater than 1 mm but less than or equal to 2 mm discrepancy between retruded contact position and intercuspal position
- 3.d Contact point displacements greater than 2 mm but less than or equal to 4 mm
- 3.e Lateral or anterior open bites greater than 2 mm but less than or equal to 4 mm
- 3.f Deep overbite complete on gingival or palatal tissues but no trauma

Grade 2 (little)
- 2.a Increased overjet greater than 3.5 mm but less than or equal to 6 mm with competent lips
- 2.b Reverse overjet greater than 0 mm but less than or equal to 1 mm
- 2.c Anterior or posterior cross-bites with less than or equal to 1 mm discrepancy between retruded contact position and intercuspal position
- 2.d Contact point displacements greater than 1 mm but less than or equal to 2 mm
- 2.e Lateral or anterior open bites greater than 1 mm but less than or equal to 2 mm
- 2.f Increased overbite greater than or equal to 3.5 mm without gingival contact
- 2.g Pre-normal or post-normal occlusions with no other anomalies (includes up to half a unit discrepancy)

Grade 1 (none)
- 1 Extremely minor malocclusions including contact point displacements less than 1 mm

(P. Brook and W. Shaw 1989. Reproduced with kind permission of the Editor of the *European Journal of Orthodontics*.)

treatment on dental health grounds, while those in grades 4 and 5 are considered to have a definite need for treatment. The borderline cases in grade 3 require a degree of judgement when deciding upon their need for treatment, and the appearance of the dentition can be taken into account using the Aesthetic Component of the IOTN.

2. *The Aesthetic Component* of the IOTN uses a scale of 10 photographs showing different levels of dental attractiveness (Fig. 13.1). The patient and the

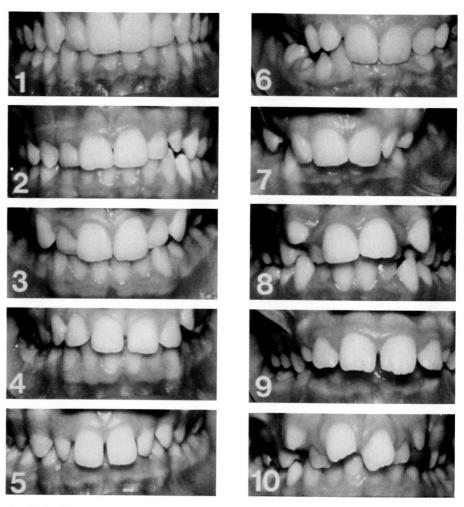

Fig. 13.1 The Aesthetic Component of the Index of Orthodontic Treatment Need. (R. Evans and W. Shaw, 1987. Reproduced with kind permission of the Editor of the *European Journal of Orthodontics*.)

dentist together rate the appearance of the dentition using the photographs as a guideline. Grades 1–4 indicate little or no need for treatment on aesthetic grounds, grades 5–7 are borderline, and patients in grades 8–10 would clearly benefit from orthodontic treatment. It is, however, difficult to be truly objective when making judgements of this kind about an individual's appearance, and the Aesthetic Component has not achieved universal use because of its subjective nature.

Demand for orthodontic treatment is affected by many factors. Patients vary enormously in how they perceive their own dental appearance, some apparently being unaware of obvious malocclusions while others express dissatisfaction about very minor irregularities. Demand for treatment thus depends upon severity of malocclusion as perceived by patients and parents rather than by dentists. It is also affected by patients' attitudes to wearing orthodontic appliances, which are influenced by the appearance of the appliances and how acceptable they think appliance treatment is among their peers. Demand for orthodontic treatment tends to increase as appliances become more common and accepted among a population, but it is also greatly affected by the availability of treatment (geographic accessibility, waiting lists, etc.).

13.2.3   Referral for orthodontic advice

The referring dentist can give the orthodontist a lot of invaluable information.

Timing of referral

The right time for orthodontic intervention will vary according to the condition, but if specialist advice is needed it is better to refer too early rather than too late. The majority of orthodontic treatments are carried out in the late mixed and early permanent dentition, but some conditions may be treated earlier (see section 13.4), and some treatments, such as functional appliances, depend on active facial growth and should not be delayed too long before starting.

Patient and family attitudes

In many cases the dentist will have known the family for some time, and will know their level of dental awareness, their degree of concern about the malocclusion and their attendance record. This information can be difficult for the orthodontist to pick up during one or two short consultations, but is vital when assessing the likely compliance with orthodontic treatment.

Oral hygiene

Appliance therapy is inappropriate for patients whose oral hygiene is poor and in general this should be improved before referring for orthodontic treatment. However, this should not be at the expense of excessive delay in referring those patients with more severe malocclusions who may gain some benefit from simple interceptive measures.

Prognosis of teeth

The family dentist is in a much better position than the orthodontist to estimate the prognosis of restored or traumatized teeth.

Radiographs

Any relevant radiographs should be forwarded with the referral to avoid unnecessary repetition.

Key Points

Screening:
- all children should be screened for malocclusion from 8 years of age
- need for treatment is judged using Index of Treatment Need (IOTN): dental health and aesthetics
- check the oral hygiene and attitude to treatment
- refer in good time and give as much background information as possible

---

13.3   EXTRACTIONS IN THE MIXED DENTITION

The extraction of teeth in children may be needed as part of orthodontic treatment, or may be necessary because of caries, trauma, or developmental anomalies. The extraction of teeth in the mixed dentition for purely orthodontic reasons, usually crowding, can sometimes be helpful, but managing the enforced extraction of carious or poor quality teeth is a matter of damage limitation.

13.3.1 Extraction of primary teeth

In general, where a child has a tendency to dental crowding, the extraction of primary teeth will worsen this as it allows the adjacent teeth to drift into the resulting space. Usually, it is the teeth distal to the extraction which migrate forwards as a result of mesial drift. This drifting is generally unhelpful where the extraction is enforced, but in some situations it can be harnessed to help with the management of dental crowding.

As there is a significant increase in the size of the arches during the mixed dentition stage, decisions about treatment of crowding should be deferred until the permanent incisors have erupted for at least a year, usually at about 8 1/2–9 years of age. Where there is severe crowding, the extraction of primary teeth may be considered at this point as part of a programme of serial extractions, but where the crowding is mild the decision should be delayed until the permanent canines and premolars are erupting.

The term balancing extraction refers to the contralateral tooth in the same arch, while a compensating extraction refers to the equivalent tooth in the opposite arch.

13.3.2 Serial extraction

Serial extraction is a form of interceptive orthodontic treatment which aims to relieve crowding at an early stage so that the permanent teeth can erupt into good alignment, thus reducing or avoiding the need for later appliance therapy. It consists of a planned sequence of extractions:

1. *Primary canines* — extracted as the permanent lateral incisors erupt to allow them space to align.
2. *First primary molars* — about 1 year later, or when the roots of the first primary molars are half resorbed or more, to encourage eruption of the first premolars. In the lower arch these often tend to erupt after the canines.
3. *First premolars* — on eruption to make space for the eruption of the permanent canines into alignment.

In effect, the extraction of primary canines transfers the crowding from the incisors to the canine regions where it is more easily treated by extracting the first premolars (Fig. 13.2). It is essential to carry out a full orthodontic assessment before embarking on a course of serial extractions. The indications for serial extraction are:

(1) significant incisor crowding;
(2) patient aged about 9 years;
(3) class I occlusion without a deep overbite;
(4) all permanent teeth present;
(5) first permanent molars in good condition.

The intended advantage of serial extraction is to minimize or eliminate the need for appliances to align the arches after the permanent teeth have erupted. Sometimes this is very successful (Fig. 13.3), but the results can be disappointing. Where crowding is severe it may be necessary to fit a space maintainer following extraction of the first premolars, to ensure that mesial drift of posterior teeth does not leave the canines short of space (see section 13.4.4).

The great disadvantage of serial extraction is the multiple episodes of extractions, starting when the child is quite young. These may well be a child's first

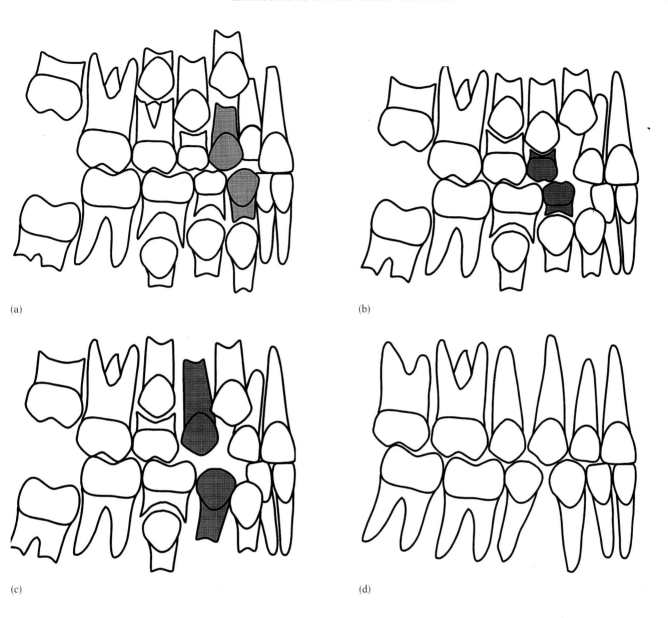

(a)

(b)

(c)

(d)

experience of dental treatment and might cause subsequent psychological problems with their attitude to dentistry, especially as the experience is to be repeated as the programme of extractions proceeds. General anaesthetics may be needed, and the likely benefit of the extractions must be considered very carefully in the present climate of concern about safety in dental anaesthesia. In practice, the extraction of the first primary molars is usually omitted, and the decision thus becomes whether the primary canines should be extracted. Extraction of these teeth might be indicated where it is clear that orthodontic appliances should be minimized or avoided for some reason, or where the crowding is obviously severe and is causing gross incisor displacement or cross-bite. It is also indicated sometimes to encourage the eruption of an ectopic permanent tooth (see section 13.5.4). However, it must always be borne in mind that the extractions will allow some mesial migration of the buccal segments, so increasing the crowding. The extractions should always be balanced by removing the contralateral canine to prevent a centreline shift, but it is not necessary to compensate by extracting the canines in the opposite arch.

Fig. 13.2 Serial extractions. (a) Class I occlusion with incisor crowding in the mixed dentition. (b) Improved incisor alignment following extraction of primary canines. The primary first molars are extracted to encourage eruption of the first premolars.
(c) First premolars are extracted on eruption to relieve crowding of the permanent canines.
(d) The result following eruption of the canines.

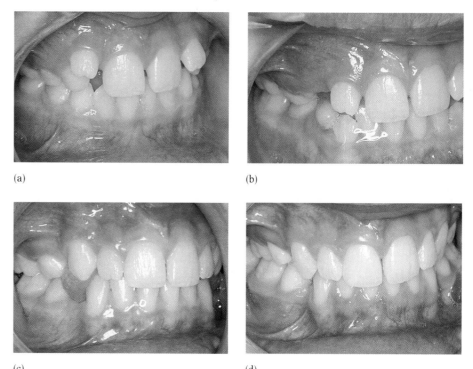

Fig. 13.3 (a) Class I occlusion with crowding of the lateral incisors in an $8^1/_2$ year old patient, before extraction of primary canines.
(b) Aged $10^1/_2$, 6 months before extraction of first premolars. Upper canines palpable in buccal sulcus, lower canines crowded buccally.
(c) Aged 13 — excess space in lower arch.
(d) Aged 15 — upper spaces closed, lower spaces reducing. (Photos courtesy of Mr T. G. Bennett.)

(a) (b) (c) (d)

13.3.3   Enforced extraction of primary teeth

The main complication of the enforced extraction of poor quality primary teeth is mesial drift of the teeth distal to the extraction space, causing crowding of the permanent successors. Mesial drift is greatest where there is a tendency to crowding, and it also becomes greater the more distal the tooth to be extracted is. It is greater in the upper arch than in the lower, as the upper permanent molars are distally inclined on eruption and readily move mesially by uprighting, whereas the lower permanent molars are mesially inclined on eruption and move forward less readily, but tilt mesially as they do so.

Extraction of *primary incisors* usually causes virtually no drifting of other teeth, but if done very early may delay the eruption of the permanent incisors. (Loss of a permanent incisor is a very different matter — see section 13.7.1.)

Extraction of a *primary canine* causes some mesial drift of the buccal segment, depending upon the degree of crowding. There is also drift of the incisors into the space, which causes a centreline shift towards the extraction site. This should be prevented by balancing the extraction with loss of the contralateral canine. In the same way the extraction of a *primary first molar* allows mesial drift of the teeth distal to it, more than with loss of a canine, and there may also be some effect on the centreline. Where the distribution of caries indicates loss of a primary canine on one side and a primary first molar on the other, these extractions can be regarded as balancing each other reasonably well and the contralateral teeth can be retained.

Extraction of a *primary second molar* allows significant mesial migration of the first permanent molar in that quadrant, causing potentially severe local crowding with displacement or impaction of the second premolar, especially in the upper arch where mesial drift is greatest (Fig. 13.4). How severe this is depends on the degree of crowding, and in a spaced arch the extraction has little effect. In principle, however, the loss of a primary second molar should be avoided if at all

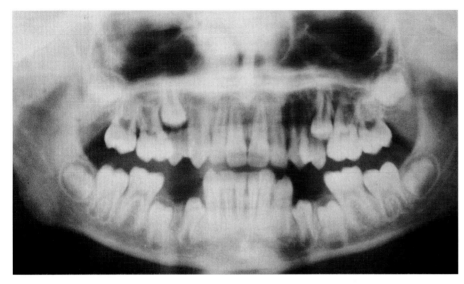

(a)

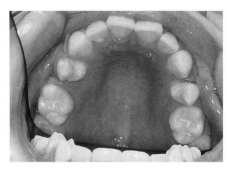

(b)

Fig. 13.4 (a) and (b) Localized crowding of upper second premolars due to early loss of primary upper second molars. (Photo courtesy of Dr J. H. Nunn.)

possible, especially in the upper arch. A space maintainer, either removable or fixed, can be considered, unless the patient's caries rate is high or the oral hygiene is poor. Primary second molar extractions should never be balanced on the contralateral side as there is very little effect on the centreline and the potential crowding becomes complicated even further.

In general, there is no need to compensate primary tooth extractions with extractions in the opposing arch.

Mixed dentition extractions: **Key Points**
- early loss of primary teeth generally worsens crowding
- extraction of primary canines may help incisor crowding
- benefit must be balanced against trauma of the extractions
- extraction of primary canines should be balanced on contralateral side
- primary second molars should be preserved if at all possible

13.3.4 Enforced extraction of first permanent molars

First permanent molars are very rarely the teeth of choice for extraction for orthodontic reasons — in practice their removal often makes treatment more difficult.

1. The space they provide is remote from the labial segments and is poorly placed either for relief of anterior crowding or for overjet reduction.
2. Depending on the timing of the extractions, much of the space is lost to mesial migration of the second molars, especially in the upper arch (see section 13.3.3).
3. The behaviour of the lower second molars is fairly unpredictable following loss of lower first permanent molars and is greatly influenced by the timing of the extractions.

In general, therefore, first permanent molars are only extracted if their long-term prognosis is felt to be poor, and the orthodontic management of these extractions aims to minimize disruption of the developing dentition. Where the loss of one or more first molars is necessary in the mixed dentition, the management of the extractions depends on whether or not the patient is likely to have active treatment with orthodontic appliances in the future — often a difficult judgement to make.

A panoramic radiograph must be taken to confirm the presence of all permanent teeth (except for third molars) before finalizing the extractions. The following discussion assumes the presence of all permanent teeth — if a premolar is congenitally absent then the first molar in that quadrant should be saved if possible.

Extraction of first permanent molars where no orthodontic treatment is planned

The objective is to minimize disruption of the occlusion. Following the extraction of a first molar, the paths of eruption of adjacent unerupted teeth alter, and erupted adjacent and opposing teeth also start to drift. Many of these changes are unhelpful but some can be used to advantage with careful planning.

In general, the most obvious change is mesial drift of the second molar, especially in the upper arch. However, in the lower arch some distal movement of premolars and canine may be also be expected, especially where the arch is crowded. The extraction of first molars can be a convenient way of relieving premolar crowding, especially in the lower arch. In the *lower arch* the timing of the extraction is important. If carried out very early the unerupted lower second premolar migrates distally, sometimes leaving a space between the first and second premolars if the arch is uncrowded (Fig. 13.5). If carried out late, as or after the lower second molars erupts, that tooth tilts mesially under occlusal forces and can cause an occlusal interference — especially if the opposing upper first molar over-erupts into the lower extraction space (Fig. 13.6 (a) and (b)). There is often residual space mesial to the tilted second molar and this poor relationship with the second premolar may cause a stagnation area. These unwanted effects can be minimized in two ways:

1. Extraction of the upper first molar — this eliminates the problem of over-eruption of the opposing first molar, and removes the occlusal contact which exaggerates mesial tilting of the lower second molar (Fig. 13.7 (a) and (b)).

2. Careful timing of the extractions — ideally when the bifurcation of the roots of the lower second molar is starting to calcify, usually at about 8 1/2–9 1/2 years of age (Fig. 13.8 (a) and (b)).

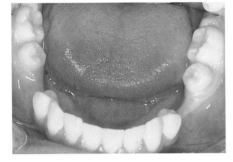

Fig. 13.5 Spaces between the lower first and second premolars resulting from very early extraction of the lower first molars.

Fig. 13.6 (a) and (b) Loss of the lower first molar after eruption of the second molars causes severe tipping of the lower second molar and over-eruption of the upper first molar.

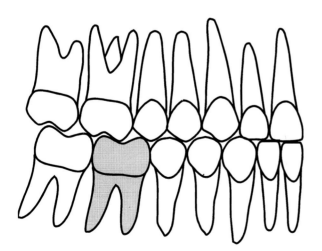

(a)

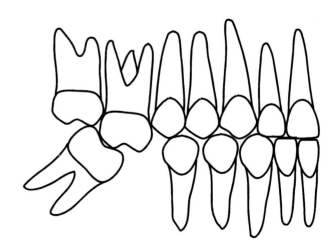

(b)

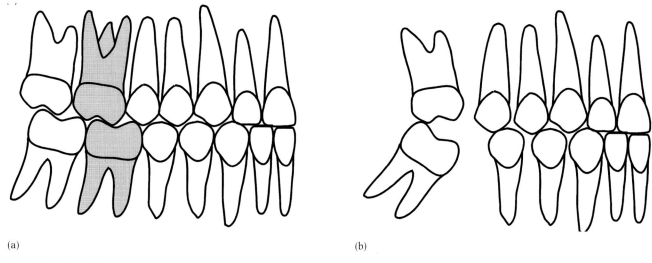

(a)

(b)

Fig. 13.7 (a) and (b) Extraction of the upper first molar as well as the lower prevents over-eruption of the opposing first molar, and reduces the mesial tilting of the lower second molar.

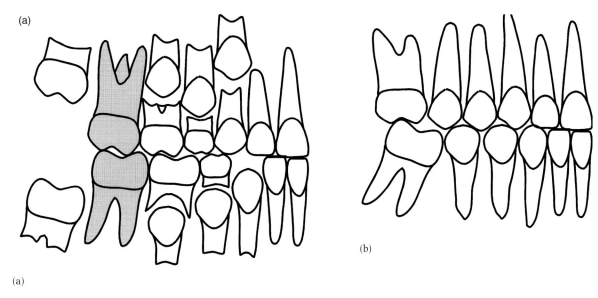

(a)

(a)

(b)

Fig. 13.8 (a) and (b) Extraction of the first molars when the bifurcation of the roots of the lower second molar is starting to calcify, usually age $8^{1}/_{2}$–$9^{1}/_{2}$ years, give the best chance of a good result.

In the *upper arch* the behaviour of the second molar is more predictable, although timing is still important. The tendency to mesial drift is much greater than in the lower arch, and there is almost no distal drift of the upper premolars. If the upper first molar is extracted early, the unerupted second molar migrates mesially so that it erupts into the position of the first molar. If the second molar has erupted before the extraction it still migrates forward, taking up most or all of the space depending on the degree of crowding, and it usually tilts mesially and rotates mesiopalatally about the palatal root. However, compensating extraction of the lower first molar is not indicated (Fig. 13.9 (a) and (b)).

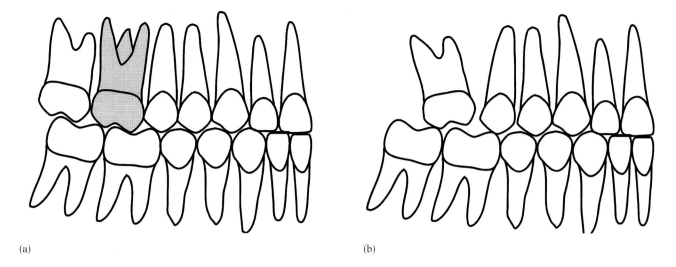

(a)   (b)

Fig. 13.9 (a) and (b) Extraction of the upper first molar does not need to be compensated with extraction of the lower first molar.

Balancing extractions of the contralateral first permanent molars are not routinely necessary unless they also are in poor condition. Where the arch is crowded an extraction on the opposite side is usually needed to relieve crowding and prevent any shift of the centreline, but if the first permanent molars are in good condition the extraction of first premolars may well be more appropriate.

Key Points	First permanent molar extractions: ● never the teeth of choice for orthodontic extraction ● best age for loss is 8 1/2–9 1/2 years ● extraction of upper first molar may reduce occlusal disturbance where lower first molar has to be extracted ● no need to extract lower first molar if upper first molar has to be extracted ● contralateral extractions depend on degree of crowding

Extraction of first permanent molars where orthodontic treatment is planned

Where future appliance treatment is anticipated, the objective is to try to avoid complicating it. It is difficult to give hard and fast rules as the management strategy will differ for each patient, but the main factor to consider is the amount of space which will be needed. Where the extraction space is to be used to relieve crowding or reduce an increased overjet, unwanted mesial drift of the second permanent molars must be minimized. On the other hand, where there will be excess space, mesial drift of the second permanent molars should be encouraged.

In the lower arch the extractions are managed according to severity of crowding. Where there is little or no crowding the extraction should if possible be carried out at the 'ideal' age of about 8 1/2–9 1/2 years, so as to encourage mesial migration of the second molar. Where there is significant crowding it is better to delay the extraction, if possible until after the lower second molar has erupted, so that the space is available for alignment of the arch.

The upper arch is also managed according to space requirements, but these are determined not only by the amount of crowding but also by the class of malocclusion. Where there is significant crowding the upper first molars should be preserved if possible until after the upper second molars have erupted and can be included in an appliance. Similarly, in a class II malocclusion space will be useful

Table 13.3 Management of enforced extraction of first permanent molars in the mixed dentition.
These guidelines are very broad and their application will vary greatly between individual patients. They assume that only one first molar is of poor prognosis, and clearly their application should be modified where more than one first molar is of poor prognosis

Extraction of lower first molar

1. Class I malocclusion
   Little or no crowding
   No appliance treatment planned

   Extract at 'ideal' age — 8 1/2–9 1/2 years. Usually compensate with extraction of opposing upper 6. Do not balance with contralateral extractions

2. Class I malocclusion
   Significant crowding
   No appliance treatment planned

   If possible delay until after eruption of second molars. Compensate with loss of opposing upper 6. Contralateral extractions usually required: 4's often better if 6's sound

3. Class I with crowding
   Later appliance treatment planned

   If possible delay extraction until after eruption of second molars. Do not compensate or balance with loss of opposing upper 6 or contralateral 6's

4. Class II
   Little or no crowding
   Later appliance treatment planned

   Extract at 'ideal' age — 8 1/2–9 1/2 years. Do not compensate with extraction of opposing upper 6. Do not balance with contralateral extractions

5. Class II
   Later appliance treatment planned

   If possible delay extraction until after eruption of second molars. Do not compensate or balance with loss of opposing upper 6 or contralateral 6's

6. Class III
   Both where appliance treatment is and is not planned

   Extract at 'ideal' age — 8 1/2–9 1/2 years. Do not compensate or balance with extraction of further 6's

Extraction of upper first molar

7. Class I malocclusion
   Little or no crowding
   No appliance treatment planned

   Extract at 'ideal' age — 8 1/2–9 1/2 years. Do not compensate or balance with extraction of opposing lower 6 or contralateral extractions

8. Class I malocclusion
   Significant crowding
   No appliance treatment planned

   If possible delay extraction until after eruption of second molars. Plan lower arch extractions on their own merits. Balancing contralateral upper arch extraction required but 4 may be more suitable if 6 is in good condition.

9. Class I malocclusion
   Significant crowding
   Later appliance treatment planned

   If possible delay extraction until after eruption of upper second molars. leave other extractions until ready for orthodontic treatment

10. Class II
    Little or no crowding
    Later appliance treatment planned

    Usually extract carious 6 and plan orthodontic treatment on its own merits. Do not compensate or balance the extraction

11. Class II with crowding
    Later appliance treatment planned

    If possible delay extraction until after eruption of upper second molars. Do not compensate or balance the extraction

12. Class III
    Both where appliance treatment is and is not planned

    Extract carious 6 and plan orthodontic treatment on its own merits. Do not compensate or balance the extraction

to reduce an increased overjet and, again, where possible the extractions should be delayed. If the upper first molar has to be removed earlier it is sometimes possible to start appliances before the upper second molars have erupted, but the treatment tends to be more complex, with headgear to move the upper premolars distally.

Conversely, excess upper arch space in a class III malocclusion complicates treatment, as proclining the upper incisors is a form of expansion which itself creates more space.

Clearly, where active orthodontic treatment is planned the loss of a lower first molar is not automatically compensated by the extraction of the opposing upper first molar.

The broad principles of management of enforced extraction of first molars are summarized in Table 13.3.

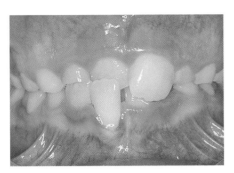

Fig. 13.10 Localized gingival recession associated with incisor cross-bite.

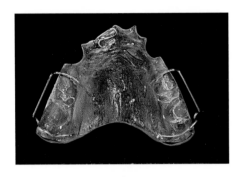

(a)

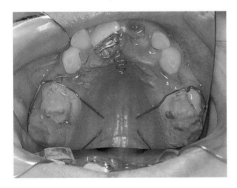

(b)

Fig. 13.11 (a) and (b) Appliance to procline upper incisor. Note posterior capping to disengage occlusion, and retention anterior to 6 | 6 to resist the displacing force generated by the Z-spring.

13.4   APPLIANCE TREATMENT IN THE MIXED DENTITION

The great majority of orthodontic treatments are carried out during the late mixed and early permanent dentitions, in order to avoid prolonged appliance wear while permanent teeth erupt. However, a few conditions can benefit from earlier intervention.

13.4.1   Anterior cross-bite

Although it may be a sign of a developing class III problem, a local anterior cross-bite involving one or two incisors is often simply due to the positions of the developing tooth germs causing the teeth to erupt into cross-bite. Possible complications of a localized anterior cross-bite include a premature contact with the tooth in cross-bite which causes the mandible to displace forwards as the teeth come into maximum intercuspal position, or one lower incisor in cross-bite may be driven labially through the supporting tissues, causing localized gingival recession (Fig. 13.10). Early correction encourages development of a class I occlusion, and treatment in the mixed dentition is often straightforward provided that these criteria are met:

1. *Normal skeletal pattern.* Treatment of frank class III problems should be delayed until the nature of the patient's growth pattern becomes clearer. However, it is essential to check for the presence of a forward displacement of the mandible, as this can make a normal facial pattern appear to be slightly prognathic.

2. *Adequate space in the arch.* There must be enough space to accommodate the tooth in alignment. In a crowded upper arch, space may be made for alignment of upper lateral incisors by extracting the primary upper canines (see serial extraction, section 13.3.2). This treatment must be started fairly early while the permanent canine is still high, because labial movement of the lateral incisor will be prevented if the canine crown is labial to the root of the lateral. It is therefore essential to palpate the position of the permanent canine crown, and, if it has come down too far, treatment must be delayed until the first premolars have erupted.

3. *Adequate overbite.* Stable correction of the cross-bite depends on there being positive overbite after treatment. Labial tipping of upper incisors with a removable appliance tends to reduce overbite, and specialist advice should be sought where lack of overbite is a problem.

There are many designs of removable appliance to correct anterior cross-bites and a typical example is shown in Fig. 13.11(a) and (b). Its essential features are:

1. *An active component* such as a Z-spring or a screw palatal to the tooth to be moved.

2. *Retention* as far anteriorly as possible to resist the tendency of the spring to displace the front of the appliance.

3. *Posterior capping* to open the occlusion while the upper incisor moves labially over the lowers.

13.4.2   Posterior cross-bite with displacement

Bilateral posterior cross-bites are often accepted as they usually reflect a transverse skeletal discrepancy and cause no functional problem. Where the upper arch is slightly narrow, the buccal teeth may initially occlude cusp to cusp and

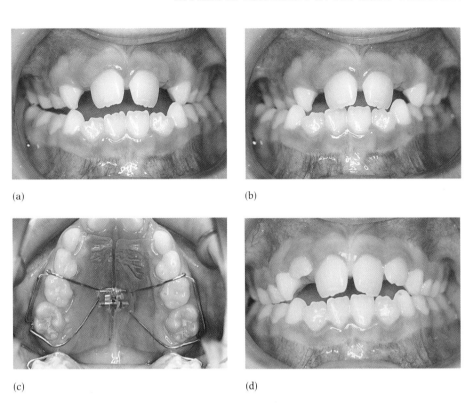

(a)

(b)

(c)

(d)

Fig. 13.12 Unilateral posterior cross-bite with lateral mandibular displacement: (a) initial contact on closure; (b) lateral displacement of the mandible on closure into maximum intercuspal position, causing unilateral posterior cross-bite; (c) upper expansion appliance; (d) displacement has been eliminated after upper arch expansion.

only achieve full intercuspation when the mandible displaces laterally (Fig. 13.12 (a) and (b)), causing a unilateral posterior cross-bite. This can be difficult to detect if the patient cannot relax the jaw muscles fully during examination, but it is important to determine whether or not there is a lateral displacement. A unilateral posterior cross-bite with a displacement is easily corrected during the mixed dentition, but one without an associated displacement is probably skeletal in origin and correction should not be attempted.

A unilateral posterior cross-bite with a displacement is treated by expansion of the upper arch to remove the initial cusp to cusp contact, using an appliance such as that in Fig. 13.12 (c). It has a mid-line expansion screw which is turned by the parent once or twice a week, and double Adams clasps on 6e|e6. The d|d are usually unsuitable for clasping as they have little or no undercut. The appliance should contact c|c as these usually need to be expanded, but need not contact the incisors unless a bite plane is required.

13.4.3 Increased overjet

The incidence of trauma to the upper incisors is greater where the overjet is increased, to the extent that among 13 year olds twice as many children with overjets of 10 mm or more have traumatized upper incisors compared with children with overjets of less then 5 mm. Boys are at greater risk than girls. Reducing the risk of trauma is a good reason for early reduction of a large overjet, even without cosmetic considerations.

In the mixed dentition this is usually done with a functional appliance. Details of the management and effects of these appliances can be found in orthodontic texts, but they induce correction of the incisor and molar relationships by a combination of dento-alveolar and skeletal changes. This is not done by active components such as springs, but instead the appliances harness forces generated by the masticatory and facial musculature. They achieve this by holding the

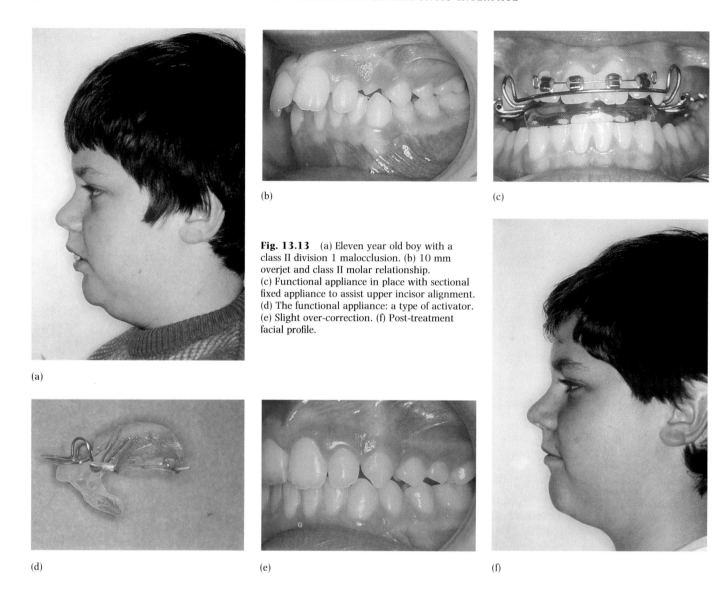

(a)

(b)

(c)

Fig. 13.13 (a) Eleven year old boy with a class II division 1 malocclusion. (b) 10 mm overjet and class II molar relationship. (c) Functional appliance in place with sectional fixed appliance to assist upper incisor alignment. (d) The functional appliance: a type of activator. (e) Slight over-correction. (f) Post-treatment facial profile.

(d)

(e)

(f)

mandible in a forward postured position, and all designs of functional appliance are similar in that they engage both dental arches and cause mandibular posturing and displacement of the condyles within the glenoid fossae (Fig. 13.13 (a)–(f)).

Functional appliances have two main limitations: they only work in growing children, most effectively during rapid growth; and, while they change the occlusion between the arches, they cannot treat irregularities of arch alignment such as crowding.

In practice these limitations mean that functional appliance treatment can become very lengthy when started early. Progress can be slow in prepubertal children because of their relatively slow growth rate, and dwindling co-operation with these demanding appliances can become a real problem during prolonged treatments. The appliance should be worn as a retainer until after the pubertal growth spurt, which in boys may be 15 or 16 years of age — a long time if treatment started at the age of 9. Treatment for crowding can usually only begin after the premolars start to erupt, and the patient effectively has two courses of treatment — one to reduce the overjet and one to align the arches. A potential difficulty of this approach is that the overjet reduction must be retained while the crowding is being treated, which can make management complex.

Early treatment is often justifiable for patients with severe overjets, but the possible disadvantages must be balanced carefully against the potential benefits.

13.4.4 Space maintenance

It is often important that drifting of teeth into an extraction space is prevented, such as: following loss of a primary molar (section 13.3.3); following loss of an upper incisor (section 13.7.2); where the crowding is severe enough that extractions give only just enough space.

In these situations a space maintainer is indicated. In the upper arch this can be a simple acrylic appliance with clasps, but in the lower a lingual arch is better tolerated (Fig. 13.14 (a) and (b)).

13.4.5 Digit sucking habits

Thumb and finger sucking habits which persist into the mixed dentition may cause: anterior open bite; increased overjet; unilateral posterior cross-bite with displacement.

A unilateral posterior cross-bite can occur because during digit sucking the tongue position is low, allowing activity of the buccal musculature to narrow the upper arch slightly (see section 13.4.2).

Although a few children continue the habit into their teenage years, nearly all grow out of it by about 10 years of age. An anterior open bite caused by a sucking habit (Fig. 13.15 (a) and (b)) will usually then resolve, but it may persist and require treatment if the tongue has adapted to the open bite by contacting

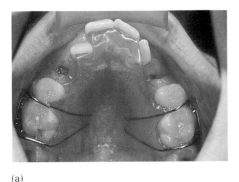

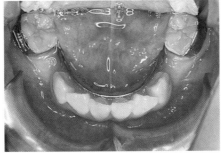

(a)   (b)

Fig. 13.14 (a) Simple upper removable appliance maintaining space following extraction of 4 | 4 while 3 | 3 erupt. (b) Lower lingual arch serving as a space maintainer.

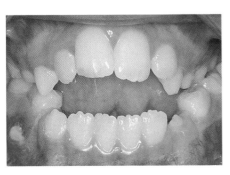

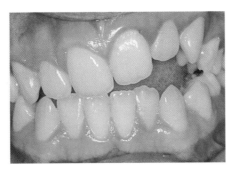

(a)   (b)

Fig. 13.15 (a) Nine year old child with anterior open bite associated with thumb sucking. (b) Sixteen year old girl with continuing digit sucking habit causing localized open bite.

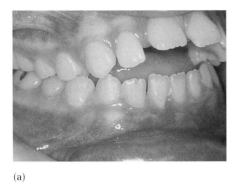

(a)

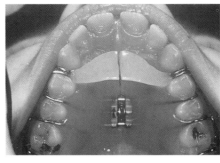

(b)

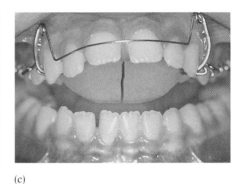

(c)

Fig. 13.16 (a) Twelve year old girl whose digit sucking habit has caused anterior open bite and increased overjet. (b) and (c) Split plate with steep anterior bite plane to break the habit while the overjet is being reduced.

the lower lip to make an anterior seal during swallowing. Correction of an increased overjet or a posterior cross-bite will need active treatment, and in most cases the presence of an appliance in the mouth finally breaks the habit. For these reasons a sucking habit in a young child is rarely a cause for concern, and parents can be reassured that drastic measures to stop the habit are unnecessary.

'Habit-breaking' appliances are thus rarely indicated and do not always work, but may be considered if the effect on the occlusion is severe or if the habit is unusually persistent. There are many designs of habit-breakers, some quite barbaric, but a common one is an upper removable appliance with a steeply inclined anterior bite plane (Fig. 13.16 (a)–(c)). The mid-line split in the acrylic of an expansion appliance may also help by breaking the suction.

13.4.6   Incisor spacing — mid-line diastema

This is mentioned only to point out that treatment just for spacing is rarely indicated in the mixed dentition stage. Parents are often concerned about spacing of the upper incisors, and they can be reassured that it will often reduce as the permanent upper canines erupt. It is, however, important to ensure that an upper mid-line diastema is not due to a supernumerary tooth (see section 13.6.1). A diastema may also be due to generalized spacing, diminutive teeth, congenital absence of upper lateral incisors, or to a fleshy upper labial fraenum. There is some disagreement about the role of fraenectomy in the treatment of diastemata, but it is very rarely indicated in the mixed dentition stage and is probably best carried out during active orthodontic treatment.

Key Points	Mixed dentition:
	• cross-bites with displacement may be treated in mixed dentition
	• treatment of increased overjet can become lengthy
	• persistent digit sucking habits usually resolve when appliance treatment is started
	• upper incisor spacing usually reduces as the permanent canines erupt
	• an upper mid-line diastema may be a sign of an anomaly of tooth size or number

13.5 ANOMALIES OF ERUPTION — THE ECTOPIC MAXILLARY CANINE

The path of eruption of any tooth can become disturbed. Sometimes the reason is obvious, such as a supernumerary tooth impeding an upper incisor (see section 13.6.1), but often it is obscure. In clinical orthodontics, the most common problem of aberrant eruption is the impacted maxillary canine, which is second only to the third molar in the frequency of impaction.

13.5.1 Prevalence of ectopic maxillary canines

Ectopic maxillary canines occur in about 2 per cent of the population, of which about 85 per cent of canines are palatal and 15 per cent buccal to the line of the upper arch. The risk of impaction of the upper canine is greater where the lateral incisor is diminutive or absent — the lateral incisor root is known to guide the erupting canine. An impacted canine can sometimes resorb adjacent incisor roots, and this risk may be as high as 12 per cent. Incisor resorption is sometimes quite dramatic (Fig. 13.17).

13.5.2 Clinical assessment

During the mixed dentition stage the normal path of eruption of the maxillary canines is slightly buccal to the line of the arch, and from about 10 years of age the crowns should be palpable as bulges on the buccal aspect of the alveolus. If not, an abnormal path of eruption should be suspected, particularly where eruption of one canine is very delayed compared with the other side. Unerupted maxillary canines should be palpated routinely on *all* children from the age of 10 years until eruption.

13.5.3 Radiographic assessment

Where the canine is not palpable it should be assessed radiographically. A periapical radiograph shows whether the primary canine root is resorbing normally and whether the canine follicle is enlarged. If the apex of the primary canine is not resorbing, with either no root resorption or only lateral resorption, the path of eruption of the permanent canine may be abnormal. However, a single radiograph cannot fully determine the unerupted canine's position relative to the other teeth. Two views are needed for this, either at right angles to each other or for the parallax technique.

Parallax technique

This method, also known as the tube-shift method, compares two views of the area taken with the X-ray tube in two different positions. Figure 13.18(a) shows a palatal canine on a periapical film being taken with the tube positioned forward or mesially. A second film taken with the tube positioned further distally gives an image which apparently shows the canine crown in a different position relative to the adjacent roots (Fig. 13.18b). In this case the image of the canine appears to have shifted distally when compared with the first film, that is in the same direction that the tube was moved, which indicates that the canine is palatal to the other teeth. An apparent shift in the opposite direction to the tube shift would indicate that the tooth is lying buccally to the other teeth.

The parallax technique works best using two periapical views, but with care it can also be applied to a panoramic tomogram with a standard occlusal view, using vertical shift (Fig. 13.19 (a) and (b)). The tube position is low down for the panoramic tomogram and much higher for the occlusal view, and so in this example the palatal canine appears to be nearer the incisor apices in the occlusal view, i.e. its apparent movement is upwards *with* the tube. The size of the image of a displaced tooth on a panoramic radiograph is another indicator, being enlarged if it is palatal and reduced if it is labial or buccal. However, a periapical view is still necessary to check for associated pathology, and can be used with the occlusal view to make another parallax pair. The combination of panoramic, standard occlusal, and periapical views, such as that in Fig. 13.19, allows comprehensive assessment of a maxillary canine.

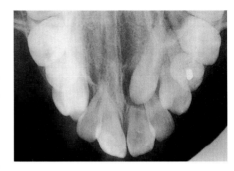

Fig. 13.17 $\underline{|\,3}$ causing root resorption of $\underline{|\,12}$.

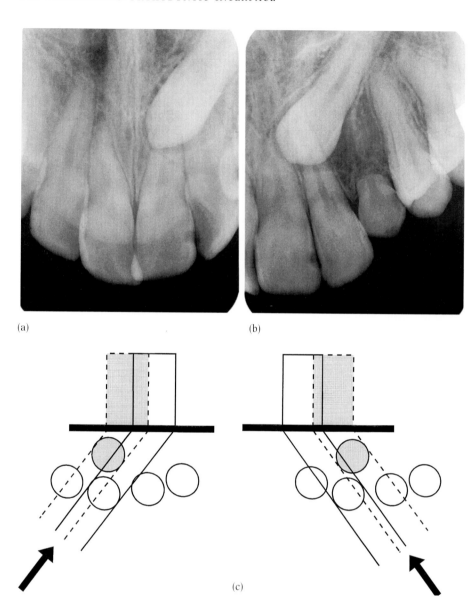

Fig. 13.18 Parallax location of ⌐3.
(a) Radiograph taken with tube positioned
forward shows image of canine crown is slightly
mesial to image of ⌐1 root. (b) Radiograph
taken with tube positioned further distally
shows image of ⌐3 is further distally. Image of
⌐3 has shifted in the same direction as the tube
shift: ⌐3 is therefore nearer to film than ⌐1,
i.e. it is palatal to the line of the arch.
(c) Diagrammatic representation of how a
palatally positioned tooth moves 'with' the tube
from left to right.

Two films at right angles

This method is more applicable to the specialist as it involves a taking lateral skull
view and a postero-anterior (p-a) view, possibly a p-a skull but more commonly
using a panoramic radiograph for the same purpose (Fig. 13.20 (a) and (b)). The
lateral skull view shows whether the canine crown is buccal or palatal to the
incisor roots, and the p-a or panoramic view shows how close it is to the mid-line.
The angulation of the tooth and its vertical position are assessed using both views.
An intra-oral view must also be taken to check for any associated pathology.

   The position of the impacted canine's crown should be determined as being
buccal, palatal, or in the line of the arch. The degree of displacement should be
assessed horizontally, that is how close it is to the mid-line, in terms of how far it
overlaps the roots of the incisors. The canine crown's vertical position is assessed
relative to the incisor apices. An estimate should also be made of the tooth's
angulation and the position of its apex relative to the line of the arch.

   Other radiographic signs which may suggest an abnormal path of eruption are
obvious asymmetry between the positions of the two upper canines, lack of

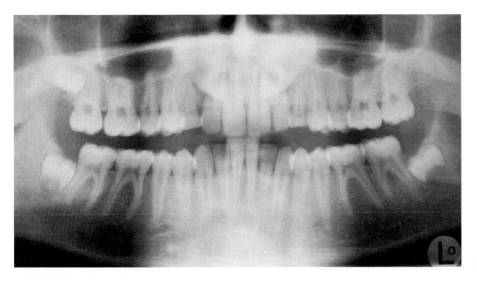

(a)

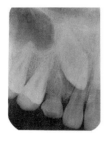

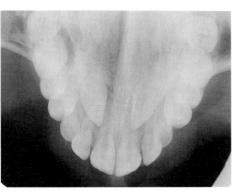

(b)

Fig. 13.19 (a) and (b) This combination of views allows use of vertical and horizontal parallax to assess ectopic canines.

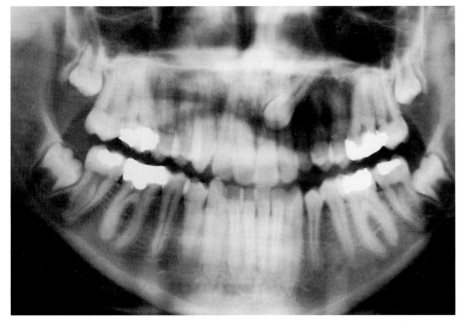

(a)

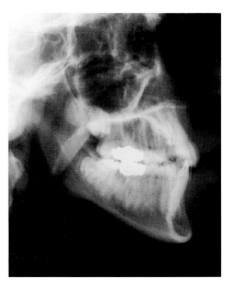

(b)

Fig. 13.20 (a) The panoramic view shows that the crown of the 3⌋ is close to the mid-line. (b) The lateral view shows that it is palatal to the roots of the incisors.

resorption of the root of the primary canine on the affected side (Fig. 13.19), and resorption of permanent incisor roots (Fig. 13.17). If there are signs of incisor resorption, urgent advice and treatment should be sought.

13.5.4 Early treatment

During the later mixed dentition, if an upper canine is not palpable normally and is found to be ectopic, extraction of the primary canine has a good chance of correcting or improving the path of eruption of the permanent canine provided it is not too severely displaced. Extraction of the primary canine is only appropriate under these conditions:

(1) early detection — mixed dentition;
(2) canine crown overlap of no more than half the width of the adjacent incisor root;
(3) canine crown no higher than the apex of the adjacent incisor root;
(4) angle of 30° or less between the canine's long axis and the mid-sagittal plane;
(5) reasonable space available in the arch — no more than moderate crowding.

Unless the upper arch is spaced, the contralateral primary canine should also be removed to prevent the upper centreline shifting. Eruption of the permanent canine should be monitored clinically and if necessary radiographically, and specialist advice sought if it fails to show reasonable improvement after a year.

The main disadvantage of extracting the primary canine is losing the option of retaining it if the permanent canine fails to erupt. It may also allow forward drift of the upper buccal teeth where there is a tendency to crowding, and if space is critical a space maintainer should be fitted.

13.5.5 Later treatment

The treatment options in the permanent dentition are:

(1) expose the canine and align it orthodontically;
(2) transplant the canine;
(3) extract the canine;
(4) leave the impacted canine *in situ*.

Exposure and orthodontic alignment

This is the treatment of choice for a well motivated patient, provided the impaction is not too severe. The canine should lie within these limits:

(1) canine crown overlapping no more than half the width of the central incisor root;
(2) canine crown no higher than the apex of the adjacent incisor root;
(3) canine apex in the line of the arch.

The tooth can either be exposed into the mouth and the wound packed open, or a bracket attached to a gold chain can be bonded to it and the wound closed. An orthodontic appliance, usually fixed, then applies traction to bring the tooth into alignment. This treatment can take up to 2 years, depending on the severity of the canine's displacement. Exposure works well for palatally impacted canines, but buccally impacted canines usually have a poor gingival contour following exposure, even when an apically repositioned flap procedure has been used. For this reason some operators prefer to attach a chain to buccally impacted canines and to close the wound, so that the unerupted canine is brought down to erupt through attached, rather than free, gingiva.

Transplantation

The attraction of transplantation is that orthodontic treatment is avoided and yet the canine is brought into function. Two criteria must be met: the canine can be removed intact with minimum of handling of the root, and there must be adequate space for the canine in the arch.

The major cause of failure is root resorption, but the incidence of this is reduced if the surgical technique is atraumatic and the transplanted tooth is root-filled with calcium hydroxide shortly after surgery. The success rate for canine transplantation is about 70 per cent survival at 5 years, but many clinicians regard it as being appropriate in only a few cases.

Extraction of the permanent canine

This is appropriate if the position of the canine puts it beyond orthodontic correction, or if the patient does not want appliance treatment. If present the primary canine can be left *in situ*, and although the prognosis is unpredictable, a canine with a good root may last for many years. When it is eventually lost a prosthesis will be needed, and provision of this can be difficult if the overbite is deep — another factor to be taken into account when considering treatment options.

Extraction of the permanent canine may also be considered where the lateral incisor and premolar are in contact, giving a good appearance. In this case it is often expedient to accept the erupted teeth and extract the canine.

Leaving the unerupted canine *in situ*

There is a risk of resorption of adjacent incisor roots, and annual radiographic review is necessary. The onset of root resorption can be quite rapid, and most authorities advise that impacted canines should be removed. There may be a case for retaining the canine in the short term in a younger patient, in case they have a change of heart about orthodontic treatment to align it.

Key Points

Ectopic canines:
- About 2 per cent of children have ectopic upper canines of which 85 per cent are palatal
- Always palpate for upper canines from age 10 until eruption
- Upper canines which are not palpable should be located radiographically or referred for investigation
- Consider extraction of primary canine if permanent canine is *mildly* displaced
- Untreated unerupted permanent canines may resorb incisor roots and should be radiographed annually

13.5.6 Other anomalies of eruption

Three other anomalies of eruption are fairly common in the mixed dentition.

1. *Infra-occluded primary teeth* (Chapter 12) usually exfoliate provided that the permanent successors are present, but should be kept under review. If they are not shed and eruption of the permanent tooth is seriously delayed, or if the infra-occlusion becomes very marked, then they should be extracted and a space maintainer fitted if appropriate.

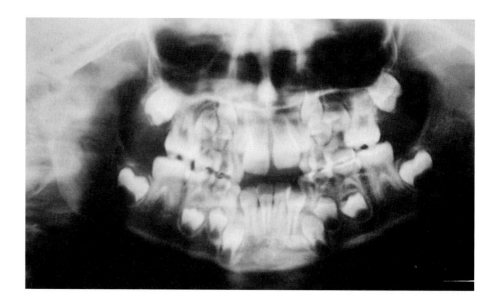

Fig. 13.21 Impaction of ⌐6 causing distal resorption of ⌐e.

2. *Impaction of the upper first permanent molar* into the distal of the upper second primary molar causing resorption (Fig. 13.21). It is possible to disimpact the tooth with an appliance, but the problem usually resolves spontaneously when the primary molar is shed. The resorption may cause pain if it involves the pulp, in which case the primary molar should be removed. This allows the permanent molar to move rapidly mesially, and a space maintainer or an active appliance to move it distally should be considered (see section 13.3.3).

3. *Second premolars* in unfavourable positions are sometimes seen as incidental findings on panoramic radiographs, but fortunately they usually correct spontaneously and eventually erupt satisfactorily. Very occasionally this does not happen and a few cases have been reported of a lower second premolar migrating towards the mandibular ramus. Upper or lower second premolars which are blocked out of the arch because of crowding usually erupt, but displaced lingually.

13.6   ANOMALIES OF TOOTH SIZE AND NUMBER

These anomalies are discussed in Chapter 12, but their clinical management often has orthodontic implications.

13.6.1 Supernumerary teeth

Supernumerary teeth are very common in the premaxilla, and can interfere with the eruption of normal teeth, or cause localized crowding if they erupt. In terms of clinical management, supernumeraries in the upper labial segment fall into three groups.

1. *Conical supernumeraries* are usually close to the mid-line between the central incisors (mesiodens), and are usually one or two in number. They are sometimes inverted, and their positions can range from having erupted to lying above the incisor apices. The majority do not prevent eruption of incisors, but may cause some displacement or a median diastema, in which case they should be extracted (Fig. 13.22). They should also be extracted if they erupt or if the adjacent

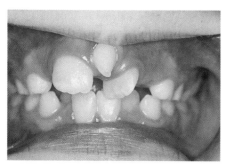

Fig. 13.22 Erupted conical mid-line supernumerary which has not prevented eruption of 1⌐1, but has displaced ⌐1.

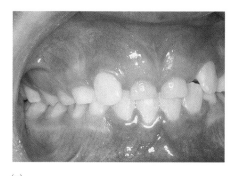

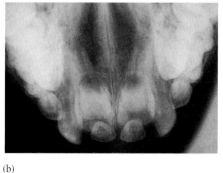

(a)

(b)

Fig. 13.23 (a) and (b) Failure of eruption of 1 | 1 due to the presence of two tuberculate supernumerary teeth. (Photos courtesy of Mr T. G. Bennett.)

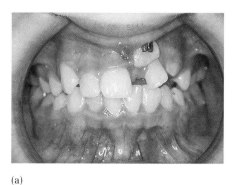

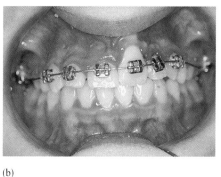

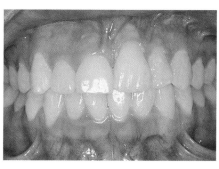

(a)

(b)

(c)

incisors are to be moved orthodontically. However, they can otherwise be left *in situ* if high and symptom-free.

2. *Tuberculate supernumeraries* are the main cause of failure of eruption of upper permanent incisors (Fig. 13.23 (a) and (b)). Early detection improves the prognosis for treatment, and a central incisor which fails to erupt before the adjacent lateral incisor should be radiographed, and any supernumerary teeth localized (see section 13.5.3). These should be removed surgically as soon as possible, and it is *essential* that the space is maintained or, if already lost, re-opened with an appliance. About 75 per cent of unerupted incisors erupt spontaneously within 2 years of removal of supernumeraries, and it is worth waiting for at least 18 months before considering surgical exposure. Even if the incisor has not erupted it has usually come down such that the crown is just sub-mucosal and only requires minimal exposure of the incisal edge, aiming to minimise loss of attached gingiva (Fig. 13.24 (a)–(c)).

3. *Supplemental teeth* of normal morphology cause localized crowding unless there is generalized spacing in the arch. Figure 13.25 shows a supplemental upper lateral incisor, and treatment consists of extracting one of the two lateral incisors in that quadrant. One is often smaller than the other and if possible the tooth which matches the contralateral incisor should be retained, but the severity of displacement and difficulty of orthodontic alignment must also be taken into account.

Fig. 13.24 (a) Surgical exposure of unerupted | 1. (b) Orthodontic alignment of | 1 — note poor gingival contour as a result of exposure. (c) Poor gingival contour persists several years after treatment.

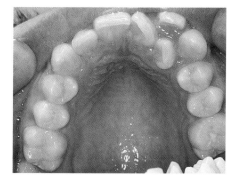

Fig. 13.25 Supplemental lateral incisor causing localized crowding.

13.6.2 Hypodontia

Any tooth in the arch can be congenitally absent but, aside from third molars, the teeth most commonly affected are lower second premolars and upper lateral incisors (Chapter 12). Where one or two teeth are absent the orthodontic options are to open, maintain, or close the space. Where multiple teeth are absent orthodontic treatment may be able to give a more favourable basis for restorative replacement.

Second premolars

Where the arch is aligned or spaced the primary second molar should be left *in situ*, but where there is crowding the space can be used for arch alignment. In the upper arch, and in a significantly crowded lower arch, the primary second molar should be retained until the start of orthodontic treatment. Where there is mild lower arch crowding which is to be treated, the primary second molar can be extracted earlier to allow some of the space to be lost to mesial drifting of the first molar.

Upper lateral incisors

Where one or both upper lateral incisors are absent in an uncrowded arch the excess space is often distributed as generalized anterior spacing (Fig. 13.26 (a)–(e)). An upper fixed appliance can be used to localize the space in the lateral incisor area prior to provision of bridgework. Some overbite reduction is often needed to create enough interocclusal space for the retaining wings of the bridge. The bridge should not be made for at least 6 months after removal of the fixed appliance, during which time a removable retainer should be worn which has wire spurs to prevent any drifting into the re-opened space. The bridge itself often acts as a permanent orthodontic retainer, and careful thought should be given to this aspect of its design. For example, if an upper canine has been moved distally, a fixed–fixed design ensures that the canine cannot relapse mesially. A cantilever design might allow relapse, causing the lateral incisor pontic to overlap the central incisor.

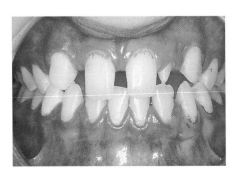

(a)

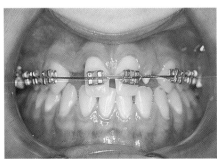

(b)

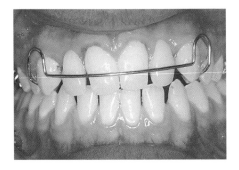

(c)

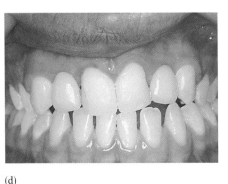

(d)

(e)

Fig. 13.26 (a) Spaced arch complicated by absence of 2| and very diminutive |2. (b) |2 to be extracted and fixed appliance opening space for replacement 2|2. (c) Removable retainer — note wire spurs to ensure space is maintained. (d) Adhesive bridges in place, and composite additions to enlarge 1|1. (e) Bridge design incorporates flexible wire for permanent orthodontic reten-

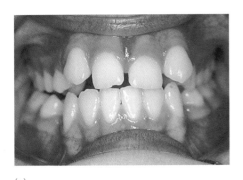 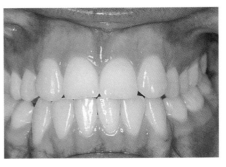

(a) (b)

Fig. 13.27 (a) Congenital absence of 2 ⫶ 2 where crowding tendency indicates space closure. (b) After alignment, with 31|13 in contact.

Where the upper arch is inherently crowded, the lateral incisor space could be closed. There is some debate as to the merits or otherwise of the resulting aesthetics, but it in general it seems unfortunate to extract a sound premolar in order to open space for a prosthesis, and in the long term the appearance following space closure is usually acceptable (Fig. 13.27 (a) and (b)). The quality of the appearance depends on the shape of the canine, but pointed canines can be made to look more like lateral incisors by reducing the cusp tip and adding composite mesio-incisally.

More severe hypodontia *with multiple missing teeth*

This often needs complex treatment. Preliminary orthodontic treatment can often help restoration by making the space distribution more favourable, uprighting tilted teeth and reducing the overbite. Fixed appliances are usually needed and orthodontic retention requires careful management (Fig. 13.28 (a)–(f)).

Supernumary teeth: • variations from the normal sequence of eruption should be investigated • supernumerary teeth which interfere with eruption of permanent teeth should be removed • the space for the permanent tooth should be maintained while it erupts • give the permanent tooth at least 18 months to erupt before considering surgical exposure • spacing due to congenitally absent teeth may be opened or closed depending on the degree of crowding	**Key Points**

13.6.3 Anomalies of tooth size

Anomalies of tooth size are discussed in Chapter 12. Any tooth may be affected, but the upper lateral incisor is most commonly involved.

Megadontia

If the upper and lower teeth do not match for size it is impossible for them to be both aligned and in normal occlusion. An abnormally large upper incisor is associated with crowding or increased overjet, or both. A grossly oversize tooth may have to be extracted and replaced with a pontic after completion of any orthodontic treatment. In milder cases it is possible to narrow the tooth by reducing the enamel interdentally. Up to 1 mm may be removed after the teeth have been aligned but before appliances are removed, so that the resulting spaces can be closed.

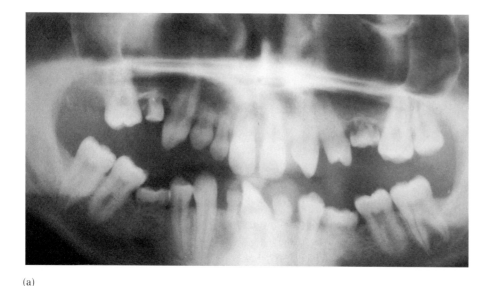

(a)

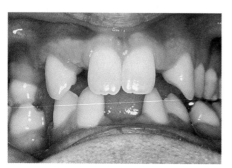

(b)

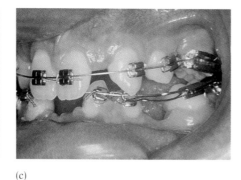

(c)

Fig. 13.28 (a) Severe hypodontia. (b) Note tilted teeth and unfavourable space distribution. (c) Fixed appliances to upright teeth and redistribute space. (d) Result of orthodontic treatment. (e) Initial retention with partial dentures incorporating spurs to prevent any orthodontic relapse. (f) Definitive fixed restorations.

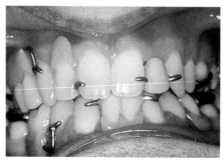

(d)

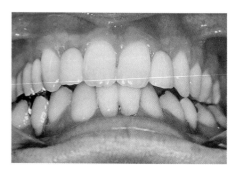

(e)

(f)

Microdontia

Upper lateral incisors are most commonly affected. Any orthodontic treatment should precede restoration of a diminutive tooth, and should leave adequate space for it to be enlarged (Fig. 13.29 (a)–(c)). The retainer should carry interdental spurs to prevent adjacent teeth from drifting into the space, and it should be worn for at least 3 months before the tooth is built up. Where the upper arch is inherently crowded but the lateral incisors are diminutive on one side and congenitally absent on the other, it may be appropriate to extract the diminutive tooth and close the spaces. This relieves the crowding and gives a symmetrical appearance.

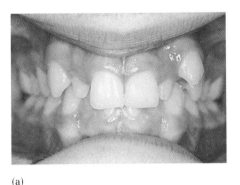
(a)

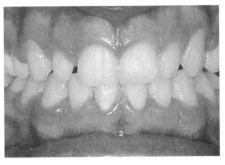
(b)

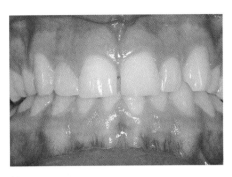
(c)

Fig. 13.29 (a) Patient with crowding and diminutive 2 ¦ 2. (b) Following orthodontic treatment to align the arches. (c) Diminutive 2 ¦ 2 enlarged with composite.

13.7 ORTHODONTICS AND DENTAL TRAUMA

Orthodontic brackets are often used as an immediate measure after trauma to stabilize loosened or reimplanted teeth, to realign displaced teeth, or to extrude teeth which have been intruded (Chapter 11). Teeth which have been fractured at gingival level may require extrusion later, to facilitate restoration.

13.7.1 Orthodontic considerations for the missing upper incisor

Upper central incisor

The space starts to close very quickly, within days of losing the tooth, and it should be maintained by inserting a partial denture *immediately* (Fig. 13.30). In a crowded arch it is often possible to move the lateral incisor into the central space, but the resulting appearance is usually very poor. Building up or crowning the lateral incisor to mimic the central is rarely satisfactory as it gives the tooth a very triangular shape, and it is difficult to maintain periodontal health around the enlarged crown.

   Where a premolar is to be extracted for orthodontic reasons it can sometimes be transplanted into the central incisor site, and then restored to mimic the missing incisor (Chapter 14).

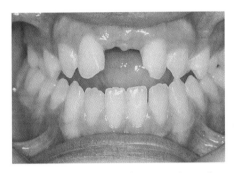

Fig. 13.30 Space loss following avulsion of 1 ¦ 1.

Upper lateral incisor

Lateral incisor spaces can be either maintained or closed, depending on the amount of crowding in the arch (see section 13.6.2).

13.7.2 Orthodontic movement of traumatized teeth

In general, root-filled teeth can be moved orthodontically quite normally, with no increased risk of external root resorption compared with normal teeth. The risk factors associated with root resorption during orthodontic treatment are discussed in section 13.8.3. Traumatized teeth, however, are already at increased risk of root resorption, especially those which have been displaced or reimplanted, and orthodontic treatment increases the risk further. In these cases the need for orthodontics should be assessed very carefully, but where it is needed the risk of resorption during tooth movement should be minimized by: (a) maintaining a calcium hydroxide dressing in the root canal during orthodontic treatment, and (b) ensuring that orthodontic forces are as light as possible.

   Fixed appliances should be used with great care as they can easily generate high forces, and treatment with them should be kept to a minimum. Functional appliances are useful for overjet reduction as they do not apply high forces to individual teeth.

A tooth which has become ankylosed cannot be moved orthodontically and will eventually be lost, but in the shorter term it will serve as a space maintainer unless the ankylosis causes excessive infra-occlusion.

Key Points	Trauma:
	• a space maintainer should be fitted *immediately* if an upper incisor is lost.
	• traumatized teeth may resorb during orthodontic treatment. This is minimized by putting calcium hydroxide in the root canal, and keeping orthodontic forces light
	• teeth of poor prognosis serve as useful space maintainers in the short term

13.8   COMPLICATIONS OF ORTHODONTIC TREATMENT

The most common problem with orthodontic treatment is lack of co-operation by the patient, which in some cases can lead to the treatment conferring no benefit or even making the malocclusion worse (see section 13.2.2). Four issues are discussed here which may concern the paediatric dentist.

13.8.1   Post-orthodontic decalcification

White spots of enamel decalcification are sometimes left after orthodontic treatment if the patient's compliance with oral hygiene and preventive advice has been poor (Fig. 13.31 (a) and (b)). The problem is greatest with fixed appliances, and decalcification is mostly related to areas of plaque accumulation around brackets, commonly involving the labial surfaces of anterior teeth. The lesions can develop very quickly, within a few weeks, and consist of some softening of the enamel surface with progressive mineral loss of the subsurface layer to a depth of up to 100 µm.

Prevention of the problem starts with careful patient selection, but if oral hygiene during treatment is poor, and especially if there are signs of decalcification, preventive measures should be implemented immediately, These include:

(1) regular reinforcement of oral hygiene (see section 13.8.2);

(2) dietary advice;

(3) prescription of daily sodium fluoride mouthwashes.

If the patient does not respond the orthodontic treatment should be stopped as quickly as possible, and it is often better to leave some residual malocclusion than to continue and risk severe damage.

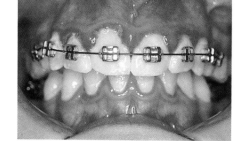 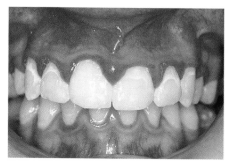

Fig. 13.31   (a) Neglected fixed appliance with associated gingival inflammation and enamel decalcification. (b) The decalcification is obvious following bracket removal.

(a)   (b)

If white enamel lesions are present on appliance removal, a daily sodium fluoride mouthwash should be started if not already in use. This encourages remineralization, and the chalky appearance and degree of opacity of the lesions usually reduce during the 3 months following appliance removal. The majority of lesions which remain unsightly respond to the hydrochloric acid-pumice microabrasion technique (Chapter 9), but severe lesions and those with surface breakdown may require localized composite restorations or even veneers.

13.8.2 Orthodontics and periodontal health

Fixed appliances

Gingival inflammation is a frequent complication of fixed appliances (Fig. 13.31), and the patient must be encouraged to maintain good oral hygiene. They must recognize that it takes longer to clean the teeth with fixed appliances than without. A standard toothbrush with a fairly small two or three row head is suitable in most cases, or special orthodontic brushes are available with a groove which is intended to facilitate cleaning behind the archwire. Some patients find interspace brushes helpful, especially for local problem areas.

Marginal gingival inflammation resolves when the brackets and bands are removed, and there is no evidence that orthodontic treatment causes clinically significant long-term damage to the periodontium (Chapter 10). However, excessive arch expansion or proclination of teeth, especially the lower incisors, should be avoided as there is a risk of fenestration of the buccal alveolar bone or even gingival clefting.

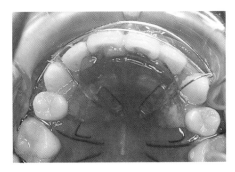

(a)

Removable appliances

Mild palatal marginal gingivitis is quite common under removable appliances, and resolves at the end of treatment. Good oral and appliance hygiene is very important, and the patient should take the appliance out to brush it and to clean the teeth at least twice a day, and to rinse it after meals. More widespread candidal infection occasionally occurs under the acrylic, but usually resolves if the patient wears the appliance part-time for a few days. Severe inflammation palatal to the upper incisors can occur during overjet reduction, due to compression of the tissues between the acrylic and the teeth (Fig. 13.32 (a) and (b)). This should be avoided by keeping the appliance under frequent review, and ensuring at each visit that enough palatal acrylic has been trimmed away to allow tooth movement.

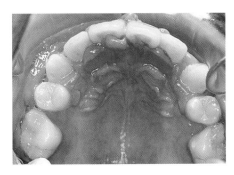

(b)

Fig. 13.32 (a) Upper removal appliance for retraction of the upper incisors.
(b) Severe gingival inflammation resulting from compression of the gingival tissues under the appliance during incisor retraction.

13.8.3 Root resorption

Most orthodontic treatments probably cause some resorption of root apices. In most cases it is slight, but significant apical resorption does occur in a few patients (Fig. 13.33 (a) and (b)). Any tooth can be affected but studies have focused on the maxillary incisors. The aetiology is multifactorial and individual susceptibility to resorption is very variable, but factors associated with increased risk include:

(1) history of trauma to maxillary incisors;

(2) signs of pre-existing resorption: short roots or blunted apices;

(3) thin, pipette-shaped root apices;

(4) prolonged use of fixed appliances, especially intermaxillary elastics,

(5) intrusive forces and torquing of apices;

(6) reduction of large overjets, other than with functional appliances;

(7) treatment to align impacted maxillary canines.

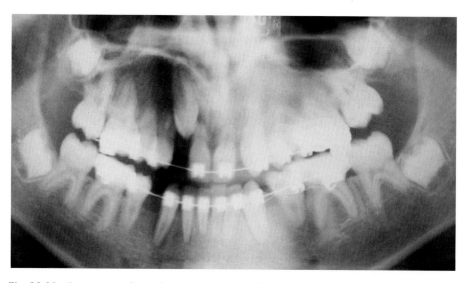

Fig. 13.33 Panoramic radiograph showing widespread root resorption during fixed appliance orthodontic treatment.

Orthodontic treatment for patients in the first three categories should be as short and simple as possible, keeping fixed appliances to a minimum and ensuring that forces are very light. Functional appliances avoid applying high forces to incisors during overjet reduction. Mild malocclusions are better left untreated in these circumstances.

13.8.4   Orthodontics and temporomandibular joint (TMJ) disorders

In general the presence of malocclusion is not associated with an increased prevalence of TMJ disorders. There is a slightly greater prevalence in subjects with malocclusions of the type which often have associated occlusal interferences, including class III cases, cross-bites, and open bites, but the correlation is weak. Even so, simple orthodontic treatment, often in the mixed dentition, to correct a crossbite with an associated mandibular displacement is well worthwhile. In older patients, orthodontic treatment to remove the interference can be complex and an alternative approach may be better, such as occlusal adjustment, unless treatment is needed anyway for other aspects of the malocclusion. Orthodontic treatment should always aim to leave the occlusion with no interferences.

It has been claimed that orthodontic treatment causes TMJ disorders, but at present there is no hard scientific evidence to support this view. Many forms of orthodontic treatment have been accused of inducing TMJ disorders, but premolar extractions have come under greatest attack. However extensive studies have found no evidence of increased prevalence of TMJ disorders in subjects who have had orthodontic treatment, including extractions, compared with untreated controls. Large prospective studies of this issue are currently in progress.

13.9   TEMPOROMANDIBULAR JOINT (TMJ) DISORDERS

Although several studies include children aged 5–7 years, most observations have been made on the young adolescent. A small number of temporomandibu-

Orthodontic injury:

● teeth with blunted or thin roots have greater risk of resorption during orthodontic treatment

● prolonged treatment with high forces increases risk of root resorption

● little evidence that malocclusion or orthodontic treatment are associated with temporomandibular joint disorderst

● no evidence of significant long-term periodontal disease

● daily fluoride mouthwashes reduce enamel decalcification

lar problems are associated with functional malocclusion (occlusal interferences) and morphological malocclusion such as cross-bite and anterior open bites, but bruxism and muscular hyperactivity probably play an important part in the development of TMJ disorders in childhood.

The commonest clinical symptoms in children and adolescents are clicking (10–30 per cent) and muscle tenderness on palpation (20–60 per cent). Clinical signs such as reduced opening, pain and movement, and tenderness of the joints on palpation are less frequent than in adults. There seems to be no consistent pattern in the development of either subjective symptoms or clinical signs during growth. Headache is common in children (girls more than boys) and its prevalence increases with age. The connection between headache, bruxism, hyperactivity of jaw muscles, and mandibular dysfunction is well recognized and should not be missed.

Children with TMJ symptoms and those starting orthodontic treatment should have a full examination of occlusion, toothwear, mandibular mobility, TMJ function and palpation, and jaw musculative function and palpation. One clinical symptom that has consistently disclosed the presence of a TMJ dysfunction is reduced opening.

Treatment principles used in adults can be broadly applied to children and adolescents after taking into account the dynamic changes in occlusion in connection with tooth eruption and facial growth. The majority of treatment is by activators and/or splints. Occlusal adjustment is not generally undertaken in the young permanent dentition as most occlusal displacement in growing individuals will change with time. However, selective grinding may be necessary when a direct causal connection is suspected. Jaw exercises may be difficult to motivate in children and adolescents compared with adults. Training of one or two movements against resistance is usually accepted.

The TMJ can also be affected by diseases or conditions which might influence mandibular growth. The most frequent are juvenile rheumatoid arthritis (JRA), traumatic injuries, unilateral hyperplasia, and congenital aplasia. JRA affects the TMJ in over 50 per cent of those with the disease. This causes destruction of the condyles and glenoid fossa leading to mandibular micrognathia, mandibular asymmetry, open bite, abnormal bite, reduced opening, and loss of muscle strength. Traumatic injuries involving the condyles can lead to abnormal growth and development and should be followed closely.

Unilateral hyperplasia of the condyle, although rare, may occur around puberty leading to cross-bite and mid-line deviation, as well as asymmetric jaw movements and tenderness and pain from muscles and joints. Congenital aplasia of the TMJ may occur in syndromes such as hemifacial microsomia and Teacher-Collins syndrome, and results in abnormal growth and function. Such cases require a combined interdisciplinary approach.

13.10   CLEFT LIP AND PALATE

Patients with clefts of the lip and palate commonly need extensive and specialized treatment, provided by a multidisciplinary team of specialists including plastic surgeon, orthodontist, paediatric dentist, speech therapist, maxillofacial surgeon, ENT surgeon, and others. Approaches to management vary greatly. It is not the purpose of this section to discuss the details of the condition or its treatment, for which the reader is referred to specialist texts, but rather to highlight the crucial part of the dentist in maintaining dental health throughout the prolonged period over which the treatment usually extends.

Management begins at birth with counselling of the parents, to reassure them, explain the likely course of events, and to give practical advice on feeding. Sometimes pre-surgical intra-oral appliances are fitted to try to reduce the size of the defect and facilitate surgical repair. The lip is repaired within the first few weeks or months, followed later by closure of the palate. The primary repairs are followed by a period of observation, usually in multidisciplinary clinics which are attended by the various specialists. As well as observing facial development, speech is monitored and corrective measures, such as speech therapy or palatopharyngeal surgery, instituted where necessary. These children often suffer middle ear infections for which ENT advice will be needed. As with all children, advice on preventive dental care should be given to the family and reinforced regularly.

A complication of surgical repair is that scar contraction in the palate causes narrowing of the upper arch. Sometimes this is quite dramatic, although modern techniques are reducing the severity of this problem. Orthodontic treatment often begins during the mixed dentition stage, at about 8 or 9 years, with expansion of the upper arch in preparation for a bone graft into the alveolar defect at about the age of 10 years. Grafting at this age provides bone into which teeth can erupt, particularly the adjacent canine, and greatly aids occlusal development. Clefts are often associated with other dental anomalies such as supernumerary, microdont, or impacted teeth.

Further orthodontic treatment, normally with fixed appliances, is needed when the permanent dentition has erupted. If this includes significant arch expansion, the patient will have to wear an appliance permanently to prevent relapse of the expansion. Secondary surgery to the lip and palate repairs may be needed, and if scarring has restricted forward growth of the maxilla, surgical correction of a class III facial deformity may be considered in the late teenage years after growth is complete. This usually requires orthodontic preparation to give a satisfactory postoperative occlusion. Finally, restorative treatment may be needed because of missing teeth or other defects, and often to provide permanent retention of the orthodontic tooth movement.

It is obvious that the success of all this treatment depends on the maintenance of a sound dentition over many years, and that the loss of teeth due to caries greatly complicates and hinders treatment. The dentist thus has a vitally important part in maintaining continuity of routine preventive and restorative care. It is well recognized that patient compliance with long and complex treatments dwindles, and unfortunately many patients with clefts, and their families, do not give routine dentistry a high enough priority by comparison with other aspects of their treatment such as surgery. An enthusiastic and supportive dental team must therefore play a central part in the multidisciplinary management of clefts of the lip and palate.

13.11 SUMMARY

1. All children from the age of 8 years should be screened for malocclusion.

2. Unerupted maxillary canines should be palpated routinely on all children from the age of 10 years until eruption.

3. A maxillary canine which is not palpable should be investigated.

4. Significant variation from the normal sequence of eruption should be investigated, e.g. upper lateral incisor erupting before upper central incisor.

5. Refer for orthodontic advice in good time and give as much background information as possible.

6. Good oral hygiene and co-operation are essential for successful orthodontic appliance treatment.

7. Consider orthodontic aspects when extractions in the mixed dentition are necessary.

8. A space maintainer should be fitted *immediately* if a traumatized upper incisor is lost.

9. Cross-bites with displacement may be treated in the mixed dentition.

10. Treatment of increased overjet in the mixed dentition can become lengthy.

11. Persistent digit sucking habits usually resolve when appliance treatment is started.

13.12 FURTHER READING

Andreason, J. O. and Andreason, F. M. (1994). *Textbook and color atlas of traumatic injuries to the teeth* (3rd edn). Munksgaard, Copenhagen. (*Comprehensive coverage of the management of dental trauma, including the role of orthodontics.*)

Houston, W. J. B., Stephens, C. D., and Tulley, W. J. (1992). *A textbook of orthodontics* (2nd edn). Wright, Oxford. (*An excellent introductory textbook*).

Isaacson, K. G., Reed, R. T., and Stephens, C. D. (1990). *Functional orthodontic appliances.* Blackwell Scientific, Oxford. (*A clear and thorough review of the role, management and effects of functional appliances.*)

Proffitt, W. R. (1993). *Contemporary orthodontics* (2nd edn). Mosby, St. Louis. (*A superb, comprehensive orthodontic textbook.*)

Okeson, J. P. (1989). *Temporomandibular disorders in children. Pediatric Dentistry* **11**, 325–9. (*A useful short summary on the subject.*)

Richardson, A. (1989). *Interceptive orthodontics* (2nd edn). BDJ Publications, London. (*A concise handbook of the role of orthodontics in the mixed dentition.*)

Shaw, W. C. (ed.) (1993). *Orthodontics and occlusal management.* Butterworth–Heinemann, London. (*An authoratative orthodontic textbook, including cleft lip and palate, and risk/benefit of treatment.*)

14 Oral pathology and oral surgery

14 Oral pathology and oral surgery

J. G. MEECHAN

14.1 ORAL PATHOLOGY

The incidence of pathological conditions of the mouth and peri-oral structures differs between children and adults. For example mucoceles are much more common in the young whereas squamous cell carcinomas are commoner in older individuals. The management of pathology in the child differs from that in the adult in that growth and development may be affected by the disease, or its treatment, and on a more practical basis anaesthetic considerations for surgical treatment of simple pathological conditions can make management more complex. This chapter deals with those conditions which occur exclusively, or more commonly in children. It is not an exhaustive guide to paediatric oral pathology for which readers should refer to oral pathology textbooks. Surgical treatment of the simpler conditions is discussed in the oral surgery section of this chapter.

14.2 LESIONS OF THE ORAL SOFT TISSUES

Conditions affecting the oral mucosa and associated soft tissues can be divided into: infections, ulcers, white lesions, vesiculobullous lesions, cysts, and tumours.

14.2.1 Infections

Infections of the oral mucosa may be caused by viruses, bacteria, fungi, or protozoa. Odontogenic infections will be discussed under 'oral surgery' later in this chapter.

Viral infections

Herpetic infections

Primary herpes simplex infection
This condition presents usually between the ages of 6 months and 5 years. Young babies are usually protected by circulating maternal antibodies. The symptoms, signs, and treatment are covered in Chapter 10.

Secondary herpes simplex infection
Secondary infection with herpes simplex usually occurs at the labial mucocutaneous junction and presents as a vesicular lesion which ruptures and produces crusting (Chapter 10).

Herpes varicella zoster

Shingles is much more common in adults than children. The vesicular lesion develops within the peripheral distribution of a branch of the trigeminal nerve.

Chicken-pox, a more common presentation of varicella zoster in children, produces a vesicular rash on the skin and intra-oral lesions, which resemble those of primary herpetic infection. The condition is highly contagious.

Mumps

Mumps produces a painful enlargement of both parotid glands commonly. The causative agent is a myxovirus. Associated complaints include headache, vomiting, and fever. Symptoms last for about a week and the condition is contagious.

Measles

The intra-oral manifestation of measles (Koplick's spots) occur on the buccal mucosa as white speckling surrounded by a red margin. They usually precede the skin lesions and disappear early in the course of the disease. The skin rash of measles normally appears first in the form of a red maculopapular lesion. Fever is present and the disease is contagious.

Rubella

German measles does not usually affect the oral mucosa; however, the tonsils may be affected.

Protection against the diseases of mumps, measles, and rubella can be achieved by vaccination of children in their early years.

Herpangina

This is a coxsackie A infection which can be differentiated from primary herpetic infection by the different location of the vesicles. These are found in the tonsillar or pharyngeal region and in addition herpangina lesions do not coalesce to form large areas of ulceration. The condition is short-lived.

Hand foot and mouth disease

This coxsackie A infection produces a maculopapular rash on the hands and feet. Intra-orally vesicles rupture to produce painful ulceration. The condition lasts for 10–14 days.

Infectious mononucleosis

This condition, caused by the Epstein–Barr virus, is not uncommon among teenagers and the usual form of transmission is by kissing. Oral ulceration and petechial haemorrhage at the hard/soft palate junction may occur. There is lymph node enlargement and associated fever. There is no specific treatment; however, it should be noted that the prescription of ampicillin and amoxycillin can cause a rash in those suffering from this condition and so these antibiotics should be avoided during the course of the disease.

Treatment of the above viral illnesses is symptomatic and relies on analgesia and maintenance of fluid intake.

Human papillomavirus

This is associated with a number of tumour-like lesions of the oral mucosa discussed below.

Bacterial infection

Staphylococcal infections

Impetigo may be caused by staphylococci and streptococci and can affect the angles of the mouth and the lips (Fig. 14.1). It presents as crusting vesiculobullous lesions. The vesicles coalesce to produce ulceration over a wide area. Pigmentation may occur during healing. The condition is self-limiting, although antibiotics may be prescribed in some cases.

Staphylococcal organisms can cause osteomyelitis of the jaws in children. Although the introduction of antibiotics has reduced the incidence of severe forms of the condition it can still be devastating. In addition to aggressive antibiotic therapy surgical intervention is required to remove bony sequestra.

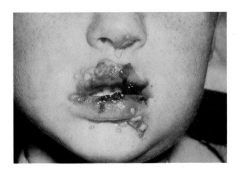

Fig. 14.1 Bacterial infection on the lip of an immunocompromised child. (By kind permission of *Dental Update*.)

Streptococcal infection

Streptococcal infections in childhood vary from a mucopurulent nasal discharge to tonsillitis, pharyngitis and gingivitis.

Scarlet fever is β-haemolytic streptococcal infection consisting of a skin rash with maculopapular lesions of the oral mucosa associated with tonsillitis and pharyngitis. The tongue shows characteristic changes from a strawberry appearance in the early stages to a raspberry-like appearance in the later stages.

Congenital syphilis

Congenital syphilis is caused by transmission from an infected mother. As well as producing oral mucosal changes such as rhagades, which is a pattern of scarring at the angle of the mouth. The condition causes characteristic dental changes such as Hutchinson's incisors (the teeth taper towards the incisal edge rather than the cervical margin) and mulberry molars (globular masses of enamel over the occlusal surface).

Tuberculosis

Tuberculous lesions of the oral cavity are rare; however, tuberculous lymphadenitis affecting submandibular and cervical lymph nodes is occasionally seen. These present as tender enlarged nodes which may progress to abscess formation with discharge into the skin. Surgical removal of infected glands produces a much neater scar than that of spontaneous rupture through skin if the disease is allowed to progress.

Cat-scratch disease

This is a self-limiting disease which presents as an enlargement of regional lymph nodes. It is caused by a *Rickettsiae bacillus* (Rochilamea Quintana). The nodes are painful and enlargement occurs up to 3 weeks following a cat scratch. The nodes become suppurative and may perforate the skin. Treatment often involves incision and drainage.

Fungal infections

Candida

Neonatal acute candidiasis (thrush) contracted during birth is not uncommon. Likewise young children may develop the condition when resistance is lowered or after antibiotic therapy (Fig. 14.2). Clinically easily removed white patches on an erythematous or bleeding base are found. Treatment with nystatin or miconazole is effective (those under 2 years of age should receive 2.5 ml of miconazole gel

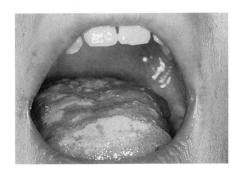

Fig. 14.2 Oral candidiasis in an immuno-compromised child undergoing chemotherapy for acute lymphoblastic leukaemia. (By kind permission of *Dental Update*.)

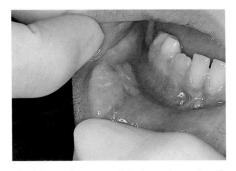

Fig. 14.3 Ulceration of the lower lip produced by biting while still anaesthetized from an inferior dental block.

[25 mg/ml] twice daily; 5 ml twice daily is prescribed for those under 6 years of age, and 5 ml four times a day for those over 6 years of age).

Actinomycosis

Actinomycosis can occur in children and may follow intra-oral trauma including dental extractions. The organisms spread through the tissues and can cause dysphagia if the submandibular region is involved. Abscesses may rupture onto the skin and long-term antibiotic therapy is required. Penicillin should be prescribed and maintained for at least 2 weeks following clinical cure.

Protozoal infections

Infection by *Toxoplasma gondii* may occasionally occur in children. The principle reservoir of infection being cats. Glandular toxoplasmosis is similar in presentation to infectious mononucleosis and is found mainly in children and young adults. There may be a granulomatous reaction in the oral mucosa and there can be parotid gland enlargement. The disease is self-limiting, although in severe infection an antiprotozoal such as pyrimethamine may be used.

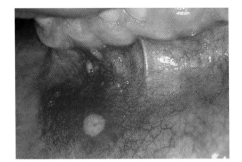

Fig. 14.4 Minor aphthous ulceration. (By kind permission of Wolfe Publishing.)

14.2.2   Ulcers

Traumatic ulceration of the tongue, lips, and cheek may occur in children especially after local anaesthesia has been administered (Fig. 14.3).

Recurrent aphthous oral ulceration unassociated with systemic disease is often found in children (Fig. 14.4). One or more small ulcers in the non-attached gingiva may occur at frequent intervals and in the young child the symptoms may be mistaken for toothache by a parent. The majority of aphthous ulcers in children are of the minor variety (less than 5 mm in diameter) which usually heal within 10–14 days. Treatment other than reassurance is often not necessary; however, in severe cases the use of topical steroids (adcortyl in orobase or corlan pellets) may be prescribed. Older children may benefit from the use of antiseptic rinses to prevent secondary infection. In the absence of a history of major apthous ulceration any ulcer lasting for longer than 2 weeks should be regarded with suspicion and biopsied.

14.2.3   Vesiculobullous lesions

Vesiculobullous lesions cause ulcers in the later stages of the condition. Viral causes have been mentioned above. Similarly, conditions such as epidermolysis bullosa and erythema multiforme can produce oral ulceration in children. The major vesiculobullous conditions such as pemphigus and pemphigoid are rare in young patients.

Epidermolysis bullosa is a term which covers a number of syndromes some of which are incompatible with life. The skin is extremely fragile and mucosal involvement may occur. The act of suckling may induce bullae formation in babies and in older children effective oral hygiene may be difficult as even mild trauma can produce painful lesions.

The oral lesions of erythema multiforme usually affect the lips and anterior oral mucosa (Fig. 14.5). There is initial erythema followed by bullae formation and ulceration. The pathogenesis of the condition is still unclear; however, precipitating factors include drug therapy and infection. Treatment includes the use of steroids and oral antiseptic and analgesic rinses to ease the pain.

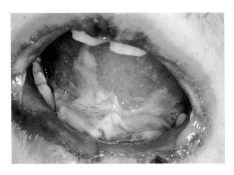

Fig. 14.5 Erythema multiforme in a teenager.

14.2.4 White lesions

Trauma of either a chemical or physical nature, e.g. burns and occlusal trauma can cause white patches intra-orally.

White spongy naevus

The white spongy naevus (also known as the oral epithelial naevus) is a rough folded lesion that can affect any part of the oral mucosa. It often appears in infancy. It is benign.

Leukoedema

This is a folded white translucent appearance that is found in children of races who exhibit pigmentation of the oral mucosa. It is considered a variation of normal.

Candidiasis

The white patches of acute candidiasis were mentioned above, and differ from the others discussed here as they are readily removed.

Geographic tongue

This condition may be seen in children. It is normally symptomless, although, some patients complain of discomfort with spicy foods. Areas of the tongue appear shiny and red due to loss of filiform papillae (Fig. 14.6). These red patches are surrounded by white margins. These areas disappear to reappear in other regions of the tongue. The condition is benign and requires no treatment apart from reassurance to child and parent.

14.2.5 Cysts

Mucoceles

The peak incidence of mucoceles is in the second decade; however, they are not uncommon in younger children (Fig. 14.7) and have even been noted in neonates. Mucoceles are caused by trauma to minor salivary glands or ducts and are most commonly located on the lower lip. They are the commonest non-infective cause of salivary gland swelling in children as salivary tumours are rare in this age group.

Ranula

This is a bluish swelling of the floor of the mouth (Fig. 14.8). It is essentially a large mucocele and may arise from part of the sublingual salivary gland.

Bohn's nodules

These gingival cysts arise from remnants of the dental lamina. They are found in neonates and usually disappear spontaneously in the early months of life.

Epstein's pearls

These small cystic lesions are located along the palatal mid-line and are thought to arise from trapped epithelium in the palatal raphe. They are present in about 80 per cent of neonates and disappear within a few weeks of birth.

Dermoid cysts

These are rare lesions of the floor of mouth. They appear as intra-oral and sub-mental swellings (Fig. 14.9), and are derived from epithelial remnants remaining from fusion of the mandibular processes.

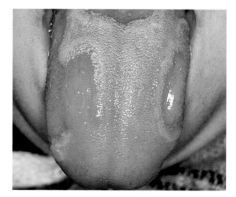

Fig. 14.6 Geographic tongue. (By kind permission of Wolfe Publishing.)

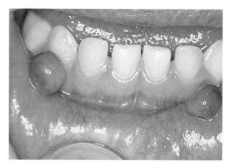

Fig. 14.7 Bilateral mucoceles in a 3 year old child. (By kind permission of *Journal of Dentistry for Children*.)

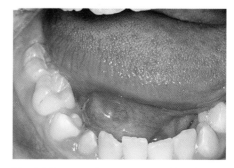

Fig. 14.8 A ranula in a 14 year old girl.

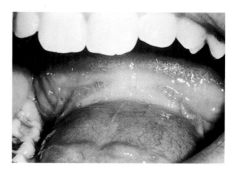

Fig. 14.9 A dermoid cyst.

Lymphoepithelial cyst

In the past this was termed branchial arch cyst as it was thought it arose from epithelial remnants of the branchial arch. They are normally found in the sternomastoid region, although can present in the floor of the mouth. Histologically, the cyst wall contains lymph tissue. The tissue of origin is now thought to be salivary epithelium.

Thyroglossal cyst

This cyst arising from the thyroglossal duct epithelium may rarely present intra-orally, but most arise in the region of the hyoid bone.

14.2.6   Tumours

Congenital epulis

This is a rare lesion which occurs in neonates and normally presents in the anterior maxilla. It consists of granular cells covered by epithelium and is thought to be reactive in nature. It is benign and simple excision is curative.

Melanotic neuro-ectodermal tumour

This rare tumour occurs in the early months of life usually in the maxilla. The lesion consists of epithelial cells containing melanin with a fibrous stroma. Some localized bone expansion may occur. The condition is benign and simple excision is curative.

Squamous cell papilloma

This is a benign condition which occurs in children. The small cauliflower-like growths which vary in colour from pink to white (Fig. 14.10) are usually solitary lesions and may be due to human papillomavirus.

Verruca vulgaris

This condition also known as the common wart may present as solitary or multiple intra-oral lesions and may be associated with skin warts. They are probably caused by the human papillomavirus.

Focal epithelial hyperplasia

This is a rare condition also known as Heck's disease. It is associated with human papillomavirus and presents as multiple small elevations of the oral mucosa especially in the lower lip.

Fibro-epithelial polyp

This is a fairly common lesion that presents as a firm pink lump. It normally affects the buccal mucosa at the occlusal level and trauma is thought to be the aetiological factor. They are usually symptomless unless further traumatized and are easily removed.

Fibrous epulis

This presents as a mass on the gingiva that varies in colour from pink to red depending upon the degree of vascularity of the lesion (Fig. 14.11). It consists of an inflammatory cell infiltrate and mature fibrous tissue, occasionally a calcified variant is found. Surgical excision is curative.

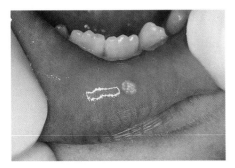

Fig. 14.10 Squamous cell papilloma in a 9 year old girl. (By kind permission of *Dental Update*.)

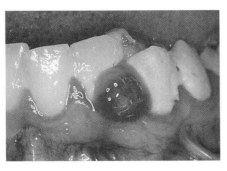

Fig. 14.11 A fibrous epulis in a 10 year old girl (a pyogenic granuloma appears similar).

Pyogenic granuloma

These commonly occur on the gingiva and are mostly found in the anterior maxilla. They are probably a reaction to chronic trauma especially from subgingival calculus. Owing to their aetiology they have a tendency to recur after removal.

Peripheral giant cell granuloma

This dark red swelling of the gingiva can occur in children. It often arises interdentally and radiographs may reveal some loss of the interdental crest. The central giant cell granuloma (see below) shows much greater bone destruction. This condition is thought to be a reactive hyperplasia. Unless excision is complete they will recur.

Haemangiomas

Haemangiomas are relatively common in children. They are malformations of blood vessels and are divided into cavernous and capillary variants, although some lesions contain elements of both. Capillary haemangiomas may present as facial birthmarks. The cavernous haemangioma is a hazard during surgery if involved within the surgical site as it is a large blood filled sinus which will bleed profusely if damaged (Fig. 14.12). The extent of a cavernous haemangioma can be established prior to surgery using either angiography or magnetic resonance imaging.

Small haemangiomas are readily treated by excision or cryotherapy. Larger lesions are amenable to laser therapy.

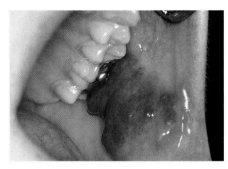

Fig. 14.12 Cavenous haemangioma of the right buccal mucosa. (By kind permission of Wolfe Publishing.)

Sturge–Weber syndrome

Sturge–Weber angiomatosis is a syndrome consisting of a haemangioma of the leptomeninges with epithelial facial haemangioma closely related to the distribution of branches of the trigeminal nerve. Mental deficiency, hemiplegia, and occular defects can occur. Intra-oral involvement may interfere with the timing of eruption of the teeth (both early and delayed eruption have been reported).

Lymphangiomas

Lymphangiomas are benign tumours of the lymphatics. The vast majority are found in children and the head and neck region is a common site (Fig. 14.13).

The cystic hygroma is a variant, which appears as a large neck swelling that may extend intra-orally to involve the floor of mouth and tongue.

Neurofibromas

These may present as solitary or multiple lesions. They are considered hamartomas and present intra-orally as mucosal swellings on the tongue or gingivae. Multiple oral neuromas are a feature of the multiple endocrine neoplasia syndrome, and as the oral signs may precede the development of more serious aspects of the condition (such as carcinoma of the thyroid), children presenting with multiple lesions should be further investigated by an endocrinologist.

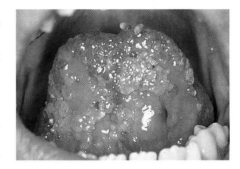

Fig. 14.13 Lymphangioma of the tongue and floor of mouth. (By kind permission of Professor C. Scully.)

Orofacial granulomatosis (OFG)

OFG is not a tumour in the true sense nor a distinct disease entity but describes a clinical appearance. Typically, there is diffuse swelling of one or both lips and cheeks, folding of the buccal reflected mucosa and occasionally gingival swelling and oral ulceration (Figs 14.14a and b). This may represent a localized disturbance due to an allergic reaction to foodstuffs, toothpaste, or even dental

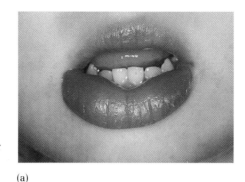
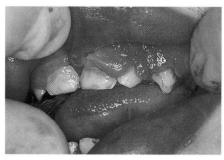

(a)   (b)

Fig. 14.14 (a) and (b) Swelling of the lower lip and attached mucosa and gingiva in a 3 year old girl with orofacial granulomatosis.

materials. Alternatively, the appearance may be due to an underlying systemic condition such as sarcoidosis or Crohn's disease.

Melkersson–Rossenthal syndrome

This is a condition which generally begins during childhood and consists of chronic facial swelling (usually the lips), facial nerve paralysis, and fissured (scrotal) tongue.

Malignant tumours of the oral soft tissues

Epithelial tumours

Malignant tumours of the oral epithelium such as squamous cell carcinoma are rare in children. Malignant salivary neoplasms are also rare, although muco-epidermoid carcinomas have been reported in young patients.

Lymphomas

Hodgkin's and non-Hodgkin's lymphomas do occur in children but not as frequently as other childhood cancers (Chapter 15). An exception is Burkitt's lymphoma, which is endemic in parts of Africa and occurs in those under 14 years of age; indeed in these areas the condition accounts for almost half of all malignancy in children. Burkitt's lymphoma is multifocal, but a jaw tumour (more often in the maxilla) is often the presenting symptom. Burkitt's lymphoma is strongly linked to the Epstein–Barr virus as a causal agent.

Rhabdomyosarcomas

These malignant tumours of skeletal muscle present in patients at about 9–12 years of age. The usual site is the tongue. Metastases are common and the prognosis is poor.

14.3   LESIONS OF THE JAWS

These can be divided into: cysts, developmental conditions, osteodystrophies, and tumours.

14.3.1   Cysts

Eruption

Eruption cysts are really dentigerous cysts (see below), which present as swellings of the alveolar mucosa. They may precede the eruption of both primary and permanent teeth (Fig. 14.15). When filled with blood they are often called eruption haematomas.

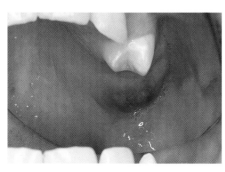

Fig. 14.15 Eruption cyst prior to appearance of upper permanent first molar.

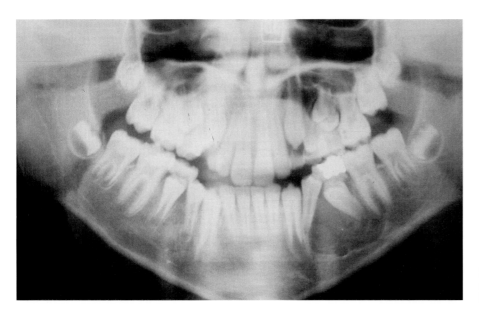

Fig. 14.16 Radiographic appearance of a dentigerous cyst associated with a lower second premolar. (By kind permission of *Dental Update*.)

Dentigerous

This is the commonest jaw cyst in children (Fig. 14.16). Its origin is the reduced enamel epithelium and attachment to the tooth occurs at the amelo-cemental junction. There are often no symptoms but eruption of the affected tooth will be prevented. Treatment of eruption and dentigerous cysts is discussed in the oral surgery section of the chapter.

Radicular

These cysts related to the apex of a non-vital tooth do occur in children, although they are rare in the primary dentition. They are often symptomless and are discovered radiographically. Extraction, apicectomy, or conventional endodontics will effect a cure.

Lateral periodontal cysts are very rare in children.

Odontogenic keratocysts

The odontogenic keratocyst is the most aggressive of the jaw cysts. It has a high rate of recurrence due to the fact that remnants left after subtotal removal will regenerate. These cysts may be found in children and may be associated with the Gorlin–Goltz syndrome. Keratocysts associated with this syndrome appear in the first decade of life whereas the syndromic basal cell carcinomas are rare before puberty. Other signs and symptoms include: multiple basal cell carcinomas, bifid ribs, calcification of the falx cerebri, hypertelorism, and frontal and temporal bossing.

Non-odontogenic

These include the nasopalatine duct cyst which may occur clinically as a swelling in the anterior mid-line of the hard palate and radiographically as a radiolucency of greater than 6 mm diameter in the position of the nasopalatine duct. The anterior teeth have vital pulps. Surgical excision is curative.

The so-called globulomaxillary cyst which occurs between the lateral incisor and canine teeth is now thought to be odontogenic in origin: either a radicular cyst, or an odontogenic keratocyst.

The haemorrhagic bone cyst is a condition that may be found in children and adolescents. It occurs most commonly in the mandible in the premolar/molar region and is often a chance radiographic finding and normally asymptomatic. Radiographically, it appears as a scalloped radiolucency between the roots of the teeth and regresses either spontaneously or after surgical investigation.

14.3.2 Developmental conditions

The number of developmental conditions which may affect the oral and perioral structures are numerous. They range from minor problems such as tongue-tie, which are readily treated under local anaesthesia or by day-stay anaesthesia, to cleft lip and palate which requires more complex surgery, and severe craniofacial disorders such as Crouzon's syndrome which require a combined interdisciplinary approach between maxillofacial and neurosurgery. Readers should refer to specialized texts for a full description of congenital jaw abnormalities. It is important to remember that patients with developmental orofacial abnormalities may have other congenital disorders such as cardiac defects which may influence routine dental treatment.

14.3.3 Osteodystrophies

Fibrous dysplasia

This can occur as one of three variants namely monostotic, polyostotic, or as part of Allbright's syndrome (where associated conditions include skin pigmentation and precocious puberty in females). The monostotic type is the most common to affect the jaws, especially the maxilla. The disease presents as a slow growing bony expansion which produces facial asymmetry and mal-alignment of teeth. Radiographically, there is a fine granular radiopacity (Fig. 14.17). Surgery can correct the asymmetry.

Cherubism

In this rare condition there is a characteristic fullness of the cheeks and jaws. Initial presentation is commonly between 2 and 4 years of age and size increases during growth. However, it is self-limiting and regression occurs in adulthood. Cosmetic surgery may be employed after active growth has finished. Multilocular radiographic radiolucencies occur at the angles of the mandible (Fig. 14.18) and the maxillary tuberosities and histologically the lesion is similar to the giant cell granuloma.

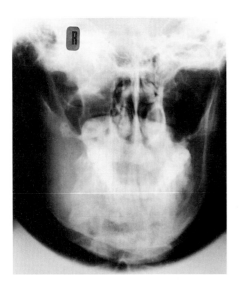

Fig. 14.17 Monostotic fibrous dysplasia of right mandibular angle and ascending ramus in a 15 year old boy.

14.3.4 Tumours of the jaws

Odontomes

Odontomes are hamartomas which contain dental calcified tissue. They are classified as compound (a collection of discrete tooth-like structures) and complex (a haphazard arrangement of dental tissue). Compound odontomes are most commonly found in the anterior maxilla (Fig. 14.19). The complex type are usually located in the premolar/molar regions of both jaws. Odontomes are usually symptomless and are diagnosed radiographically. The mean age of patients at diagnosis is 15 years. Occasionally, an odontome will become infected

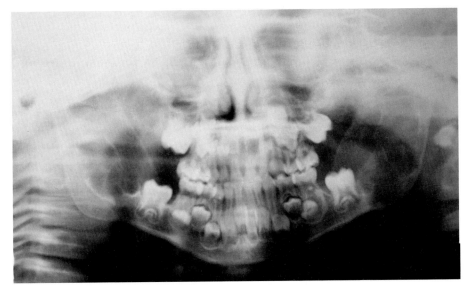

Fig. 14.18 Bilateral multilocular radiolucencies affecting the angles of the mandible in a 5 year old with cherubism.

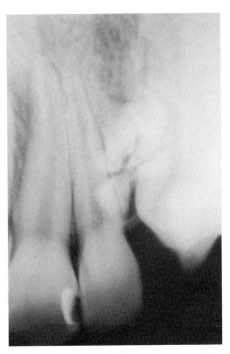

Fig. 14.19 Compound odontome in upper left canine region.

when partially erupted and surgical excision is required. Similarly, removal is indicated if an odontome is interfering with the eruption of a neighbouring tooth or as part of an orthodontic treatment plan.

Juvenile ossifying fibroma

This benign lesion differs from the adult ossifying (or cemento-ossifying) fibroma in that growth is rapid. It consists of fibrous tissue with a varying amount of mineralized material and normally affects the mandible. Radiographs show a well circumscribed radiolucency with 'speckling', and surgical excision is required.

Central giant cell granuloma

This swelling of bone usually affects the mandible (Fig. 14.20). Radiographically, there is a well defined radiolucency with occasional resorption of associated teeth. Histologically, there are large numbers of osteoclast-like cells in a vascular stroma. Surgical curettage is curative.

Histiocytoses

Langerhans cell histiocytosis, formerly known as histiocytosis X is a condition which predominantly affects children (Chapter 10). Bone is replaced by Langerhans cells producing sharply defined radiographic radiolucencies.

Ameloblastoma

Although more commonly found in adults this locally invasive neoplasm can occur in children. It is usually found in the mandible, is slow growing, and is often symptomless in the early stages. As it progresses it causes a bony swelling which appears as a multilocular radiolucency in the jaw. Surgical resection to sound bone is necessary for a cure.

Ameloblastic fibroma

This rare lesion usually affects a younger age group than the ameloblastoma. The average age of patients at diagnosis being 14 years. It is a benign tumour. A related lesion is the ameloblastic fibro-odontoma which contains dentine and enamel and occurs in children under 10 years of age.

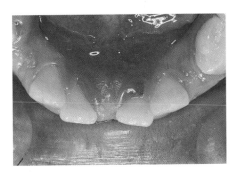

Fig. 14.20 Central giant cell granuloma in a 9 year old girl.

Primary intraosseous carcinoma

This is a very rare tumour but when it occurs it is usually in children. It is thought to arise from odontogenic epithelium and shows rapid growth.

Sarcomas

Sarcomas of the jaws are rare; however, the highly malignant Ewing's sarcoma occurs in children between the ages of 5 and 15 years of age. The mandible is usually the bone affected and the prognosis is poor.

14.4   ORAL MANIFESTATIONS OF SYSTEMIC DISEASE

In addition to specific pathological oral conditions, diseases that affect other systems of the body can present oral manifestations, for example Crohn's and coeliac disease. Other disorders such as chronic renal failure and diabetes can predispose to periodontal disease and there may be poor resistance to spread of odontogenic infection. However, not only the oral soft tissues are affected by systemic conditions. The temporomandibular joint can be involved in juvenile rheumatoid arthritis and the jaws can be affected in hyperparathyroidism (giant cell tumours).

In some cases an oral condition may be the presenting feature of a systemic disease and dental practitioners should not hesitate to refer children with abnormal oral signs for further investigation.

14.5   ORAL SURGERY

This section deals with dental extractions and minor oral surgical procedures for children. The procedures described are those which can be performed under local anaesthesia with or without sedation (normally inhalational) or day-stay general anaesthesia in healthy children. Oral surgery procedures which require in-patient facilities other than the treatment of severe infection will not be considered in this text.

14.5.1   Exodontia

Differences between primary and permanent teeth

1. *Size.* Primary teeth are smaller in every dimension compared with their permanent counterparts. Although the roots of primary teeth are smaller than those of the permanent dentition they do form a proportionately greater part of the tooth.
2. *Shape.* The crowns of primary teeth are more bulbous than the crowns of permanent teeth. The roots of primary molars are more splayed than the roots of permanent molar teeth. The furcation of primary molar roots is positioned more cervically than in the corresponding permanent teeth.
3. *Physiology.* The roots of primary teeth resorb naturally whereas in the permanent dentition resorption is normally a sign of pathology.
4. *Support.* The bone of the alveolus is much more elastic in the younger patient.

These differences mean that there are some modifications to extraction techniques in children. The type of forcep employed for the removal of primary teeth differs from that used for the removal of permanent teeth. The beaks and handles are smaller and to accommodate the more bulbous crown the beaks are more curved in primary forceps.

The wide splaying of primary molar roots means that more expansion of the socket is required for the extraction of primary teeth and the more elastic alveolus of the younger patient allows this to be achieved.

Owing to the relatively cervical position of the bifurcation in primary molars it is injudicious to use forceps with deeply plunging beaks (such as the adult cowhorn design) as these could damage the underlying permanent successors. This is especially so with the lower primary molars.

As primary roots are resorbed it is often preferable to leave small fragments *in situ* if the root fractures. When a proportion of the root fractures and it is visible then it should be removed. However, blind investigation of primary sockets should not be performed as there is a danger of damaging the underlying permanent successor. Similarly, blind investigation of the distal root socket of first permanent molar teeth must not be carried out in children with unerupted second molars as unintentional elevation of the second molar can occur.

Problems peculiar to the child patient

These will affect the way in which extractions are carried out.

Natal and neonatal teeth

Most neonatal teeth (85 per cent) are found in the mandible and only about 5 per cent of these are supernumaries (Chapter 12).

Infra-occlusion

Surgical division is usually necessary to remove these teeth (Chapter 12).

Fusion/gemination (connation)

Such teeth may not lend themselves to forceps extraction due to their unusual coronal shape. Elevators are usually employed with or without tooth division and bone removal, to effect delivery (Chapter 12).

Damage to permanent successor

This may occur if forceps with large beaks are used or during root elevation.

Dislocation of the mandible

It is very easy to dislocate a child's mandible during extraction under general anaesthesia (when the muscles are relaxed) unless adequate support is provided by the 'non-working' hand. This is because the articular eminence is not so pronounced in young patients as in adults. It is essential to verify that dislocation has not occurred before the patient is allowed to regain consciousness.

14.5.2 Extraction techniques

Patient position

The child should be seated in a dental chair reclined about 30° to the vertical for extractions under local anaesthesia. Under general anaesthesia the patient is usually supine. When removing upper teeth under local anaesthesia the operator stands in front of the patient, with straight back and the patient's mouth at a level just below the operator's shoulder.

A right-handed operator removes lower left teeth from a similar position in front of the patient except that the patient's mouth is at a height just below the operator's elbow. When removing teeth from the lower right the right-handed operator stands behind the patient with the chair as low as possible to allow good vision.

When performing extractions for the supine patient under general anaesthesia the patient's mouth is usually at a level just below the operator's elbow, once again lower right teeth are removed from behind with all others being extracted by the operator standing in front of the patient. It does save time during general anaesthesia if teeth can be removed ambidexterously as all teeth can be extracted with the operator standing in front of the patient. The removal of primary teeth with the non-dominant hand is not difficult to master and is a useful skill to acquire.

The non-working hand

The sections below describe the instruments and technique used by the operator's working hand. However, the 'non-working' hand also has an important part to play (Fig. 14.21). This hand:

(1) retracts soft tissues to allow visibility and access;
(2) protects the tissues if the instrument slips;
(3) provides resistance to the extraction force on the mandible to prevent dislocation;
(4) provides 'feel' to the operator during the extraction and gives information about resistance to removal.

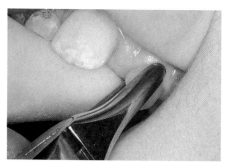

Fig. 14.21   The non-working hand supports the tooth for extraction and reflects the soft tissues.

Order of extraction

When performing multiple extractions in all quadrants of the mouth (especially if under general anaesthesia) the order of extraction is as follows:

(1) symptomatic teeth before 'balancing extractions' on the opposite side;
2) lower teeth before upper teeth (to eliminate bleeding interfering with the surgical field);
(3) if there are symptomatic teeth in all quadrants a right-handed operator should begin with lower right extractions as this minimizes the number of changes of position of the surgeon which will reduce general anaesthetic time.

Upper primary and permanent anteriors

When these teeth are in a normal position in the dental arch they should be removed by application of the forceps beaks to the root and then using clockwise and anticlockwise rotations about the long axis (the action one would employ when using a screwdriver). In older children some additional buccal expansion may be required for the removal of the permanent upper canine. When removing primary upper anteriors, upper primary anterior or upper primary root forceps are used; for the permanent maxillary anteriors upper straight forceps are employed.

Malpositioned permanent upper anteriors are frequently encountered and modifications to technique must be employed. Labially placed upper lateral incisors and canines have very little buccal support and are easily removed either by using straight forceps applied mesially and distally and using a slight rotatory movement as described earlier or by the use of elevators. The most useful elevators under these circumstances are the straight and curved Warwick-James and Couplands. The straight elevators are applied along the length of the mesial and distal surfaces of the root and directed in a rotatory manner towards the apex (Fig. 14.22). The mesiobuccal and distobuccal surfaces are used alternately, although in many instances the tooth will be elevated after application to only one of these surfaces. When the curved Warwick-James elevators are used the right-sided Warwick-James is positioned on the mesiobuccal surface of upper right teeth and the distobuccal surface of upper left teeth and then rotated towards the mid-line of the tooth. The left-sided instrument is used on the opposite root surface in a similar fashion.

Palatally positioned lateral incisors and canines are usually not accessible with forceps and thus elevators are used as described above with the exception that they are applied on the palatomesial and palatodistal surfaces. When the curved elevators are used the right-sided instrument is applied distally on the right side and mesially on the left side.

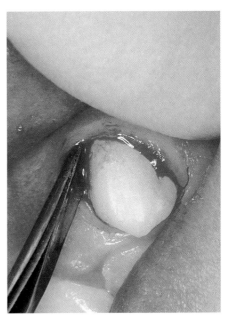

Fig. 14.22 Use of a Coupland's chisel to elevate a buccally placed upper canine.

Upper primary molars

These teeth display the most widely splayed roots found in either dentition and thus considerable expansion of the socket is required. Upper primary molar forceps are used and applied to the roots. The initial movement after application of the forceps is palatal to expand the socket in this direction. The tooth is then subjected to a continuous buccally directed force which results in delivery. Occasionally buccal movement is not adequately obtained due to gross caries on the palatal aspect causing slippage of the forceps beak on the palatal side during buccal expansion; this may be overcome by completing the extraction by continued palatal expansion, the elastic bone of younger patients allowing this to be performed.

Upper premolars

The two-rooted upper first premolar is best removed by buccal expansion using upper premolar forceps. The upper second premolar is often single rooted and although buccal expansion with premolar forceps should be attempted in the first instance this tooth can also be subjected to a rotation about its long axis to effect delivery. Palatally displaced upper premolars are difficult to remove with forceps, elevators used in a manner similar to that described for palatally placed canines are preferred.

Upper permanent molars

These teeth are removed using left and right upper molar forceps. Following application of the forceps to the roots of the tooth (the pointed beak being driven towards the buccal root bifurcation) the tooth is delivered by expanding the socket in a buccal direction. The use of palatal expansion is not as successful in the removal of permanent molars but may be worth attempting if buccal expansion fails to deliver the tooth. The problem with palatal expansion when extracting permanent molars is that it can cause fracture of the palatal root which is usually the most closely associated with the maxillary antrum.

Lower primary anteriors

These teeth are extracted in the same manner as their upper counterparts in that rotation about the long axis using lower primary anterior or root forceps is employed.

Lower permanent anteriors

Permanent lower incisors are not readily removed by rotation as their roots are thin mesiodistally and rotation is likely to cause root fracture. The most effective method of removal is to apply lower root forceps and expand the socket labially.

Permanent lower canines may be delivered by a rotatory movement about the long axis or by buccal expansion.

Labially displaced lower canines are removed in a manner similar to that described for buccally placed upper anteriors. Mesial and distal application of forceps or straight elevators are used. Straight elevators are used on lower incisors which are labially placed.

The position of lingually placed lower anteriors normally precludes the use of forceps and straight elevators applied mesially and distally should be employed.

Lower primary molars

These teeth are removed by buccolingual expansion of the socket. They can be extracted using either lower primary molar or lower primary root forceps. The lower primary molar forcep is similar in design to the permanent molar forcep and has two pointed beaks which engage the bifurcation. Lower primary root forceps are used by applying the beaks to the mesial root of the primary molar. Lower first primary molars are usually more easily removed with lower primary root forceps. After application of the forceps a small lingual movement is followed by a continuous buccal force which delivers the tooth.

Lower premolars

When these teeth are fully erupted in the arch of the young patient they are usually simply removed by a rotatory movement around the long axis of the root using lower premolar forceps. Malpositioned lower second premolars are normally lingually positioned and can be difficult to remove with lower forceps. When lingually placed, lower premolars may be extracted using straight elevators applied mesially, lingually, and distally. Alternatively, it is often possible to apply the beaks of upper fine root forceps mesially and distally to the crown of the lingually placed tooth when the forceps are directed from the opposite side of the jaw. Gentle rotation of the tooth with the forceps may then effect removal.

Lower permanent molars

Two designs of forceps are used to extract lower molar teeth. The lower molar forcep has two pointed beaks which are applied in the region of the bifurcation buccally and lingually. Once applied the forceps are used to move the tooth in a buccal direction to expand the buccal cortical plate. When buccal expansion is not sufficient to deliver the tooth then the forceps should be moved in a figure of eight fashion to expand the socket lingually as well as buccally and this is generally successful.

A different technique is used with forceps of the cowhorn design. These forceps have two beaks which taper to a point. The points are applied to the bifurcation of the lower molar in a manner identical to that described above. The next movement is to squeeze the forceps handles together which results in the beaks approaching one another at the base of the bifurcation. The only way the beaks can approach each other is by displacing the tooth in an occlusal direction resulting in extraction of the tooth.

Both of the above methods are successful in removing permanent molar teeth in children and the choice of technique depends mainly on the preference of the operator.

Management of buried teeth

Buried teeth (including supernumaries) are treated in children for several reasons:

(1) symptomatic (e.g. pain);
(2) radiographic signs of pathology (e.g. dentigerous cyst formation);
(3) part of an orthodontic treatment plan.

If buried teeth are symptomless, have no associated pathology and are not causing orthodontic problems (either by their absence or in preventing the orthodontic movement of erupted teeth) they should be left alone. However, such teeth should be kept under clinical and radiographic review so that any developing pathology may be detected and treated.

In cases where unerupted teeth are to be removed the first step in management is to localize the buried tooth by clinical examination and radiographic techniques. A number of radiographic views may be used:

(1) parallax periapicals;
(2) orthopantomogram;
(3) occlusal views;
(4) true lateral facial bones.

In practice parallax periapicals and an orthopantomogram are usually sufficient; the periapical films will help to establish the buccolingual position of the buried tooth in relation to the erupted dentition and the orthopantomogram will supply information concerning the overall shape of the tooth, its relationship to neighbouring structures (such as the antrum, inferior dental canal, other unerupted teeth) and the extent of any associated pathology. Once the tooth has been located and the difficulty of removal and patient co-operation assessed then the method of anaesthesia should be determined.

Extraction of buried teeth

When removing buried dental tissue in children it is imperative to have an excellent view of the operative field, especially when removing unerupted teeth or supernumeraries closely associated with other unerupted teeth that are to be retained. In these circumstances the tooth of interest and its unerupted neighbours must be very clearly identified.

Flap design

Flaps should be mucoperiosteal, be cut at 90° to bone, have a good blood supply, avoid damage to important structures, allow atraumatic reflection, provide adequate access, allow good visibility, and permit reapposition of wound margins over sound bone.

Flaps for buccally placed teeth

Two designs of flap may be used for the removal of buccally placed teeth.

The first of these includes the gingival margin as the horizontal component and a vertical relief incision into the depth of the buccal sulcus (Figs 14.23a–g). It allows good exposure, easy orientation, can be readily extended and, for the most part the wound edge will be replaced over sound bone at the end of the procedure. Care must be taken if this design is used in the mandible in the region of the mental foramen to ensure that the vertical relief is at least one tooth in front

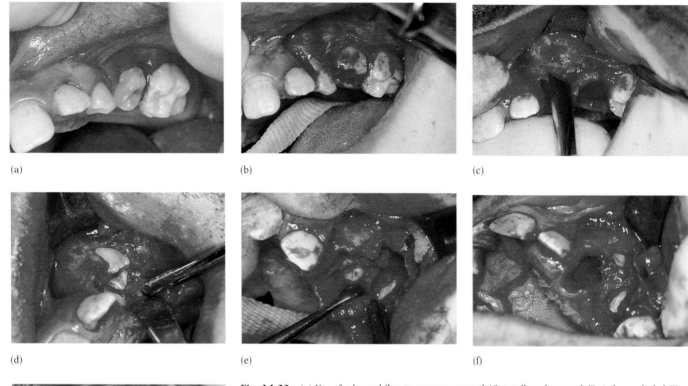

(a)   (b)   (c)

(d)   (e)   (f)

(g)

Fig. 14.23 (a) Use of a buccal flap to remove erupted /C, totally submerged /D, infra-occluded /E and unerupted ⌊4. (By kind permission of *Dental Update*.) (b) The buccal flap is raised. (By kind permission of *Dental Update*) (c) Bone is removed with a chisel following removal of /CE. (By kind permission of *Dental Update*.) (d) Totally submerged /D is identified by occlusal amalgam. (By kind permission of *Dental Update*.) (e) /45 are identified. (By kind permission of *Dental Update*.) (f) /4 removed /35 remain. (By kind permission of *Dental Update*.) (g) Wound closure. (By kind permission of *Dental Update*.)

of the mental foramen (which will have been localized from the orthopantomogram). The only problem with this type of flap is that it may disrupt gingival contour but this is not a major long-term problem in the child.

The second design of flap for buccally placed teeth is a semilunar incision. At least 5 mm of attached gingiva should be maintained at the narrowest point to ensure a good blood supply to the marginal gingivae. This flap does not provide such good exposure or orientation as the previous design, and it is easy at the end of surgery to be left with a large part of the wound margin over a bony defect. This can lead to wound breakdown.

Flaps for palatally/lingually placed teeth

Palatally positioned teeth are best removed via an incision that follows the palatal gingival margin (Fig. 14.24a–g). Such an incision maintains the integrity of the greater palatine nerves and blood vessels. It is often possible to raise this flap without sacrificing the neurovascular bundle that leaves the incisive foramen as this bundle will stretch to a certain degree; however, if access demands it should be cut (this rarely results in any postoperative complications). The extent of the palatal incision depends upon the surgery involved. A flap extending between the mesial aspect of both first permanant molars is not unusual for the removal of bilateral impacted maxillary canines, although smaller flaps may be sufficient to remove palatally placed teeth or supernumeraries near the mid-line.

In the lower jaw adequate access to the lingual side is obtained by raising the normal buccal flap and then elevating the lingual gingiva and reflected mucosa via an incision run around the lingual gingival margin.

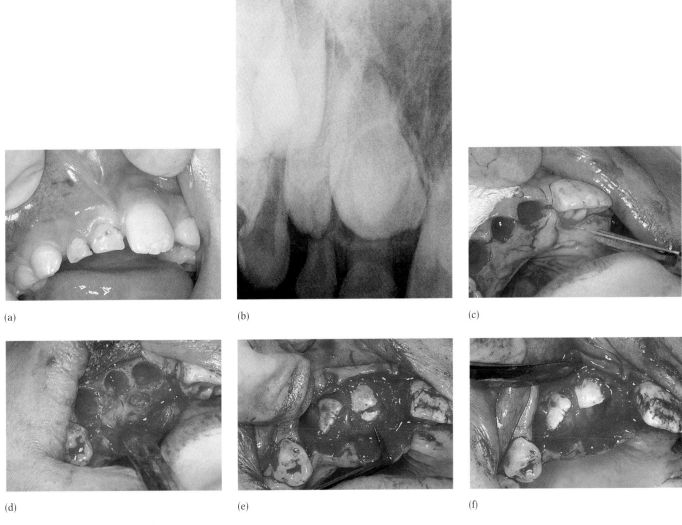

(a) (b) (c)

(d) (e) (f)

(g)

Fig. 14.24 (a) Pre-operative view prior to removal of palatal supernumerary (+ CBA/C) in a 9 year old child via a small palatal flap. (By kind permission of *Dental Update*.) (b) Unerupted 21\ and supernumerary obvious on radiograph. (c) Erupted teeth extracted and palatal gingival margin being incised. (By kind permission of *Dental Update*.) (d) Small palatal flap raised. (By kind permission of *Dental Update*.) (e) 21\ and supernumerary identified after bone removed. (By kind permission of *Dental Update*.) (f) 21\ remain. (By kind permission of *Dental Update*.) (g) Wound closure. (By kind permission of *Dental Update*.)

Bone removal

When working close to buried teeth that are to be retained it is essential that bone is removed with care. This may be carried out using a handpiece and bur very slowly, but the use of chisels with hand pressure (mallets are not used unless working under general anaesthesia and are seldom required in children) is much safer because this is unlikely to damage coronal tissue.

Tooth removal

Once sufficient bone removal has been removed to allow identification of the tooth to be extracted and exposure of the greatest diameter of its crown the tooth should be elevated. If this is likely to produce undue pressure on neighbouring erupted or buried teeth then the tooth should be divided and removed in parts. Mandibular teeth that are impacted within the line of the arch are best removed by the so-called 'broken instrument technique' in which pressure is applied from one side of the tooth (for example using a straight Warwick-James elevator) to force it out of the other side.

Suturing

Resorbable sutures should be used in children whenever possible: 3/0 or 4/0 softgut is ideal.

Discharge

Any bleeding should be arrested before the patient is allowed to leave the surgery and the patient and parent instructed in simple methods of haemorrhage control. The patient is encouraged to maintain good oral hygiene and may be given an antiseptic mouthwash. The problem of self-inflicted trauma in anaesthetized areas is stressed at this stage.

Pain relief

Simple analgesics are usually required but aspirin must be avoided in those under 12 years of age due to its association with Reye's syndrome (a neurological disorder characterized by encephalopathy). Paracetamol elixir (120 mg/5 ml four times daily for those under 6; 250 mg/5 ml four times daily, 6–12 years) is ideal. The patient is given a review appointment but should return sooner if there are any problems with bleeding, excessive pain or swelling. A telephone number for contact in an emergency must be provided.

Review

The patient should be reviewed 1 week after surgery, at which stage resorbable sutures will invariably have disappeared. The area of surgery should be examined for undue swelling, the area of local anaesthesia examined for evidence of self-inflicted trauma, and the patient questioned about any residual altered sensation. It is often necessary to reinforce good oral hygiene at this stage.

Post-extraction problems

Fortunately, post-extraction problems are rare in children. Dry socket does not seem to occur after the removal of primary teeth but it can affect older children following permanent molar extractions, although the incidence is not as great as in adults. Local measures such as irrigation and dressing with a sedative pack, plus the prescription of an analgesic are sufficient.

Postoperative haemorrhage is an occasional problem with children and can be impressive following multiple extractions under general anaesthesia. Usually pressure applied with gauze or a handkerchief is effective, if not sutures with or without haemostatic gauze must be used. Severe blood loss is very rare, but if this occurs it is important to exclude a systemic cause to ensure subsequent treatment can be performed safely.

14.5.3 Surgical exposure of teeth

The exposure of buried teeth may involve either the extraction of erupted teeth or the removal of buried dental elements, but in some cases all that is required is excision of overlying soft tissue. If the tooth can be exposed adequately through a collar of attached gingiva then the procedure is quite simple:

1. Erupted primary predecessors may be extracted.

2. A flap is raised in the manner described above.

3. Any unerupted supernumeraries or buried teeth are extracted.

4. The bony impaction is relieved and the widest diameter of the crown exposed. At this stage it may be possible to place an orthodontic bracket to aid eruption, although this is by no means essential.

5. A pack, for example Whitehead's varnish on 1/2 inch or 1/4 inch ribbon gauze, is then placed around the tooth and the flap replaced around the pack. It is not always necessary to sacrifice soft tissue if the tooth is exposed, and the pack can be placed via primary tooth sockets. Alternatively, it is possible in some cases (such as the exposure of a palatally placed canine) to incorporate a periodontal pack on to the acrylic of an upper removable orthodontic appliance to maintain exposure during healing.

6. The use of non-resorbable sutures to maintain the pack is recommended, although other parts of the incision can be closed with resorbable sutures.

7. In cases in which the removal of soft tissue from the palate or crest of the ridge is all that is required to expose a tooth then it is not necessary to raise a full flap. All that is needed is to sacrifice the overlying tissue and pack the wound (Fig. 14.25a and b). Occasionally, this can cause excessive bleeding in the palate, which is controlled by passing a non-resorbable suture across the full thickness of the palatal mucoperiosteum just posterior to the wound edge; this ligates the greater palatine artery.

8. When an unerupted tooth, classically a canine, is palpable high in the buccal sulcus under reflected mucosa it should not be exposed by sacrificing the overlying soft tissue as this would result in the cervical collar of the tooth being surrounded by non-keratinized mucosa. To overcome this problem a flap containing keratinized gingiva must be raised coronal to the impacted tooth, bone removed if necessary, and the flap replaced in a more apical position to allow a collar of attached gingiva around the tooth at eruption.

9. The pack and any remaining non-resorbable sutures should be removed after 7–10 days.

14.5.4 Apical surgery

Apicectomy is rarely performed in children; however, there are some indications for the technique, most commonly teeth with intransigent open apices. A number of different flap designs may be used — the best being the triangular flap involving the gingival margin and vertical relief incision described above for the removal of buccally placed buried teeth. Principally, this is because the extent of apical pathology is often more extensive in children than is suggested radiographically and use of the semilunar flap can lead to parts of the incision being left over a bony defect at the end of surgery.

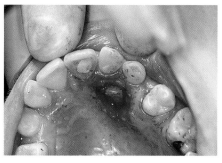

(a)

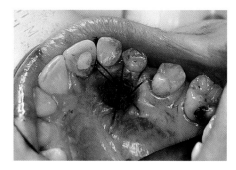

(b)

Fig. 14.25 (a) Exposure of palatal canine by tissue sacrifice. (By kind permission of *Dental Update.*) (b) Ribbon gauze pack sutured in defect. (By kind permission of *Dental Update.*)

Technique

The surgical technique is identical to that used in adults but there are a number of points of difference when placing the apical seal. In teeth with immature open apices through and through root fillings are unsatisfactory as the apex may be wider than the bulk of the canal, thus some form of retrograde restoration is required. However, it is often difficult to secure undercuts at the apex when dealing with a tooth that has an open apex, but this can be overcome by placing a large retrograde filling and relying on multiple microscopic undercuts to secure it.

14.5.5 Cysts interfering with eruption

Eruption and dentigerous cysts can interfere with the eruption of teeth. Eruption cysts in the young child are simply incised (when occluding teeth are present this can be achieved by the patient themselves on biting).

Dentigerous cysts may be marsupialized to the oral mucosal lining following the removal of any overlying primary predecessor and the permanent tooth allowed to erupt. Some authorities advocate more aggressive treatment involving enucleation of the cyst (with or without removal of the tooth) to ensure that epithelial remnants are not left behind.

Fissural cysts (such as the nasopalatine cyst) are rare in children; when found they should be enucleated.

14.5.6 Treatment of acute orofacial infection

At this point it is relevant to discuss the treatment of orofacial infection. The major cause of this condition is dental in origin and thus the minor oral surgical treatments discussed above may all be employed definitively to treat the source of an orofacial infection. Alternatively, conservative treatments such as endodontic therapy may be appropriate. However, a rapidly spreading extra-oral infection is a surgical emergency which merits immediate treatment and may require admission for in-patient management. Two areas of extra-oral spread are of special importance. These are the submandibular region and the angle between the eye and nose. Swelling in the submandibular region arising from posterior mandibular teeth can produce raising of the floor of the mouth. This can cause a physical obstruction to breathing and spread from this region to the parapharyngeal spaces may further obstruct the airway. The advance from dysphagia to dyspnoea can be rapid and a submandibular swelling should be decompressed as a matter of urgency in children. A child with raising of the floor of the mouth requires immediate admission to hospital. The fact that trismus is invariably an associated feature makes expert anaesthetic help essential for safe management.

Infection involving the angle between the eye and nose has the potential to spread intracranially and produce a cavernous sinus thrombosis (Fig. 14.26). This is a potentially life-threatening complication. The angular veins of the orbit which have no valves, connect the cavernous sinus to the face and if the normal extra-cranial flow is obstructed due to pressure from an extra-oral infection then infected material can enter the sinus by reverse flow. To prevent this complication infection in this area (which arises from upper anterior teeth, especially the canine) must be treated expeditiously.

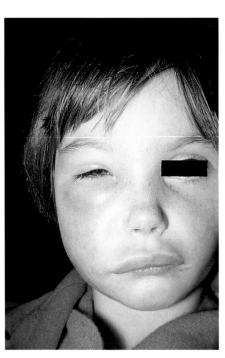

Fig. 14.26 Infection in this region can spread intracranially. (By kind permission of *Dental Update*.)

The principles of the treatment of acute infection are:

(1) remove the cause;
(2) institute drainage;
(3) prevent spread;
(4) restore function.

In addition, analgesia and adequate hydration must be maintained. Removal of the cause is essential to cure an orofacial infection arising from a dental source. This may involve extraction or endodontic therapy.

Institution of drainage and prevention of spread are supportive treatments; they are not definitive cures. Drainage may be obtained during the removal of the cause, for example a dental extraction, or may precede definitive treatment if this makes management easier, for example incision and drainage of a sub-mandibular abscess. Drainage may be intra or extra-oral. When an extra-oral incision is made it is made in a skin crease parallel to the direction of the facial nerve. In the submandibular region the incision is made more than one finger's breadth below the angle of the mandible to avoid the mandibular branch. Once skin has been incised the dissection is carried out bluntly until the infection has been located. Locules of infection are then ruptured using blunt dissection and a drain secured to the external surface. Depending on the amount of drainage the drain is secured for 24–48 h. Any pus should be sent for culture and sensitivity testing to the microbiology laboratory.

Prevention of spread may be achieved surgically or by the use of antibiotics. In severe cases intravenous antibiotics will be used. The antibiotic of choice in children is a penicillin.

It is important to remember that acute infections are painful and that analgesics, as well as antibiotics, should be prescribed. The use of paracetamol elixir is usually sufficient. Similarly, it is important that a child suffering from an acute infection is adequately hydrated. It the infection has restricted the intake of oral fluids due to dysphagia then admission to hospital for intravenous fluid replacement is required.

14.5.7 Autotransplantation of teeth

Replantation of an avulsed tooth due to trauma has been discussed in Chapter 11. In this section autotransplantation of teeth is discussed. Autotransplantation of teeth in children may be considered as a treatment for the following: (a) repositioning of an ectopic tooth, or (b) replacement of an unrestorable tooth with a redundant member of the dentition.

The ectopic tooth most commonly repositioned by surgical means is the unerupted palatally placed upper permanent canine. An example of using autotransplantation as a means of tooth replacement is the substitution of an upper incisor that is undergoing resorption by a premolar tooth, which is scheduled for extraction as part of an orthodontic treatment plan (Fig. 14.27a–j). The management regimen for both treatments is similar and is as follows:

(1) assesment of donor tooth and recipient site;
(2) atraumatic extraction of donor tooth;
(3) preparation of recipient site;
(4) transplantation;
(5) splinting of transplanted tooth;
(6) root treatment of transplanted tooth.

344

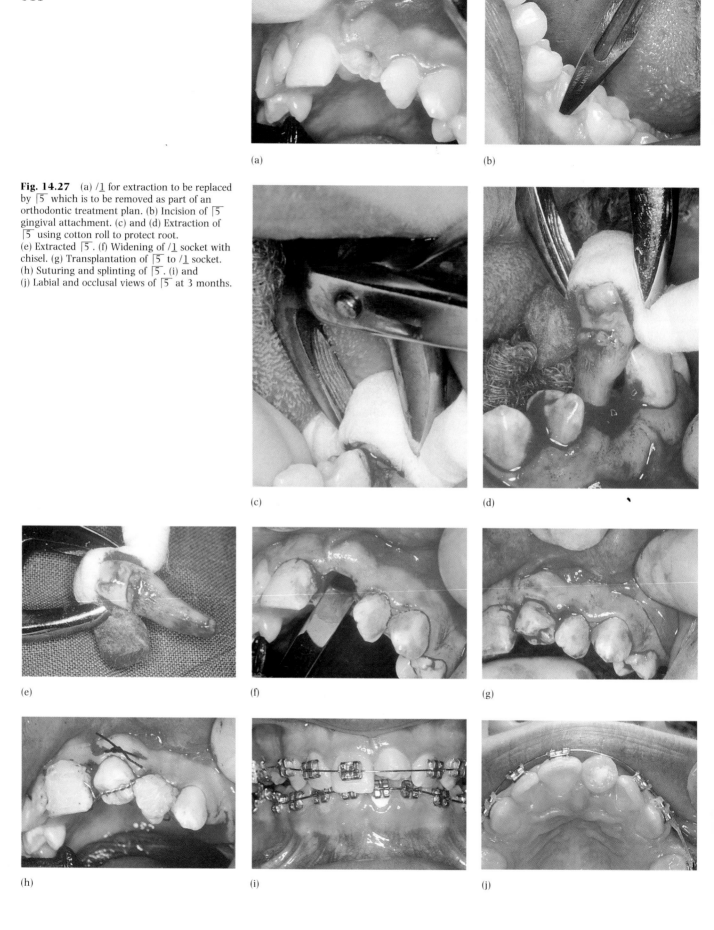

Fig. 14.27 (a) /1 for extraction to be replaced by 5̄ which is to be removed as part of an orthodontic treatment plan. (b) Incision of 5̄ gingival attachment. (c) and (d) Extraction of 5̄ using cotton roll to protect root. (e) Extracted 5̄. (f) Widening of /1 socket with chisel. (g) Transplantation of 5̄ to /1 socket. (h) Suturing and splinting of 5̄. (i) and (j) Labial and occlusal views of 5̄ at 3 months.

(a)

(b)

(c)

(d)

(e)

(f)

(g)

(h)

(i)

(j)

In addition, when autotransplantation is used to replace a tooth in the arch some coronal preparation and orthodontic movement of the donor tooth may be required.

Transplantation surgery is usually performed under antibiotic prophylaxis (either oral or intravenous amoxycillin) as the use of systemic antibiotics has been shown to decrease the incidence of root resorption.

Assessment of donor tooth and recipient site

The tooth to be transplanted has to be appraised clinically and radiographically prior to surgery. The crown of an erupted tooth can be assessed for caries and its dimensions measured. Root status and shape will be determined using periapical radiographs. Donor teeth should have an open apex with at least three-quarters of the root formed. The morphology of unerupted teeth for transplantation can only be determined radiographically. Teeth with severe root curvature are not suitable for transplantation as it is unlikely that they can be removed intact without trauma. In addition, the production of a donor site suitable for a dilacerated tooth may be difficult to produce without damaging neighbouring vital teeth.

It is important to evaluate the recipient site both clinically and radiographically. The space available for the transplanted tooth must be assessed both in the horizontal and vertical dimensions. It may be necessary to create sufficient space using pre-operative orthodontics. Periapical radiographs will alert the clinician to the presence of any bony pathology or retained dental remnants at the recipient site.

Atraumatic extraction of donor tooth

It is essential to remove the donor tooth using minimal trauma and avoiding contact with the root surface. Damage to the root surface will lead to resorption or ankylosis. Thus when removing an erupted tooth for transplantation the usual rules concerning the application of forcep beaks to the root surface do not apply, the beaks being positioned on the crown. Prior to the application of the forceps a scalpel should be run around the gingival margin to the crest of the ridge to sever gingival attachments.

When an unerupted tooth is being used as a donor great care must be exercised during its removal. The entire crown must be exposed. As mentioned earlier bone removal with hand chisels is less likely to damage the donor than use of a bur. Once the crown has been exposed elevators or forceps (again confined to the crown) are used to extract the tooth as gently as possible. When the tooth has been extracted it should be replaced gently into its socket and maintained there until the recipient site is prepared. This is to ensure that a satisfactory tooth is obtained before recipient site surgery is performed.

Preparation of recipient site

The recipient site may or may not contain a tooth. Following extraction of the tooth at the recipient site the socket is enlarged if necessary using either a chisel or a bur (an implant bur is ideal). Some workers recommend that the socket is enlarged following flap raising and removal of the buccal plate of bone which is stored in saline prior to being replaced with the cortical surface against the root. It is thought that this might decrease the incidence of ankylosis.

Transplantation

Once the socket has been prepared the donor tooth is gently placed in its new position. The occlusion is assessed to ensure that it is not traumatic to the transplanted tooth and the gingival margin is held around the tooth with a horizontal mattress suture. It is usual to use black silk sutures in this instance.

Splinting of transplanted tooth

The donor tooth should be splinted at the time of transplantation. However, it is important to stress that rigid splinting should not be employed as this will lead to ankylosis. A simple splint using orthodontic wire bonded to the tooth and its neighbours with composite resin is sufficient. It is essential that splinting is not maintained for too long a period as this may also lead to ankylosis. Three weeks is the maximum length of time, indeed in some cases the splint can be removed at 1 week.

Root treatment of transplanted tooth

The pulp of the transplanted tooth is extirpated after 3 weeks and the root canal filled with non-setting calcium hydroxide. The calcium hydroxide is replaced with gutta percha at about 6 months post-transplant as long as there is no evidence of root resorption.

Follow-up of transplanted teeth

At the time of discharge the patient should be given an antiseptic mouthwash to maintain good hygiene in the surgical site. The first review is at 1 week at which stage sutures are removed and a 'base-line' periapical radiograph may be taken. It may be possible to remove the splint at this stage.

The next review is at 3 weeks for splint removal and endodontic treatment. Another periapical film should be taken at this stage.

Further reviews should be undertaken at 3 and 6 months and then annually. Coronal reshaping can be performed at any stage.

Orthodontic movement of transplanted teeth

Transplanted teeth can be moved orthodontically. This should begin 3 months following transplantation and be completed within 9 months of the transplant.

14.6   IMPLANTOLOGY

The use of dental implants in children is contra-indicated except under circumstances where severe psychological stress merits such treament. There are three reasons for avoiding implants in young patients:

1. The implant does not move with the growing alveolus — it acts as an ankylosed tooth. Thus implants should not be placed until vertical growth of the jaws is virtually complete (about 18 years of age). The exception to this rule is the lower intercanine region which can receive implants earlier in exceptional cases of hypodontia, e.g. X-linked ectodermal dysplasia.
2. Implants can interfere with normal growth of the jaws.

3. Young bone does not behave in the same way as mature bone. Due to squashing and crushing the axis of an inserted implant may deviate widely from the axis of tap.

In addition, the use of teeth for autotransplantation is often a viable alternative in young patients.

14.7   SOFT TISSUE SURGERY

The following short synopsis covers the important functional and orthodontic problems in the child and adolescent.

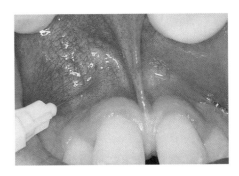

(a)

14.7.1   Labial fraenae

A prominent mid-line fraenum in the maxilla may be present in association with a diastema. Whether or not the fraenum is the cause of the diastema is open to question as a fleshy fraenum does not always produce an aesthetic defect. Nevertheless, the excision of a mid-line maxillary fraenum is often requested as part of an othodontic treatment plan. This procedure is very simply performed under local anaesthesia (Fig. 14.28a–d). Before surgery a radiograph of the upper incisor area should be taken to eliminate other possible causes of a mid-line diastema (such as a mesiodens). A mid-line maxillary fraenum should not be removed before the permanent canines have erupted, as the space may close spontaneously when these teeth appear.

Surgical removal is achieved by dissecting the mid-line tissue via incisions parallel to the fraenum from the labial mucosa at a point beyond the prominent fibrous tissue through the interdental space to palatal mucosa. The part of the incision in attached gingiva is mucoperiosteal. The surface of the exposed bone in the interdental space should be curetted or gently burred to remove residual fibrous attachments. Primary closure of the labial part of the incision is achieved by suturing and the defect in attached gingiva is covered by a pack such as Whitehead's varnish on ribbon gauze held in place by sutures. The pack is removed 7–10 days after surgery.

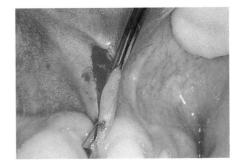

(b)

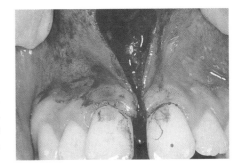

(c)

14.7.2   Lingual fraenae

A prominent lingual fraenum should be excised if it is interfering with speech or oral hygiene. This is simply performed under local anaesthesia. The fraenum is held by a pair of haemostatic forceps, a triangular section of tissue is removed and the wound ends sutured.

14.7.3   Mucoceles

Mucoceles are common in the second decade of life, although they occasionally occur in younger children including the newborn. If these lesions cause functional or emotional problems they should be excised, but if there is no disturbance removal may be delayed until the child is older.

An incision is made next to the lesion, which is removed by a blunt dissection under the epithelium. Invariably, a number of minor salivary glands are obvious during surgery (they often appear like a bunch of grapes around the mucocele) and these should be removed in view of the fact that mucoceles are produced as a result of trauma. Any obvious dental cause of trauma, for example a sharp tooth, should be remedied.

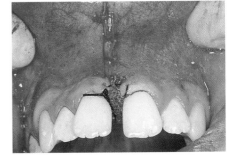

(d)

Fig. 14.28 (a) Patient for upper mid-line labial fraenectomy. (b) Incisions parallel to fraenum. (c) Defect at end of removal. (d) Wound closure with resorbable sutures in reflected mucosa and silk suture holding pack interdentally.

One type of mucocele that is best referred for specialist treatment is that found in the floor of the mouth, the so-called 'ranula' (Fig. 14.8). This lesion is often more extensive than is at first apparent and complete cure occasionally involves removing the sublingual gland.

14.7.4   Incisional biopsy

Incisional biopsies are performed to confirm a diagnosis by removing part of a lesion. It is preferable that the surgeon who is going to treat the lesion performs the incisional biopsy and therefore this procedure is best performed by an oral surgeon.

14.7.5   Excision biopsies of non-attached mucosa

Small lesions of the oral mucosa are removed by excisional biopsy, which involves the removal of an ellipse of tissue including the lesion. The long axis of the ellipse is made parallel to the direction of muscle pull and it is best to hold the specimen with a suture passed through it to avoid crushing, which could render the specimen useless for histological examination (Fig. 14.29). All tissue surgically removed should be sent for histological examination by placement in a solution of 10 per cent formal saline (not in water) for transport to the laboratory. Lesions that are obviously benign and are not interfering with function or causing emotional distress can be left in the young child and removed, if necessary, at a later date (Fig. 14.30a and b).

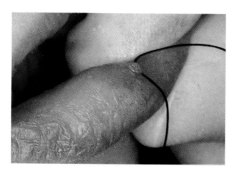

Fig. 14.29   Lip lesion held by suture. (By kind permission of *Dental Update*.)

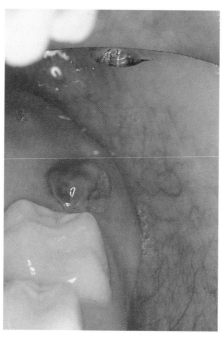

(a)

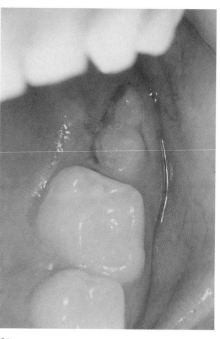

(b)

Fig. 14.30   (a) and (b) Lump related to erupting /7. and view 1 week later — the lump has disappeared and the /7 has erupted — no treatment was given. (By kind permission of *Dental Update*.)

14.7.6 Excision biopsy of attached gingiva/palate

These procedures leave a defect that is not readily treated by primary closure. Following the biopsy it is useful to lay a haemostatic material over the defect to arrest bleeding and then the area is covered either by a periodontal dressing or by securing a Whitehead's varnish ribbon gauze pack in the defect with non-resorbable sutures.

14.7.8 Suturing

Resorbable sutures should be used to close soft tissue wounds in children whenever possible; however, in mobile structures such as the tongue and lip these may be lost shortly after surgery as their knots may be less secure than those obtained with black silk. To overcome this problem it is useful to bury knots by taking the first bite of tissue from within the wound rather than from the mucosal surface and the second bite beginning on the mucosal surface of the opposite wound edge, thus ensuring that the knot disappears into the wound when it is tied (Fig. 14.31).

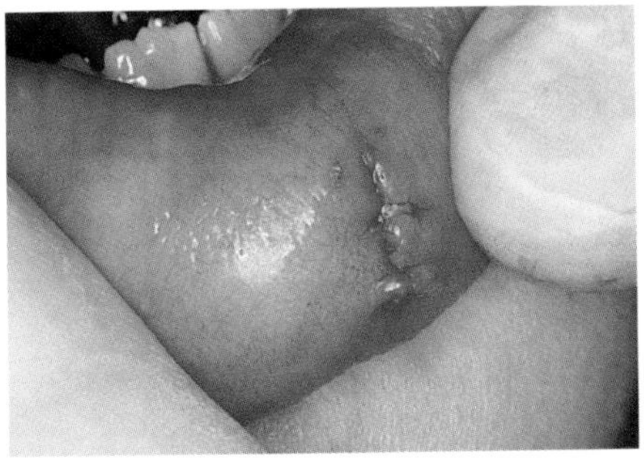

Fig. 14.31 Same patient as in Fig. 14.29 showing buried knots with softgut sutures. (By kind permission of *Dental Update*.)

14.8 SUMMARY

This chapter has considered:

1. Pathological conditions of the oral and perioral structures in children.

2. Dental extractions in children.

3. Minor oral surgical procedures which can be performed without in-patient anaesthetic facilities in healthy children.

4. The management of acute spreading infection from a dental focus in children.

14.9 FURTHER READING

Andreasen, J. O. (1992). *Atlas of replantation and transplantation of teeth*. Mediglobe, Fribourg. (*A beautifully illustrated guide to tooth transplantation.*)

Gorlin, R. J., Cohen, M. M., and Levin, L. S. (1990). *Syndromes of the head and neck* (3rd edn). Oxford University Press, Oxford. (*A valuable reference text.*)

Soames J. V. and Southam, J. C. (1993) *Oral pathology* (2nd edn). Oxford University Press, Oxford. (*A comprehensive oral pathology text.*)

15 Medically compromised children

15 Medically compromised children
L. SHAW

15.1 INTRODUCTION

There are many general medical conditions which can directly affect the provision of dental care and some where the consequences of dental disease, or even dental treatment, can have life-threatening implications. An increasing number of children who now survive with complex medical problems due to improvements in medical care, present difficulties in oral management. The remarkable decline in childhood mortality has led to increasing emphasis on maintaining and enhancing the quality of the child's life and ensuring that children reach adult life as physically, intellectually and emotionally healthy as possible. Dental care can play an important part in enhancing the quality of life.

Even though the infant mortality rates (deaths under 1 year of age) have declined dramatically in the United Kingdom in the twentieth century, the death rates are still higher in the first year of life than in any other single year below the age of 55 in males and 60 in females. The main causes of death in the neonatal period (the first 4 weeks of life) are associated with low birth weight, pregnancy complications, and congenital malformations. In the remainder of the first year, however, the main causes of death are respiratory and other infective diseases, congenital malformations, the sudden infant death syndrome (cot death), and accidents.

15.1.1 The medical history (see also Chapter 3)

All patients should have an accurate medical history taken before any dental treatment is undertaken. This is important for several reasons:

1. To identify any medical problems that might require modification of dental treatment.
2. To prioritize children who require intensive preventive dental care.
3. To identify those requiring prophylactic antibiotic cover for potentially septic dental procedures.
4. To check whether the child is receiving any medication which could result in adverse inter-reaction with drugs or treatment administered by the dentist. This would include past medication that could have had an effect on dental development.
5. To identify systemic disease that could affect other patients or dental personnel; this is usually related to cross-infection potential.
6. To establish good rapport and effective communication with the child and their parents.
7. To facilitate communication with medical colleagues.
8. Medico-legal requirement.

Many dental practitioners use standard questionnaires to obtain a medical history; it has been found that one of the most effective methods is to use a questionnaire followed by a pertinent personal interview with the child and their parent or guardian.

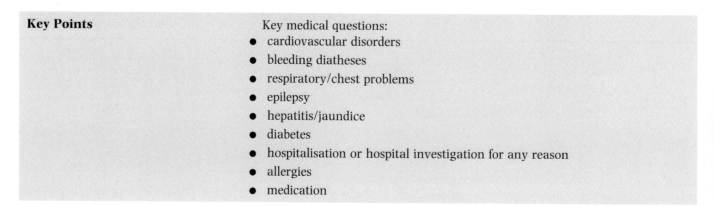

Key Points	Key medical questions:
	• cardiovascular disorders
	• bleeding diatheses
	• respiratory/chest problems
	• epilepsy
	• hepatitis/jaundice
	• diabetes
	• hospitalisation or hospital investigation for any reason
	• allergies
	• medication

15.1.2   The general examination

General observation of the child is invaluable and can provide vital information. The child's demeanour is important in assessing their potential co-operation for dental treatment but assessment of general outward appearance can be helpful in determining their state of health. Visually accessible areas such as skin and nails can reveal cyanosis, jaundice, and petechiae from bleeding disorders. The hands particularly are worthy of inspection and can also show alterations in the fingernails such as finger-clubbing from chronic cardiopulmonary disorders, as well as infections and splinter haemorrhages. Overall shape and symmetry of the face may be significant and there may be characteristic facies that are diagnostic of some congenital abnormalities and syndromes.

15.2   CARDIOVASCULAR DISORDERS

These can be divided into two main groups, congenital heart disease (existing before or at birth) and those disorders which are acquired after birth. Congenital heart disease occurs in approximately eight children in every 1000 live births. There is a wide spectrum of severity but two to three of these children will be symptomatic in the first year of life.

15.2.1   Congenital heart defects

The cause is rarely known in individual cases but multifactorial inheritance patterns are mainly responsible. Several chromosomal abnormalities, such as Down syndrome, are associated with severe congenital heart disease but these represent fewer than 5 per cent of the total. The main types of congenital conditions are shown in Table 15.1. In most instances there is a combination of genetic and environmental influences including infections during the second month of pregnancy.

Many defects are slight and cause little disability but a child with more severe defects may present with breathlessness on exertion, tiring easily, and suffering from recurrent respiratory infections. Those children with severe defects such as tetralogy of Fallot and valvular defects including pulmonary atresia and tricuspid atresia, will have cyanosis, finger clubbing, and may have delayed growth and

Table 15.1 Prevalence of Congenital Cardiac Disease

Defect	%
Ventricular septal	28
Atrial septal	10
Pulmonary stenosis	10
Patent ductus arteriosus	10
Tetralogy of Fallot	10
Aortic stenosis	7
Coarctation of the aorta	5
Transposition of great arteries	5
Rare/diverse	15

development (Figs. 15.1–15.3). Characteristically, these children will assume a squatting position to relieve their dyspnoea on exertion.

Heart murmurs

Many parents will report that their child either has, or had, a 'heart murmur'. These may only be discovered at a routine examination and occur in over 30 per cent of all children. Most of these murmurs are functional or innocent and not associated with significant abnormalities, but are the result of normal blood turbulence within the heart. Innocent murmurs are heard most frequently from 3 to 7 years of age. In a small minority of cases a heart murmur indicates the presence of a cardiac abnormality causing the turbulence. If the dentist is in any doubt of the significance of a murmur then a cardiological opinion should be sought. Normally contact with the child's medical practitioner will clarify the situation. Innocent murmurs do not require any special precautions or treatment.

Ventricular septal defects (VSD)

These are the most common of the cardiac malformations. Small defects are asymptomatic and may be found during a routine physical examination. Large defects with excessive pulmonary blood flow are responsible for symptoms of breathlessness, feeding difficulties, and poor growth. Between 30 and 50 per cent of the small defects close spontaneously, usually within the first year of life. Larger defects are usually closed surgically in the second year of life, but defects involving other cardiac structures may require complex surgery or even transplantation.

Atrial septal defects (ASD)

Not as common as the VSD in children, but proportionately more significant in adults and more frequent in females. An isolated patent foramen ovale is of no clinical significance and not considered to be an ASD. Even an extremely large ASD rarely produces heart failure in children but symptoms usually appear in the third decade. Surgery is usually carried out before school-age.

Pulmonary stenosis

With mild to moderate stenosis of the pulmonary valve there are usually no symptoms, but exercise intolerance and cyanosis may occur if this is severe. Treatment is required for the moderate to severe forms but relief of this obstruction is now carried out in the majority of children by balloon dilatation rather than surgery.

Patent ductus arteriosus

During fetal life most of the pulmonary arterial blood is shunted through the ductus arteriosus into the aorta, thus bypassing the lungs. Functional closure of the ductus arteriosus usually occurs at birth. Virtually all pre-term babies weighing less than 1750 g have a patent ductus arteriosus in the first 24 h of life but this usually closes spontaneously. Ductus arteriosus patency is mediated by prostaglandins and administration of inhibitors of prostaglandin synthesis such as indomethacin is effective in closing the ductus in a significant number of babies. Surgical ligation, however, is a safe and effective back-up if indomethacin is contra-indicated or has not been successful.

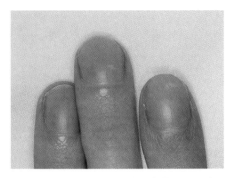

Fig. 15.1 This shows the hand of a boy with Down syndrome and Fallot's tetralogy. The cyanosis and finger-clubbing associated with his severe cardiac disease are obvious.

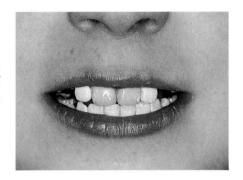

Fig. 15.2 Cyanosis affecting the lips in a boy with Fallot's tetralogy. The mucous membranes appear bluish.

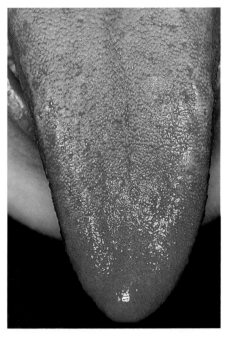

Fig. 15.3 Central cyanosis affecting the tongue of the boy shown in Fig. 15.2.

Tetralogy of fallot

This classically consists of the combination of:

(1) obstruction to right ventricular outflow (pulmonary stenosis);
(2) VSD;
(3) dextroposition of the aorta;
(4) right ventricular hypertrophy.

Cyanosis is one of the most obvious signs of this condition but it may not be present at birth. As the child grows, however, the obstruction to blood flow is further exaggerated. The oral mucous membranes and nail-beds are often the first places to show signs of cyanosis. Growth and development may be markedly delayed in severe untreated tetralogy of Fallot and puberty is delayed. Early medical management involves the use of prostaglandins so that adequate pulmonary blood flow can occur until surgical intervention can be carried out. Initially, a shunt procedure (usually the Blalock–Taussig shunt) is performed to anastomose the subclavian artery to the homolateral branch of the pulmonary artery. Later in childhood total surgical correction is undertaken but the mortality rate from this procedure is 5–10 per cent.

15.2.2   Acquired cardiovascular disease

Rheumatic fever

Rheumatic fever follows a group A streptococcal infection of the upper respiratory tract, especially in developing countries, and may occur at all ages but usually between 5 and 15 years. Environmental factors such as overcrowding promote the transmission of streptococcal infections and the incidence of rheumatic fever is higher among lower socio-economic groups. The clinical onset is usually acute and occurs 2–3 weeks after a sore throat. Joint pains are common and of a characteristic migratory polyarthralgia or polyarthritis. Carditis is the most serious manifestation, occurring in 40–50 per cent of initial attacks, especially in young children. Fever is usually present but in an insidious onset of the condition it may be low grade. Most of the carditis resolves except the lesions on the cusps of the heart valves which become fibrosed and stenotic. Rheumatic heart disease is the most important manifestation of rheumatic fever and may affect mitral, aortic, tricuspid, and pulmonary valves.

Diseases of the myocardium and pericardium

Major diseases involving the myocardium and pericardium include bacterial infections such as diphtheria and typhoid, tuberculous, fungal, and parasitic infections, rheumatoid arthritis, systemic lupus erythematosus, uraemia, thalassaemia, hyperthyroidism, neuromuscular diseases such as muscular dystrophy, and glycogen storage diseases. They are relatively rare in children in developed countries.

Other cardiovascular problems

There are several other important conditions which are common in adults but not in children. These include coronary artery disease (ischaemic heart disease), cardiac arrhythmias, and hypertension. In children, secondary hypertension is more common than essential hypertension and is associated with renal abnormalities in 75–80 per cent of those affected.

15.2.1 Dental care for children with cardiovascular disorders

The most important consideration in planning dental care for children with cardiovascular disorders is the prevention of dental disease. As soon as a child is diagnosed as having a significant cardiac problem they should be referred for dental evaluation and an aggressive preventive regimen commenced to include dietary counselling, fluoride therapy, fissure sealants, and oral hygiene instruction. Regular monitoring both clinically and radiographically, with reinforcement of the preventive advice is essential. Active dental disease should be treated before cardiac surgery is undertaken.

Treatment planning

If the child and parents are seen in infancy and effective preventive dental procedures are instituted, then theoretically operative dentistry should not be necessary. In practice, the situation may be very different. If invasive operative procedures are required then antibiotic prophylaxis will be necessary (see p. 358 and Table 15.2), which influences treatment planning. Ideally, treatment in children should be carried out during short appointments so that

Table 15.2 Prophylactic regimen for dental procedures

Under local anaesthesia
Adults: Amoxycillin 3 g orally 1 h pre-operatively
Children: 50 mg/kg body weight orally 1 h pre-operatively (or under 10 years — half adult dose; under 5 years — quarter adult dose)
If allergic to penicillin:
Adults   Clindamycin 600 mg orally 60 min pre-operatively
Children   6 mg/kg body weight 60 min pre-operatively (or under 10 years — half adult dose; under 5 years — quarter adult dose)
Under general anaesthesia
Adults   Amoxycillin 1 g, i.m. or i.v. at induction then 0.5 g Amoxycillin by mouth 6 h later
Children   Under 10 years — half adult dose
             Under 5 years — quarter adult dose
Special risk patients
Including patients who have:
1. Previous history of endocarditis
2. Prosthetic heart valves and require a general anaesthetic:
    (a)   adults: Amoxycillin 1 g, i.m. or i.v. plus Gentamicin 120 mg i.m. or i.v. at induction: then 0.5 g Amoxycillin by mouth 6 hours later.
    (b)   children: (i)   under 10 years: Amoxycillin, half adult dose, Gentamicin 2 mg/kg;
                       (ii) under 5 years: Amoxycillin, quarter adult dose, Gentamicin 2 mg/kg
3. Had penicillin in previous month and require a general anaesthetic.
4. An allergy to penicillin and require a general anaesthetic.
    (a)   adults   Vancomycin 1 g by slow intravenous infusion over 100 min plus Gentamicin 120 mg, i.v. just before induction or 15 min before procedure.
    (b)   children   Under 10 years:Vancomycin 20 mg/kg, Gentamicin 2 mg/kg
or
    (a)   adults   Teicoplanin 400 mg, i.v. plus Gentamicin 120 mg i/v at induction or 15 min before procedure
    (b)   children   Under 14 years:Teicoplanin 6 mg/kg, Gentamicin 2 mg/kg
or
Adults: Clindamycin 300 mg, i.v. over at least 10 min at induction or 15 min before procedure then oral or i.v. Clindamycin 150 mg, 6 h later
Children: Under 10 years–half adult dose
             Under 5 years–quarter adult dose

co-operation is maximized. However, if prophylactic antibiotics are required it is important to carry out as much treatment as possible under each cover but this has to be balanced against the stress of longer appointments. If multiple appointments with prophylaxis are required, then 2–4 weeks should be allowed between appointments to allow penicillin-resistant organisms to disappear from the oral flora.

Other problems may include prolonged bleeding following scaling or surgical procedures due to thrombocytopenia and anticoagulant medication. It is essential to check the platelet count and prothrombin time (INR) if dental extractions are planned. The patient's prothrombin time is compared with normal and called the international normalized ratio (INR).

No child with symptomatic cardiac problems should have any routine dental procedures until details of the condition have been obtained and the patient's physician consulted.

Antibiotic prophylaxis

If dental procedures are likely to induce a bacteraemia then prophylactic antibiotic therapy is required to prevent the development of endocarditis. Any procedure that breaches the integrity of the oral mucosa or exposes pulpal tissue is a risk. This includes extractions, scaling, surgery involving gingival tissues, and restorative procedures where the gingival margins are likely to be traumatized either during cavity preparation or during matrix band placement. Endodontic treatment should only be carried out on teeth where there is a very high probability of success. This is usually confined to permanent incisor teeth with straight canals and closed apices and is carried out as a single visit procedure under appropriate antibiotic cover. Endodontic treatment on multirooted teeth and on primary teeth is contra-indicated in patients with cardiovascular disease.

Antibacterial prophylaxis recommendations are constantly updated and revised as new scientific evidence and drugs become available. The latest American Heart Association guidelines and the British National Formulary should be checked. The medication should be taken under supervision.

There is still some controversy over which conditions do or do not require prophylactic antibiotic therapy. If any doubt exists then the paediatrician or cardiologist should be consulted before invasive dental procedures are undertaken. Children who have had corrective surgery for a patent ductus arteriosus are considered to have normal hearts and only require prophylactic antibiotics for the initial 6 months following surgery. Prophylaxis is not required for functional heart murmurs or isolated secundum atrial septal defects. It is, however, necessary for most other congenital cardiac malformations, for those with mitral valve prolapse and for those who have had prosthetic cardiac valves. It is essential also for patients who have had rheumatic fever induced dysfunction and with previous infective endocarditis. At present there are insufficient scientific data to support specific recommendations for endocarditis prevention in people with cardiac transplants and the cardiologist responsible for the patient's care should be consulted.

Key Points

Antibiotic prophylaxis:
- congenital heart defects
- rheumatic fever
- previous infective endocarditis
- previous heart surgery (with exceptions)

15.3 DISORDERS OF THE BLOOD

15.3.1 Bleeding disorders

The blood is in a dynamic equilibrium between fluidity and coagulation but the haemostatic mechanism is more complex than just alterations in this equilibrium. It involves local reactions of the blood vessels, platelet activities, and the interaction of specific coagulation factors that circulate in the blood.

In early childhood many of the bleeding disorders have a genetic background but with increasing age more become iatrogenic — usually due to anticoagulant medication. Patients who have had cardiac surgery for some congenital abnormality, those who have had a recent myocardial infarction, and those who have had cerebrovascular accidents may all be receiving long term anti-coagulant therapy. Table 15.3 gives a classification of bleeding disorders which is based on disorders of coagulation, bleeding problems due to decreased numbers of platelets, and disorders of bleeding where there are normal numbers of platelets. Many of these conditions are very rare and will not be considered further.

Haemophilia

Haemophilia A is an X-linked recessively inherited condition caused by deficiency of factor VIII. The degree of severity is very varied but tends to be consistent within the same family. Children with over 25 per cent of normal levels of circulating factor VIII may lead normal lives, those with between 1 and 5 per cent are moderately to severely affected by minor trauma etc., while those with under 1 per cent have multiple bleeds into joints (haemarthroses) and may be severely physically handicapped as a result.

Factor VIII level:

Key Points

- > 25 per cent — mild
- 1–5 per cent — moderate to severe
- < 1 per cent — severe

Obviously, prevention of trauma to those who have this condition is extremely important but the availability of concentrates of factor VIII has revolutionized the quality of life of haemophiliacs. Unfortunately, some of these blood replacement products have been contaminated in the past with hepatitis and HIV viruses and, therefore, cross-infection control is a high priority.

It was found that a number of patients who were thought to be haemophiliacs did not respond to replacement with factor VIII (antihaemophiliac globulin) but

Table 15.3 Classification of bleeding disorders

1. Coagulation defects
   (a) inherited: (i) haemophilia A: factor VIII deficiency; (ii) Haemophilia B: factor IX deficiency (Christmas disease)
   (b) Acquired: (i) liver disease; (ii) vitamin deficiency; (iii) anticoagulant drugs (heparin, warfarin); (iv) disseminated intravascular coagulation (DIC)
2. Thrombocytopenic purpuras
   (a) Primary: (i) idiopathic thrombocytopenic purpura (ITP); (ii) pancytopenia, Fanconi syndrome
   (b) Secondary: systemic disease–leukaemia: (ii) drug induced; (iii) physical agents–radiation
3. Non-thrombocytopenic purpuras:
   (a) Vascular wall alteration: (i) scurvy; (ii) infections; (iii) allergy
   (b) Disorders of platelet function: (i) inherited: Von Willebrand's disease; (ii) drugs: aspirin, non-steroidal anti-inflammatories, alcohol, penicillin; (iii) allergy; (iv) auto-immune disease; (v) uraemia

were deficient in another factor — factor IX. This is known as Christmas disease or haemophilia B. This is also transmitted as an X-linked recessive trait with a wide range of clinical severity but female carriers of this condition also have a tendency to bleed.

Key Points

Genetic coagulation disorders:
- haemophilia A (VIII) — 80 per cent
- haemophilia B (IX) — 13 per cent
- factor XI — 6 per cent

Von Willebrand's disease

This is a dominantly inherited, complex, and variable condition characterized by a vascular abnormality of large irregular capillaries, defective platelets which do not adhere to each other, and decreased levels of factor VIII. Common clinical manifestations are nose bleeds and spontaneous gingival haemorrhage. Von Willebrand's disease is the most common inherited bleeding disorder affecting approximately one in every 1000 individuals in the United States United and United Kingdom.

Key Points

Bleeding disorders:
- haemophilia A 1:20 000
- von Willebrand's disease 1:1000

Thrombocytopenia

This is caused by a reduction in the numbers of circulating platelets in the bloodstream. Normal levels are between 150 and 400×10^9 per litre. The platelet count should be at least 50×10^9 per litre before surgery is attempted. Clinical signs are petechial haemorrhages into the skin and mucous membranes with haematemesis (blood in the vomit), haematuria (blood in the urine), and melaena (blood in the faeces).

In children the usual causes of thrombocytopenia are idiopathic, an acute immune response usually following an upper respiratory tract infection, leukaemic infiltration of the bone marrow, or following the administration of various drugs.

15.3.2 Dental management of bleeding disorders

A good history is the best screening device but a bleeding tendency may only become manifest after a surgical procedure or trauma. Effective communication with the child's physician or haematologist is important, not only to establish the aetiology of any bleeding tendency but also to liaise over any necessary medical treatment that is required to replace reduced levels of clotting factors etc.

The cornerstone of dental care must remain preventive procedures and regular reviews so that if disease does occur it can be treated at an early stage. Local anaesthetic infiltrations or intraligamentous injections are unlikely to cause problems if given carefully. Regional anaesthesia such as an inferior dental block, is contra-indicated as bleeding in the pterygomandibular region may result in asphyxia.

Pulp treatment of primary molar teeth may be required to avoid extractions. Most primary teeth exfoliate spontaneously with little haemorrhage; however, occasionally when they are very mobile the soft tissues develop an inflammatory hyperplastic response and bleeding may be a problem. In these situations extraction may be necessary with the appropriate haematological replacement therapy. If dental extractions or surgery do become necessary then the patients are usually best managed in the hospital situation.

Haemophilia

Adequate replacement and careful monitoring of factor VIII and factor IX levels are required. This is usually done with fresh frozen plasma or freeze dried concentrate. Patients with mild to moderate haemophilia A can often be managed on an out-patient basis using replacement therapy or DDAVP (1 desamino–8, d-arginine vasopressin) which stimulates release of factor VIII. Antifibrinolytic agents such as EACA (Epsilon–amino caproic acid) and tranexamic acid are also given to prevent lysis of the clot. They also significantly reduce the requirement for replacement of factor VIII. Medications containing non-steroidal anti-inflammatory drugs or aspirin should not be given (aspirin should not be given anyway to a child under 12 years because of the risk of developing Reye's syndrome).

Von Willebrand's disease

Factor VIII concentrates are not usually effective but DDAVP is used in combination with EACA or tranexamic acid. Patients with more severe types of von Willebrand's disease will require fresh frozen plasma or cryoprecipitate replacement.

Thrombocytopenia

The platelet count should be at least 50×10^9 per litre before surgery is attempted and continuous infusion of platelets may be required. In children with the idiopathic form of this condition, prednisolone (4 mg/kg per day for 1 week, given orally) will increase the platelet count to over 50×10^9 per litre within 48 h in about 90 per cent of cases. The necessary treatment can then be carried out.

15.3.3 Blood dyscrasias

There are several relatively common disorders of the red and white blood cells that may influence dental care in the child. Many of these conditions also give rise to abnormal bleeding but in addition, may lead to delayed healing, infection, or mucosal ulceration. An outline classification is given in Table 15.4.

Table 15.4 Classification of blood dyscrasias

1. Red blood cell disorders
(a) Anaemia:
(i) iron deficiency; (ii) glucose 6-phosphate dehydrogenase deficiency; (iii) sickle cell; (iv) thalassaemia
(b) Polycythaemia
2. White blood cell disorders
(a) Leucocytosis: (i) infections–mononucleosis (glandular fever); (ii) neoplasia
(b) Leucopenia: neutropenia (i) congenital; (ii) drug induced
(c) Leukaemias: (i) acute lymphocytic (ALL); (ii) acute myeloid (AML); (iii) chronic
(d) Lymphomas: (i) Hodgkin's ; (ii) Non-Hodgkin's ; (iii) Burkitt's

Red blood cell disorders: anaemia

There is a reduction in the red cell volume or haemoglobin concentration and the oxygen carrying capacity of the blood is lowered. Anaemia is not a specific disease but a symptom of an underlying disorder. Children with anaemia may be very pale (examine the nail beds, conjunctiva, and oral mucous membranes). They may also be tired, listless, and breathless.

Iron-deficiency anaemia

This may result from chronic blood loss, possibly as a result of haemorrhagic disorders, but in children it is more commonly due to dietary deficiency (milk contains very little iron) or malabsorption. Vitamin B_{12} and folic acid are also needed for maturation of red blood cells in the bone marrow.

Glucose 6-Phosphate Dehydrogenase (G-6-PD) Deficiency

This enzyme is needed in the hexose monophosphate shunt pathway. In deficiency the accumulation of oxidants in the red blood cells causes their haemolysis and may result in jaundice, palpitations, dyspnoea, and dizziness. Drugs such as aspirin, phenacetin, and ascorbic acid, as well as infections, may precipitate haemolysis. As the gene for G-6-PD is located on the X-chromosome it is inherited as a sex-linked condition. There are many variants of the condition and it is common in certain ethnic groups; for example, type A is found in 11 per cent of American black people and G-6-PD MED is relatively common in ethnic groups of Mediterranean origin.

Sickle cell anaemia

This is an inherited autosomal recessive disorder that results in the substitution of a single amino acid in the haemoglobin chain. Sickle cell trait is the heterozygous state in which the affected individual carries one gene for haemoglobin S. Approximately 10 per cent of American black children and up to 25 per cent of central African black children carry the trait. Sickle cell anaemia is the homozygous state, with affected genes from both parents. The red blood cells containing haemoglobin S have a life of only 30–60 days and become clumped together under certain conditions, blocking small blood vessels, and leading to pain and necrosis.

Affected children may be pale, tired, weak, and breathless. They may complain of painful joints and swelling of the hands and feet. There tends to be a failure to thrive and growth retardation with an increased susceptibility to infection. Later problems include renal function impairment and retinal and conjunctival damage.

Thalassaemia

This is another inherited disorder of haemoglobin synthesis which may occur as a heterozygous trait or homozygous thalassaemia major. It occurs particularly in Mediterranean countries and in the Middle-Eastern Arab countries. It results, like Sickle cell anaemia, in a severe progressive haemolytic anaemia. Regular blood transfusions are necessary to maintain the haemoglobin level above 10 g/dl. If treatment is inadequate then hypertrophy of erythropoietic tissue occurs and this results in massive expansion of the marrow of the facial and skull bones producing maxillary hyperplasia and protrusion of the middle third of the face.

Dental management of anaemia

All anaemic children have a greater tendency to bleed after invasive dental procedures. Therefore, any signs or symptoms suggestive of anaemia should be investigated. The haemoglobin level and haematocrit are simple tests used for screening and a white blood cell and platelet count should also be obtained. If these reveal any abnormalities then further more complex tests may need to be undertaken. Ideally, the underlying defect should be corrected before embarking on a course of routine dental care.

A family history of conditions such as sickle cell anaemia and thalassaemia is significant and all black patients should be tested routinely for sickle cell disease prior to a general anaesthetic. Sickle cell crises occur due to inadequate oxygenation, and if possible, general anaesthetics should be avoided in preference to the use of local anaesthesia.

Key Point

Sickle cell disease:
- all black patients should be screened prior to general anaesthesia

White blood cell disorders: leukaemia

Leukaemia is a malignant proliferation of white blood cells. It is the most common form of childhood cancer, accounting for about one-third of new cases of cancer diagnosed each year. Acute lymphocytic leukaemia accounts for 75 per cent of cases with a peak incidence at 4 years of age. The general clinical features of all types of leukaemia are similar as all involve a severe disruption of bone marrow functions. Specific clinical and laboratory features differ, however, and there are considerable differences in response to therapy and long-term prognosis.

Acute leukaemia has a sudden onset but the initial symptoms are usually non-specific with anorexia, irritability, and lethargy. Progressive failure of the bone marrow leads to pallor, bleeding, and fever, which are usually the symptoms that lead to diagnostic investigation. The bleeding tendency is often shown in the oral mucosa (Fig. 15.4) and there may also be infective lesions of the mouth and throat. The dental practitioner may, therefore, be the first to diagnose the condition (Fig. 15.5). Bone pain and arthralgia are also important presenting complaints in about one-quarter of children. On initial haematological examination most patients will have anaemia and thrombocytopenia. A significant proportion will have white blood cell counts of less than 3000/mm3 and about 20 per cent will have counts greater than 50 000/mm3. The diagnosis of leukaemia can be suspected on seeing blast cells on the blood smear confirmed on bone-marrow biopsy which will show replacement by leukaemic lymphoblasts.

The treatment varies with the clinical risk features; children under 2 years and over 10 years with an initial white blood cell count of over 100 000/mm3 and central nervous system involvement (leukaemic cells in the cerebrospinal fluid) have the worst prognosis. The basic treatment components are:

1. Induction of remission: to remove abnormal cells from the blood and bone marrow. Drugs used: vincristine and prednisone
2. Prophylactic treatment to central nervous system. Drugs used: intrathecal methotrexate plus irradiation of central nervous system.

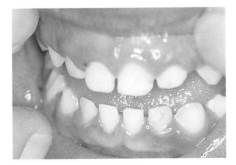

Fig. 15.4 This 3 year old was brought to the dental surgery with spontaneous bleeding from his gums. He had recently had several nose-bleeds and had become very lethargic. His skin and mucosa were very pale. Haematological investigation showed acute lymphocytic leukaemia.

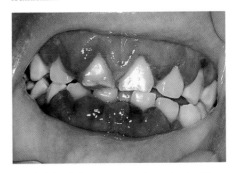

Fig. 15.5 Oral appearance of a patient with acute myeloid leukaemia, with infiltration of the gingivae and spontaneous haemorrhage. This oral presentation and type of leukaemia is less common than the lymphocytic type shown in Fig. 15.4. (Courtesy of Wolfe Publishing.)

Key Points

Childhood leukaemia:
- 75 per cent is Acute Lymphocytic leukaemia
- peak incidence 4 years

3. Consolidation. Drugs used: cytosine arabinoside plus asparaginase

4. Maintenance. Drugs used: methotrexate plus mercaptopurine for approximately 2 years.

5. If relapse occurs then bone marrow transplantation can be considered.

On this regimen over 70 per cent of children now survive and can be regarded as cured.

Dental management of leukaemia

Unless there is a major dental emergency no active dental treatment should be carried out until the child is in remission. Any dental pain should be treated conservatively by the use of antibiotics and analgesics. The drug regimen used to induce remission has numerous side-effects, including nausea and vomiting, reversible alopecia (hair loss), neuropathy and oral ulceration. It can be extremely difficult to carry out normal mouthcare for children at this stage and many have difficulty with toothbrushing due to acute nausea. Swabbing the mouth with chlorhexidine mouthwash and routine use of antifungal agents are essential. Local anaesthesia preparations such as 5 per cent lignocaine ointment or benzydamine hydrochloride (Difflam) applied before mealtimes can help to reduce pain from ulceration or mucositis.

Once the leukaemia is in remission and after consultation with the child's physician, then routine dental care can be undertaken with the following adjustments:

1. If invasive procedures are planned then current haematological information is required to assess bleeding risks.

2. Prophylactic antibiotic therapy to prevent postoperative infection should be considered. This is given if the functional neutrophil count is depressed.

3. Children who are immunosuppressed are also at risk of fungal and viral infections. Fungal infections should be treated aggressively with amphotericin B, nystatin, or fluconazole, and herpetic infections with topical and/or systemic acyclovir.

4. Regional block anaesthesia may be contra-indicated due to risk of deep haemorrhage.

5. Long-term preventive dental care is important.

Key Points	Oral side effects of chemotherapy: • mucositis, oral ulceration • infection (leucopenia) • haemorrhage (thrombocytopenia)

Key Points	Oral prophylaxis during chemotherapy: • oral hygiene • fluorides • chlorhexidine • antifungals

15.4   RESPIRATORY SYSTEM DISEASE

There are age-related disease patterns as far as the respiratory system is concerned; these patterns are also affected by sex, race, season of the year, geography, and environmental and socio-economic conditions. For example, the relatively short eustachian tube in infants and young children allows easy access to ascending infections from the pharynx. Cystic fibrosis largely affects Caucasians whereas lung infections and infarctions associated with sickle cell disease occur almost exclusively in black children. Seasonal variation in the incidence of respiratory tract infections and asthma are quite marked and certain infections have a well defined geographical distribution. The frequency of bronchitis may not be very different between socio-economic groups, but the severity is and may reflect differences in nutritional status and perhaps the availability of medical care.

15.4.1 Asthma

Asthma is a diffuse obstructive lung disease which causes breathlessness, coughing, and wheezing. It is associated with a hyper-reactivity of the airways to a variety of stimuli and a high degree of reversibility of the obstructive process.

Asthma is a leading cause of chronic illness in childhood. Prevalence data are conflicting, but 10 per cent of children will, at some time, have signs and symptoms compatible with a diagnosis of asthma. There is mounting recent evidence to suggest that the prevalence is increasing considerably in the United Kingdom. Before puberty approximately twice as many boys than girls will suffer from asthma, thereafter, the sex incidence is similar. About half of the children who are affected will be virtually free of symptoms by the time they become adults.

The aetiology is poorly understood but it is a complex disorder involving immunological, infectious, biochemical, genetic, and psychological factors. Acute episodes of coughing and wheezing are often precipitated by exposure to allergens and irritants such as cold air or noxious fumes and emotional stress. Drug therapy is now the mainstay of treatment both prophylactically and during acute exacerbations.

Dental management of asthma

Dental treatment itself can cause emotional stress which may precipitate an attack. Routine dental care with local anaesthesia is not usually a problem but severe asthmatics on steroids may need additional steroids to cover the stress of a procedure. General anaesthesia for severe asthmatics usually requires in-patient hospital admission.

15.4.2 Cystic fibrosis

Cystic fibrosis is an autosomal recessive multisystem disorder predominantly of the exocrine glands. A thick viscid mucus is produced, particularly in the lungs, which leads to chronic obstruction and infection of the airways and to malabsorption. It is the most common genetic condition in Caucasians with approximately 5 per cent of the population being carriers and 1 in 2000 of live births affected. The abnormal gene has been located on the long arm of chromosome 7.

The clinical manifestations of the condition are variable and some patients remain asymptomatic for long periods of time. Coughing is the most constant symptom of pulmonary involvement and this may lead to recurrent respiratory infections and bronchiolitis. Lung disease progresses leading to exercise intolerance and shortness of breath (Fig. 15.6). More than 85 per cent of affected children show evidence of malabsorption due to exocrine pancreatic insufficiency. Symptoms include frequent, bulky, greasy stools and a failure to thrive despite a large food intake.

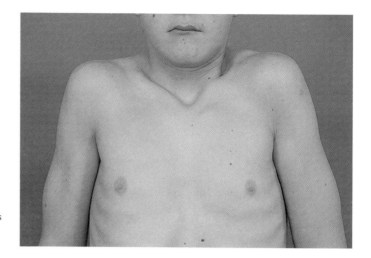

Fig. 15.6 This boy has cystic fibrosis and shows a 'barrel chest' deformity due to respiratory infections. Coincidentally he also has a deformity of his clavicles. (Courtesy of Wolfe Publishing.)

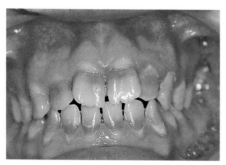

Fig. 15.7 Tetracycline was administered to this patient who has cystic fibrosis over a prolonged period. This has resulted in its incorporation into the mineral matrix with marked discoloration. Alternative antibiotics are now used; recent improvements in management of people with cystic fibrosis have meant that an increasing number are not maintained on long-term antibiotic prophylaxis.

Dental management of cystic fibrosis

These children need to have a very high calorific intake and may have frequent refined carbohydrate snacks. Preventive advice is essential. General anaesthetics should be avoided if possible in view of the pulmonary involvement. A significant proportion of affected children also have cirrhosis of the liver with resultant clotting defects and liability to haemorrhage following surgical procedures. At one time, children with cystic fibrosis were maintained on long-term antibiotic prophylaxis of tetracycline to prevent chest infections. This led to intensely intrinsically stained teeth due to tetracycline deposition in the developing dentine (Fig. 15.7).

15.5   CONVULSIVE DISORDERS

15.5.1   Febrile convulsions

Convulsions are common; about 5 per cent of children have had one or more convulsions and accurate diagnosis of the aetiology is very important. The vast majority of these are febrile convulsions and are associated with illnesses that cause high fever late in infancy such as otitis media. The seizures are usually tonic–clonic with loss of consciousness followed by sustained contractions of muscles. Respiration may be impaired which may lead to cyanosis. The teeth are often firmly clenched with possible tongue and lip biting. There may also be loss of bladder and bowel control. This tonic phase is followed by the clonic phase of intermittent muscular contraction. The duration is always less than 15 min. These convulsions occur usually early in the illness during the period of rapid temperature rise and may be the first indication that the child is ill. It is most important to eliminate the possibility of central nervous system infection and examination of the cerebrospinal fluid is essential if there is persistent drowsiness following the attack.

15.5.2   Epilepsy

It may be difficult to differentiate these simple febrile convulsions from epilepsy but it is essential that this diagnosis is made as the therapy, prognosis and implications differ enormously. Epilepsy is not a disease in itself but a term applied to recurrent seizures, either of unknown origin (idiopathic epilepsy) or

Table 15.5 Conditions commonly associated with seizures

1. Febrile convulsions

2. Idiopathic epilepsy: often genetic predisposition

3. Secondary epilepsy
   cerebral neoplasms
   cerebral vascular disorders, e.g. subdural haemorrhage, especially seen in child abuse
   cerebral malformation, e.g. Down syndrome, hydrocephalus
   neurocutaneous syndromes, e.g. Tuberous sclerosis, neurofibromatosis, Sturge–Weber disease
   nutritional disorders, e.g. Pyridoxine deficiency, lead encephalopathy, drug intoxication
   Metabolic disorders, e.g. hypoglycaemia, renal failure, phenyl-ketonuria
   atrophic cerebral lesions, e.g. Post-anoxic, post-traumatic and post-infectious
   degenerative cerebral disease, e.g. Batten's
   central nervous system infection, e.g. Meningitis, encephalitis, brain abscess

due to congenital or acquired brain lesions (secondary epilepsy). It affects about 0.5–1 per cent of the population. Table 15.5 gives a list of conditions which are commonly associated with recurrent seizures.

Dental management of epilepsy

Medical management usually consists of long-term anticonvulsant drug therapy. The choice of drug depends on the seizure type but the dosage needs to control the seizures with minimal side-effects. The child with good control of seizures needs a minimum of restrictions but the possibility of an attack occurring in the dental chair should be considered. If possible, any liquid medication should be sugar-free (Fig. 15.8). Sodium valproate fulfils this criteria and is not associated with gingival hyperplasia; however, phenytoin results in gingival hyperplasia in about half of patients. A very high standard of oral hygiene is required to minimize the development of hyperplasia and gingival surgery should never be contemplated unless the oral hygiene is good.

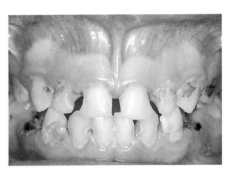

Fig. 15.8 This 3 year old child with epilepsy has rampant caries of the primary dentition with a somewhat unusual distribution of approximal lesions in both upper and lower incisors as well as molars. The child had been on long-term sucrose-based medication but has now changed to the sugar-free sodium valproate liquid. (Courtesy of Wolfe Publishing.)

Key Points

Epilepsy:
- 0.5–1.0 per cent of population
- gingival overgrowth with phenytoin

Trauma to anterior teeth is often encountered in people with epilepsy who may have frequent, unpredictable falls. Re-implantation of avulsed teeth is usually contra-indicated in those with severe learning difficulties, however, if any prostheses are required, then they should be well retained with clasps and unlikely to break or be inhaled during any subsequent attacks.

15.6 METABOLIC AND ENDOCRINE DISORDERS

15.6.1 Diabetes mellitus

Diabetes is the most common endocrine/metabolic disorder of childhood and is due to deficiency of insulin and abnormal metabolism of carbohydrate, protein and fat. Type I diabetes mellitus is insulin dependent (IDDM) and usually of juvenile onset. It is highly age related with peaks of presentation between 5 and 7 years and at puberty. The prevalence of diabetes in school-age children is approximately 2 per 1000. Although there is a genetic predisposition, there may well be a triggering effect of viral infections in the aetiology of diabetes.

The clinical manifestations are polydipsia (increased thirst), polyuria (increased urination), polyphagia (increased appetite), and weight loss. There may be an insidious onset of lethargy, weakness, and weight loss. The diagnosis is dependent on demonstration of hyperglycaemia in association with glucosuria.

The aims of treatment are to control the symptoms, prevent acute metabolic crises of hypo- and hyperglycaemia and to maintain normal growth and body weight, with an active life-style. If there is good control of blood sugar levels with insulin therapy and nutritional management, then diabetic complications are minimized. One of the major hazards of insulin treatment is the development of hypoglycaemia. It is usually of rapid onset (unlike hyperglycaemia) with sweating, palpitations, apprehension, and trembling. This progresses to mental confusion, drowsiness, and coma. Hypoglycaemia in a diabetic child indicates too much insulin relative to food intake and energy expenditure. For an acute episode a carbohydrate-containing snack or drink should be given. Another problem, particularly in adolescents, is the psychological adjustment to the condition; the rebellious teenage years may lead to non-compliance with insulin therapy and nutritional management. Many of these problems can be averted by suitable education and counselling.

Dental management of diabetes

The well controlled diabetic child with no serious complications can have any dental treatment but should receive preventive care as a priority. Uncontrolled diabetes can result in varied problems which mainly relate to fluid imbalance, altered response to infection, possible increased glucose concentrations in saliva, and microvascular changes. There may be decreased salivary flow and an increased incidence of dental caries has been reported in uncontrolled young diabetics. There is also well documented evidence of increased periodontal problems and susceptibility to infections, particularly candida.

Dental appointments should be arranged at times when the blood sugar levels are well controlled; usually a good time is in the morning immediately following their insulin injection and a normal breakfast. General anaesthetics are a problem because of the pre-anaesthetic fasting that is required and are normally carried out on an in-patient basis to enable stabilization of insulin and carbohydrate balance intravenously.

15.6.2 Adrenal insufficiency

There are a number of syndromes associated with adrenal insufficiency, such as Addison's Disease and Cushing's syndrome, but problems in dental management of patients with steroid insufficiency are more likely to occur in children who are being prescribed steroid therapy for other medical conditions; for example in the suppression of inflammatory and allergic disorders, acute leukaemia, and to prevent acute transplant rejection. In children, the risks of taking corticosteroids are greater than in adults and they should only be used when specifically indicated, in minimal dosage, and for the shortest possible time.

If a child has adrenal insufficiency and/or is receiving steroid therapy, then any infection or stress may precipitate an adrenal crisis. For routine restorative treatment no additional steroid supplementation is usually necessary. However, if extractions under local anaesthesia or more extensive procedures are planned and/or if the patient is particularly apprehensive, then the oral steroid dosage should be increased or parenteral supplementation given (Table 15.6). General anaesthesia should not be carried out on an out-patient basis.

Table 15.6 Corticosteroid cover for dental procedures

	No steroids in previous 12 months	Steroids given in previous 12 months	Steroids taken currently
Single extraction under local anaesthetic	No cover required	Hydrocortisone i.m. or i.v. pre-operatively	Hydrocortisone orally, i.m. or i.v. pre-operatively. Normal steroid medication postoperatively.
Multiple extractions or minor oral surgery or treatment under general anaesthesia	Consider cover if large doses given previously	Hydrocortisone i.v. pre-operatively. Oral or i.m. for 24 h postoperatively.	Hydrocortisone i.v. pre-operatively. Oral or i.m. for normal steroid medication

Doses of hydrocortisone: under 12 years, 50 mg; 12–16 years, 100 mg.
Oral doses given 2 h pre-operatively.
i.m. i.v. doses given 30 minutes pre-operatively.

Consultation with the child's physician is necessary before prescribing steroids and anaesthetists must be aware of such medication in order to avoid a precipitous fall in blood pressure during anaesthesia or in the immediate postoperative period.

15.6.3 Other disorders

There are many other metabolic and endocrine disorders which do occur in children but these are rare events. Thyroid disease may present in early adolescence but is generally more common in adults. Dental management should present no problems if the thyrotoxic patient is medically well controlled but liaison with the physicians is important.

15.7 NEOPLASTIC DISORDERS

Cancer causes more childhood deaths between the ages of 1 and 15 years than any other disease but is still considerably behind trauma as the most common reason for mortality. The incidence of malignant tumours in children under 15 years of age in developed countries is estimated to be in the region of one in 10 000 children per year but the mortality rate is high at between 30 and 40 per cent.

Although leukaemia is the most common form of childhood cancer tumours of the central nervous system, and neural crest cells and lymphomas also form a significant proportion (Table 15.7). Prognosis varies with the type of tumour, the stage at which it was diagnosed and upon the adequacy of treatment. Major advances have been made in the treatment of childhood malignancy in the last few decades, largely as a result of advances in chemotherapy and bone marrow transplantation. The side-effects of this treatment can have considerable repercussions intra-orally and good oral care is essential (see p. 364). The principles of dental management are very similar to those involved in the care of children with leukaemia.

Table 15.7 The major types of childhood cancer

Leukaemia	48%
Central nervous system	16%
Lymphoma	8%
Neuroblastoma	7%
Nephroblastoma	5%
Others	16%

15.8 ORGAN TRANSPLANTATION

Kidney, heart, bone marrow, liver, and pancreas transplantation are now routine procedures Most liver transplants in children occur because of biliary atresia and bone marrow transplants are the treatment of choice for children with aplastic anaemia, those who fail conventional therapy for leukaemia, and for some immune deficiency disorders. Although children with end-stage renal disease can be kept alive by haemodialysis, their quality of life is considerably improved by kidney transplantation.

15.8.1   Pre-transplant treatment planning

Any candidate for organ transplantation should be referred for dental evaluation. Whenever possible, active dental disease should be treated before the procedure and any teeth with doubtful prognoses extracted. This may present difficulties as many pre-transplant patients can be seriously ill and have various associated medical problems. Children undergoing bone marrow transplantation are prone to infection, bleeding, and delayed healing due to leucopenia and thrombocytopenia. However, the majority of children awaiting liver transplantation due to biliary atresia are of a very young age and have not experienced dental caries. This is a time at which intensive oral hygiene instruction and preventive advice and therapy are of paramount importance in helping to minimize later potential oral problems.

Before any invasive dental procedures are undertaken, consultation with the child's physician is vital in order to establish the extent of the organ dysfunction and its repercussions. Prophylactic antibiotics are likely to be required in patients with cardiac problems and depressed white blood cell counts (see Table 15.2). Any significant alterations in bleeding times and/or coagulation status must be checked. There are also certain drugs which should be avoided in patients with end-stage liver or kidney disease.

Key Points	Transplant immunosuppression:
	• leucopenia
	• thrombocytopenia
	• gingival overgrowth

15.8.2   Immediate post-transplant period

Drugs prescribed to prevent graft rejection have several side-effects. Azathioprine results in leucopenia, thrombocytopenia, and anaemia; hence, children in this immediate post-transplant phase may be even more prone to infections and haemorrhage than before. Cyclosporin and FK506 are largely replacing azathioprine but may cause severe kidney and liver changes leading to hypertension and bleeding problems. Cyclosporin is also associated with gingival hyperplasia. Steroids are prescribed at this time with the risk of adrenal suppression.

Full supportive dental care is required and children complain of nausea and may develop severe oral ulceration. Routine oral hygiene procedures can become difficult but use of chlorhexidine as a mouthwash, spray, or on a disposable sponge, together with local anaesthetic preparations is helpful.

15.8.3   Stable post-transplant period

Once healing has occurred and any acute graft rejection been brought under control then routine dental treatment can be undertaken. Reinforcement of all preventive advice and liaison with the child's dietician may be helpful as many are on high carbohydrate supplementation. Steroid therapy is discontinued in children with liver transplants after 3 months but may be continued for longer periods than this in those with other organ transplants. Antifungal prophylaxis is usually given in the first few months after transplantation to prevent oral candidal infections. Dental problems, apart from oral ulceration and those associated with immunosuppression and bleeding tendencies, include delayed eruption and exfoliation of primary teeth and ectopic eruption of permanent teeth, which are related to the gingival hyperplasia associated with cyclosporin and nifedipine medication (Fig. 15.9).

In all children who are medically compromised the dental team can play a vital part in the overall medical management and in helping these children and their parents adjust to normal life following recovery. Oral care is extremely important in enhancing the quality of life by reducing the morbidity and mortality of oral conditions and by allowing the child to eat without pain and gain optimal nutrient intake. Preventive care should be the cornerstone of any oral care programme.

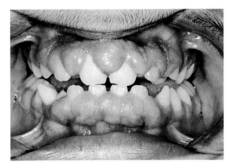

Fig. 15.9 These grossly hyperplastic gingivae are associated with cyclosporin and nifedipine medication in this 11 year old boy who has had a kidney transplant. This combination of drugs is required to prevent rejection and to control his blood pressure.

15.9 SUMMARY

1. An increasing number of children with complex medical problems now survive due to improvements in medical care, and present difficulties in oral management.

2. An accurate, detailed medical history must be obtained for all children before any dental treatment is undertaken.

3. An aggressive preventive regimen is required for all children with significant medical problems; this must encompass dietary counselling, suitable fluoride therapy, fissure sealant applications, and oral hygiene instruction.

4. Congenital heart disease is more common in children than acquired conditions. Most of these malformations require prophylactic antibiotics prior to carrying out any invasive dental procedures.

5. Children with bleeding disorders, such as haemophilia, thrombocytopenic purpura, and Von Willebrand s disease, must be haematologically investigated prior to dental treatment. Haematological replacement therapy may be required before operative treatment.

6. Children with anaemia, whether from iron deficiency or from such inherited conditions as sickle cell anaemia or thalassaemia, represent general anaesthetic risks in particular.

7. Leukaemia is the most common form of childhood cancer and the first disseminated cancer to respond completely to chemotherapy in a significant number of children. Dental management of affected children needs to consider their haematological status as well as their immunocompromised condition.

8. Asthma is a leading cause of chronic illness in childhood; severe asthmatics may be on systemic steroid therapy which has implications for dental care.

9. Convulsions are common in children, occurring in approximately 5 per cent but many of these are associated with episodes of high fever in the child and not with epilepsy.

10. Diabetes mellitus is the most common endocrine/metabolic disorder of childhood; if there is good control of blood sugar levels with insulin therapy and nutritional management, then diabetic complications are minimized and dental care should be routine.

11. Organ transplantation in children is now being increasingly undertaken; there are many side-effects of drug control of immunosuppression which affect treatment planning and oral care.

12. The participation of the dental team in the overall management of children with medical problems can significantly help to enhance the quality of life; preventive care should be the cornerstone of dental management.

15.10   FURTHER READING

Behrman, R. E. and Vaughan, V. C. (1987). *Nelson textbook of paediatrics.* (W. B. Saunders. Co. Philadelphia. *The standard paediatric 'bible'; a huge amount of information about all types of medical problems in children.*)

Gorlin, R. J., Cohen, M. M., and Levin, L. S. (1990). *Syndromes of the head and neck* (3rd ed). Oxford University Press, Oxford. (*The authoritative publication on this subject with erudite lists of references.*)

Grundy, M. C., Shaw, L., and Hamilton, D. V. (1993). *An illustrated guide to dental care of the medically compromised patient.* Wolfe, London. (*Basic information on a wider range of subjects than can be covered in the present chapter and with practical information on dental care.*)

Little, J. W. and Falace, D. A. (1993). *Dental management of the medically compromised patient.* (4th ed). Mosby Year Book, St Louis. (*Comprehensive information but with very helpful summaries on potential problems related to dental care.*)

16 Childhood disability

16 Childhood disability

J. N. NUNN

16.1 INTRODUCTION

Disabilities and impairments only become a handicap for a child if they are unable to carry out the normal activities of their peer group. For example, a child who has broken an arm is temporarily 'handicapped' by not being able to eat and write in the normal way. However, for some children disability is a permanent feature of their lives, but only becomes a handicap if they are unable to take part in everyday activities, like communicating with others, climbing stairs, and toothbrushing. The definition of Soble (1974) helps to clarify which children are 'handicapped' for the purposes of providing dental care: 'dentally handicapped' refers to patients who have some gross condition or deficit in their oral cavities, which necessitates special dental treatment consideration, for example, a cleft of the lip and palate. By contrast, children who are 'handicapped for dentistry' are those who have a physical and/or mental or emotional condition that may prevent them from being treated routinely.

There are a number of reasons why children with disabilities merit special consideration for dental care:

1. The oral health of some disabled children is different from that of their normal peers, for example,the greater incidence in Down syndrome of periodontal disease.

2. The prevention of dental disease in disabled children must be a higher priority because dental disease, its sequelae or its treatment, may be life-threatening, for example, the risk from an oral bacteraemia in congenital heart defects (Fig. 16.1).

3. Treatment planning and the provision of dental care may need modification in view of the patient's capabilities, likely future co-operation, and home care. For example, the feasibility of providing a resin-bonded bridge for a teenager with cerebral palsy, poorly controlled epilepsy, and little home oral care.

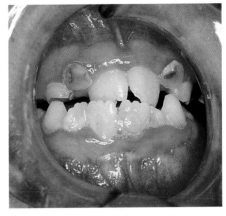

Fig. 16.1 A 13 year old Down syndrome boy awaiting a combined heart and lung transplant as well as a renal transplant, with gross caries

Key Points

The need for special dental care:
- differences in dental disease prevalence
- dental disease/treatment may be life-threatening
- modifications to treatment plans
- special facilities
- treatment may be time consuming

In the light of these considerations, do such children need special dental care? Most of the studies which have been undertaken on disabled children have indicated that the majority of children examined can in fact be treated in a dental surgery together with the rest of their family in the normal way. This normalization is desirable, provided the disabled person actually receives good dental care. The evidence from many studies is that although the overall caries experience is similar between disabled children and their so-called normal contemporaries, the type of treatment they have experienced is different; disabled children have similar levels of untreated decay, but more missing teeth and fewer restored teeth. A minority of children with complex disabilities need special facilities, usually only available in dental or general hospitals, or from specialized community dental clinics. What *is* needed by all patients with disabilities is a very aggressive approach to the prevention of dental disease. Because of the potential for dental disease, or its treatment, to handicap disabled patients in a significant way, priority must be given to preventive dental care for such individuals from a very young age.

Children with a significant degree of disability are termed children with special educational needs or children with learning difficulties. This encompasses a wide variety of impairments but three main areas, intellectual impairment, physical disability, and sensory impairments predominate and will now be considered in more detail. It is important to stress, however, that disability does not always present as a discrete entity; in any population of affected children, at least a quarter of the group will be multiply disabled, making it difficult to assign a 'label' to that child's disabilty type. The way in which some of these disabilities may present to a dentist are given below, together with the dental management issues relevant to each type of impairment. Many of the issues raised are common to a number of disabilities.

Key Points

Classification — disabled children:
- intellectually impaired: mentally retarded, learning difficulties
- physically impaired: developmental, degenerative
- sensory impairment
- medically compromised
- combination of disabilities

16.2   INTELLECTUAL IMPAIRMENT

The causes of intellectual impairment are numerous and for many children a cause for their disability may never be identified. Approximately 25 per thousand of the child population are affected, and the majority, like other disabilities, will be males. Children with intellectual impairment can be divided broadly into those who are either mentally retarded or have a learning difficulty. These are broad groups, often without a well defined aetiology or consistent presenting features, but there are two distinct subgroups where the cause is known and the features are well described, namely Down and Fragile X syndromes. Intellectual impairment may be present in some children with cerebral palsy and those who have suffered birth anoxia, and severe infections, for example, meningitis and rubella. Intellectual impairment is also a feature of autism, microcephaly, metabolic disorders, for example phenylketonuria, and may be acquired after significant trauma. Not every condition will have specific dental features like Down syndrome, but an understanding of the underlying disability will help the dentist plan treatment more effectively.

Mental retardation, pervasive developmental disorders (autism and schizophrenia), learning disabilities, dyslexia, attention deficit disorders, and hyperactivity are all controversial categories whose definition and processes of measurement are not universally agreed.

Intellectual impairment may occur in:
- cerebral palsy
- birth anoxia
- severe infections
- autism
- microcephaly
- metabolic disorders
- major trauma
- some syndromes

Mental retardation

This is sometimes called mental handicap, mental subnormality, or mental deficiency. It is a general category characterized by low intelligence, failure of adaptation, and early age of onset. Low general intelligence is the main characteristic. Affected children are slow in their general mental development and they may have difficulties in attention, perception, memory, and thinking. They may be stronger in some skills than others, for example, music and computing but generally they are of low intellectual attainment. Children with low intelligence are not called mentally retarded unless they also have some problem in adaptation. That is, they are unlikely to be able to live independently and will always depend inappropriately on others as a source of income. Five levels are traditionally described according to IQ levels. The simplicity of the classification is somewhat illusory with great individual differences among mentally retarded people.

Down syndrome

Down syndrome is a chromosomal disorder, trisomy 21, with distinct clinical features. The prevalence is approximately one in 600 births but there is variation with maternal age, so that at 40 years of age the incidence is about one in 40 births. The general physical features associated with Down syndrome are a greater predisposition to cardiac defects, leukaemia, hepatitis B infection (especially in institutionalized males), and now increasingly, Alzheimer's disease. Varying degrees of mental retardation occur and upper respiratory tract infections with an inability to withstand infections are common.

Extra-orally the predominant features are a rounded small face with an underdeveloped mid-face, especially of the nasal bridge, an upward slant of the eyes with prominent epicanthic folds, squints, cataracts, and Brushfield spots on the iris. The hands of children with Down syndrome are stubby with a pronounced transverse palmar crease. Intra-orally the tongue is large, protruding, and sometimes heavily fissured. The palate may be high vaulted and narrow. There is usually a delay in the exfoliation of primary teeth and in the eruption of permanent teeth while some teeth may be congenitally missing. Teeth that erupt are often microdont and/or hypoplastic (Fig. 16.2).

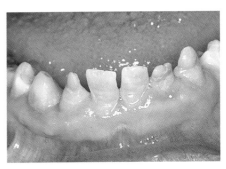

Fig. 16.2 A Down syndrome patient with marked dental hypoplasia, conical teeth, and hypodontia.

Oral features in Down syndrome:
- large fissured tongue
- narrow, high-vaulted palate
- delay in exfoliation/eruption
- congenitally absent teeth
- microdont/hypoplastic teeth
- Maxillary hypoplasia

Fragile X syndrome

Next to Down syndrome this is the commonest cause of mental retardation. This disorder is largely under-diagnosed and previously people classified as 'mental handicap of unknown origin', especially if they were male, probably had Fragile X syndrome. It is of particular significance because a high proportion of affected individuals have congenital heart defects that require antibiotic prophylaxis. Although males are predominantly affected, milder versions of the disability may be seen in females.

Pervasive developmental disorders

This group encompasses autism and childhood schizophrenia. The former is characterized by early onset, usually before 30 months of age whereas childhood schizophrenia presents later. They are rare conditions that represent profound adaptive problems in thinking, language, and social relationships. Autism in particular has the distinctive feature of restricted and stereotyped behaviour patterns. Most score below normal on IQ testing and thus experience significant developmental delay. The more severely delayed children seem oblivious to their parents or carers, express themselves minimally, show a low level of interest in exploring objects, avoid sounds, and engage in ritualistic behaviour.

These features need to be taken into consideration when attempting dental care and underlines the particular importance of acclimatization and familiarity of routine (rituals) as part of that process.

The causes of autism are unknown but are thought to be prenatal and not social in origin. A major malformation in the cerebellum has recently been implicated. The prevalence of autism ranges from 0.03 to 0.1 per cent with fluctuations that may point to an environmental cause.

Learning difficulty

Associated with learning difficulty are dyslexia, minimal brain damage, attention deficit disorder, and hyperactivity. All of these categories are controversial, mainly because they have been overextended.

Historically, a child with a learning difficulty has been defined as one whose performance in one academic area is more than 2 years behind the child's ability. Thus the disability is restricted in its range and there is a discrepancy between academic performance and tested general ability. In these two ways a learning disability differs from mental retardation because the latter is characterized by *general* delay and academic performance is usually at the level expected from ability. In practice, learning difficulty has been used to characterize any child with a learning problem who cannot be labelled mentally retarded, no matter how broad the range of disabilities and what the discrepancy from the tested ability level. This overextension of the definition has not only increased the apparent prevalence of learning disability but has also made the field confusing.

In general the prevalence is estimated on average to be about 4.5 per cent. There is overlap between learning difficulties and other problems, for example, higher levels of classroom behaviour problems and an increased risk of delinquency. In part this accounts for the greater predominance of males in groups with intellectual impairment as they are more likely than females to be disruptive at school and thus be referred for assessment by educational psychologists.

Dyslexia

This widely discussed form of learning disability is a specific problem with reading. The broadest definition of dyslexia includes those children whose reading skills are delayed for any reason and it is usually associated with a number of cognitive deficits. Prevalence varies from 3 to 16 per cent depending on the breadth of the definition and the country. For example, prevalence rates are higher in the United States than they are in Italy, perhaps due to the complexity of the English language as compared with Italian!

Minimal brain damage

This category of disability is used to describe the child who has minor neurological signs, which are often transitory. They are not reliable predictors of future behavioural and educational problems.

Attention disorder and hyperactivity

These are disorders that are often confused with one another. Children who cannot sit still are thought to be inattentive to their lessons in school. A child who does not attend often fails to finish activities, acts prematurely or redundantly, infrequently reacts to requests and questions, has difficulties with tasks that require fine discrimination, sustained vigilance or complex organization, and/or improves markedly when supervised intensively. A child who is hyperactive engages in excessive standing up, walking, running, and climbing; does not remain seated for long during tasks; frequently makes redundant movements; shifts excessively from one activity to another and/or often starts talking, asking, or making requests. This elevated activity level expresses itself differently at different ages.

Inattentive, hyperactive children are disturbing to their parents, other children, and to professionals like teachers, doctors, and dentists. They are often judged to be behaviourally disturbed. The variation in definition, age, sex, source of the data, and cultural factors produces prevalence estimates of up to 35 per cent. However, most estimates are under 9 per cent for boys and even less for girls.

Emotional and behavioural disorders

There are many manifestations of emotional disorder: fear, anxiety, shyness, aggressive, destructive or chronically disobedient behaviour, theft, having bad companions, and truancy. When parents or teachers believe that these problems interfere with the childs socialization, they are often referred for professional help. In considering the prevalence of emotional or behavioural disorders, account has to be taken of the very common, seemingly identical behaviours of normal children. Eating disorders, which may be of concern to dentists because of dental erosion, are important in the pre-school period and, in different ways, in adolescence.

16.2.1 General considerations

Access to care

Segregated special education and institutions, especially in rural areas, were characteristic of services for handicapped children until after the Second World War. During the 1950s there was a move towards *normalization* of the lives of 'handicapped' children. This movement set about making major changes in the lives of affected children and adults but cannot yet be considered as completely successful. The move to normalization came about largely for ideological and legal reasons.

The philosophy of this movement which originated in Sweden centred on the idea that a disabled person should live in an environment as near normal as possible. This involved residing in home-like residences and attending schools, working places, and recreation programmes that were part of the community. On the basis of this ideology, many mildly disabled people were moved out of long-stay institutions into community homes. This movement was fostered by the belief that institutionalization retarded emotional and cognitive growth. Deinstitutionalization would also reduce the state's expense in maintaining disabled people, and the onus would be shifted to parents, private charities, and local authorities.

While most people would agree with the principle of normalization, inadequate funding has produced a less than satisfactory alternative in community care and disasterous consequences for some mentally ill people and those they interact with. While many disabled children and adults were resident in long-stay institutions the provision of dental services was relatively efficient. With the move to normalization, children were often returned to parents or guardians, thereby placing an additional burden on these families to organize dental care.

Alongside this programme has been the move to integrate as many children as possible into mainstream education. This may mean that these children are not as readily identifiable as their peers in special schools and thus may miss out on the opportunity to receive the dental care they need.

For teenagers it has rapidly become apparent that managers of the adult training centres that they attend on a daily basis feel that, as part of normalization, their clients should receive 'normal' dental care, that is, from a general dental practitioner. This would be desirable, provided general dental practitioners were happy to provide this service. The evidence to date is that this is not generally the case. In the meantime, teenagers and young adults could lose out by not continuing to receive the special dental services that the Community Dental Service has to offer, simply because it is felt by their advocates that this runs contrary to the philosophy of 'normalization'.

Consent for dental care

A treatment plan for a child (less than 16 years) requires the consent of a parent before embarking upon active treatment. This is often by implied consent, that is, the parent brings the child to the surgery and the child sits in the chair, the implication being that the parent has consented to treatment. This is no different to the scenario with a disabled child.

Difficulty arises in adolescents with an intellectual impairment who are over the age of consent. In this situation parents or carers are unable to give a valid consent on their charges behalf. This is a matter which is being reviewed currently but until the position is clarified, dentists would be well advised to obtain a second opinion on their treatment plan before embarking on dental care for a disabled young person who is judged to be incapable of giving their own valid, i.e. informed, consent. This is particularly the case where dental care under general anaesthesia is being contemplated.

16.2.2 Oral health

Dental caries

In the absence of targeted preventive and treatment programmes, children with disabilities fare less well than their normal peers. While overall disease experience as measured using the DMF index (decayed, missing, filled teeth) is similar, for the disabled child there is often more untreated decay, more missing, and fewer filled teeth. Early studies pointed to a reduced prevalence of dental caries in Down syndrome children but this feature may have been attributable more to the later eruption of teeth relative to a control group of unaffected children so that the teeth are 'at risk' in the mouth for a shorter period of time. The relative microdontia in Down syndrome may also be a contributory factor in this supposed reduction in dental disease prevalence.

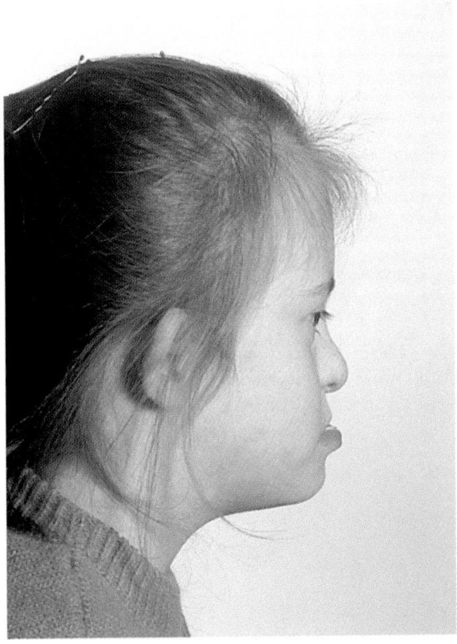

Periodontal disease

The periodontal status of children who are intellectually impaired may be compromised by their inability to comprehend and thus comply with oral hygiene measures. In these children periodontal disease is more prevalent, possibly as a result of an altered immune state. Almost universally, plaque and gingivitis scores are higher in disabled children.

Malocclusion

There are no studies that deal specifically with the problems of malocclusion in intellectually impaired children. However, in prevalence studies of general dental health, the number of orthodontic anomalies is frequently higher because many are untreated. In Down syndrome the relative mid-face hypoplasia contributes to the pseudo-skeletal class III relationship and this in combination with the narrow, high vaulted palate produces buccal cross-bites (Fig. 16.3).

Other oral defects

One feature of note is the prevalence of enamel defects often caused by the aetiological agent which produced the disability. It is possible that dentists could play a part not only in the diagnosis of some disabilities, for example coeliac disease (Fig. 16.4), but also in the timing of the insult which led to the disability. Teeth provide a good chronological record of the timing of severe systemic upsets. (Chapter 12)

16.2.3 Operative procedures

Children who are intellectually impaired may accept dental treatment but, their ability to accept specific procedures such as local anaesthetic and high-speed instruments will depend on their degree of understanding and age. Isolation may be difficult due to a large tongue and poor control of movement and in these situations it may be necessary to compromise on the treatment approach. In fissure sealing it may be more practicable to use a glass ionomer cement, protected by occlusal adjustment wax during the setting phase, rather than to struggle with all the stages of application of a conventional resin sealant (Fig. 16.5; see also Chapters 6 and 7).

Human clinical trials are now underway in both the United Kingdom and the United States to investigate the use of intra-oral fluoride releasing devices. These are small diameter, approximately 4 mm, glass devices that are attached to the

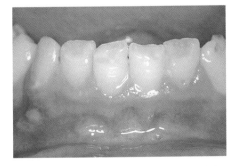

Fig. 16.3 Lateral view of a Down syndrome child to show Angles class III skeletal relationship.

Fig. 16.4 Chronological hypoplasia in a child with coeliac disease.

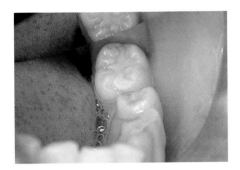

Fig. 16.5 Glass ionomer cement fissure sealant.

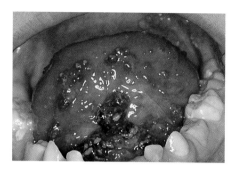

Fig. 16.6 Fluoride varnish on primary molars in a child with a mixed lymph/haemangioma and a learning disability.

surface of a tooth with composite resin. The device dissolves slowly in saliva, releasing fluoride as it does so. Those currently on trial have continued to elevate salivary fluoride levels for up to 2 years. Whether the released fluoride is equitably distributed around the mouth is not yet known.

Duraphat fluoride varnish (5 per cent sodium fluoride = 2200 p.p.m. fluoride, Inpharma A.S., Drammen, Norway) is an almost ideal preventive dental agent for children with poor tolerance of dental procedures. The amber coloured polyurethane-based material is applied to the tooth surface (preferably dry), although the varnish is water tolerant and the resulting adherent film slowly releases fluoride (Fig. 16.6). The exercise should be repeated up to four times a year depending on caries risk. A reduction of caries in permanent teeth of between 30 and 62 per cent has been reported using Duraphat varnish.

Another innovation which may be of use for disabled patients is a chlorhexidine varnish which would be applied like Duraphat. Early clinical results in trials looking at reduction of microbial counts are promising.

For some patients general anaesthesia will be necessary to provide adequate dental care (Fig. 16.7). This facility is not widely available and often means considerable disruption for the family because of the distance involved in travelling to specialist centres. Additionally, the child may be unsettled by the whole process of being starved, looked after by strange personnel, being put off to sleep, and then waking up with a sore throat and perhaps a mouth full of blood. There is evidence that this experience is only in the short-term memory as many parents comment on how much better their child is in terms of behaviour, sleeping patterns, and eating after the immediate postoperative period.

Treatment planning for dental care under general anaesthesia has to be more radical. The opportunity to reduce a 'high' restoration or to review a doubtful tooth is not necessarily available without recourse to another general anaesthetic. Radiography is an important aid in theatre, especially in the patient who is totally uncooperative in the dental chair. It is particularly important for detecting otherwise hidden pathology and for early enamel lesions. The latter cannot normally be left in the hope that they will remineralize with good preventive care. Similarly, the chances of restoration failure can be reduced by

Fig. 16.7 Day-stay general anaesthesia for a disabled child.

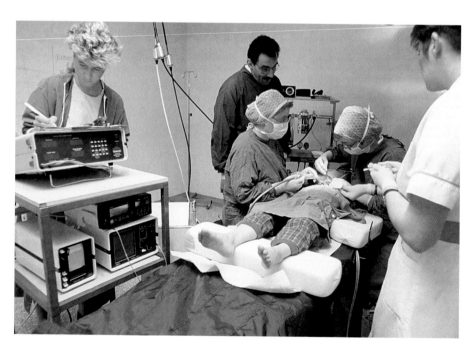

the use of pulpotomy techniques and preformed metal crowns. Most forms of treatment can be carried out under general anaesthesia provided there is sufficient operating time.

Success is dependent upon careful pre-anaesthetic assessment by dentist and anaesthetist. Appropriate perioperative care in theatre, for example steroid or antibiotic cover, and the back up of in-patient facilities where medically or socially indicated, are vital to a successful outcome.

Key Points

Pre-anaesthetic assessment — important features:
- accurate medical history
- previous anaesthetic history
- significant airways difficulties
- need for pre-medication
- transport arrangements
- home care

16.2.4   Home care

Oral hygiene

There is little to be gained in embarking on elaborate treatment plans including advanced restorative work when it will not be maintained by regular oral hygiene measures at home.

Parents/carers need specific advice and practical help in the best way to care for their child's mouth. Great reliance is thus placed on the parent or carer who must be actively involved in oral hygiene instruction and given positive suggestions for modifications to the standard techniques. Examples include advice on the way to position a child (a bean bag can be helpful), in order to clean their mouth more efficiently and less traumatically. Another aid is the use of a prop such as a toothbrush handle to gain access to tooth surfaces on the other side of the mouth. Modification of existing, often very narrow handled toothbrushes or the use of specially modified brush heads can be helpful (Fig. 16.8). For some children, the mechanical removal of plaque can be more readily accomplished using an electric or battery operated toothbrush. Once the child has become accustomed to the sensation, results in certain circumstances have been good.

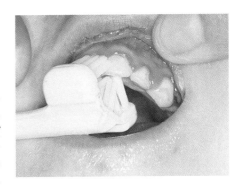

Fig. 16.8   A 'Superbrush' in use in a child with cerebral palsy.

Chemical agents are effective in reducing plaque in the short term, but not enough is known about the effects of their long-term usage. Many children and adults find the taste of 0.2 per cent chlorhexidine gluconate, either as a gel or solution, unpalatable and parents or carers are unhappy about the extrinsic brown staining. Many disabled patients may not be able to use a mouthwash correctly and either swallow or spit out anything distasteful.

Some schools for children with special educational needs provide toothbrushes for their pupils during their learning of personal hygiene skills. However, awareness of the best method of mouth cleaning is often limited among supervising staff and is more dependent on their own perceptions of oral health and the perceived difficulty, than any other factor (Fig. 16.9).

Toothbrushing can be taught in the same way as other skills but it requires time for the individual as well as committment on the part of the regular carer to ensure that all areas of the mouth are being cleaned each time. However, many disabled children are intolerant not only of toothbrushing but also of toothpaste and they may gag when toothpaste, which they cannot swallow because of poor reflexes, is introduced into the mouth. Toothpaste also obscures the view for the carer during toothbrushing and they cannot always be sure that the tooth sur-

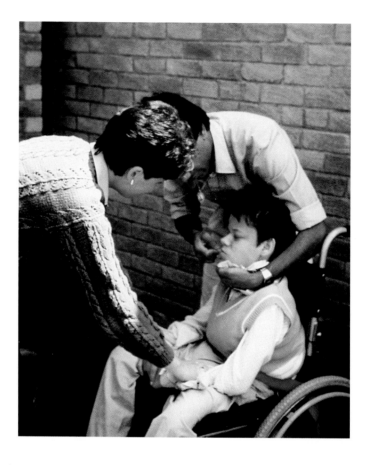

Fig. 16.9 Toothbrushing in a special school.

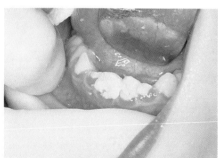

Fig. 16.10 Loose calculus deposits in a child with 4p syndrome.

faces are clean. Where toothbrushing and/or toothpaste are unacceptable, parents or carers should attempt to clean around the mouth with a piece of gauze moistened in 0.2 per cent chlorhexidine gluconate solution or a toothbrush dipped in fluoride mouthrinse (0.05 per cent sodium fluoride if used on a daily basis). Alternatively, chlorhexidene in gel form or a fluoride toothpaste can be rubbed as vigorously as possible around the tooth surfaces using a finger.

Children that are tube fed for some or all of their nutrient intake still need oral care. They will sometimes accumulate significant quantities of calculus, which if detached might be inhaled. Regular mouth cleaning and the use of a 'tartar control' toothpaste is necessary (Fig. 16.10).

Diet

More severely disabled children usually have well regulated eating times and a reduced likelihood of snacking. The food consumed may be semi-solid or even liquidized and those foods which are easily reduced to this form are often dentally undesirable. In these circumstances the dentist should offer advice on limiting the number of intakes of food, provided it conforms to the childs general nutritional and dietary needs.

For some children establishing a normal eating routine while 'growing up' becomes a battlefield and disabled children are no exception to this. It is often easier for parents to 'give in' to a child and allow them to eat a limited variety of unsuitable foods frequently. This will be justified by parents saying they are desperate to get the child to eat something, and so biscuits, and other snacks high in non-milk extrinsic sugars, become the norm. This pattern is further endorsed in some disabled children where weight gain is paramount and the dental implications are secondary (if indeed they are even considered).

Drinks can be a difficult area, particularly the use of sweetened bottles for an extended period in a child's life. It is not uncommon for children of 2 years of age or older still to be using a bottle containing milk; last thing at night before going to bed; during the night; and first thing on waking. This is an extremely difficult habit to break but the most successful approach has been to advise the parent gradually to dilute the contents with water over a period of weeks, until eventually the child is drinking water only. This not only eliminates the undesirable habit but also gives the parent of the child who is able to be toilet trained, some prospect of getting the child dry and out of nappies overnight.

For a number of disabled children the use of sweetened medication has led to an increase in dental caries (Fig. 16.11). In the past this has arisen because of a lack of sugar-free alternatives. However, with greater awareness now on behalf of the pharmaceutical industry it is often only due to ignorance among the medical profession that such outmoded prescribing continues.

Another consideration is spoiling. For any parent the birth of a disabled child is a shock. Months of eager anticipation are followed by disbelief, anger, denial, frustration, and guilt. Parents have to grieve for the normal child they will never have, before coming to terms with their new responsibilities. Parents continue to feel guilty; maybe their child is disabled because of something they have done, or something they should not have done. Either way, they can assuage that guilt by spoiling the child. This may take the form of sweet foods that are thought to be pleasurable and are welcomed by the child with a poor appetite, thus compounding the problem of poor eating.

Poor eating habits resulting in oral disease need to be tackled together with the paediatrician and dietician, as well as the parents/caregivers.

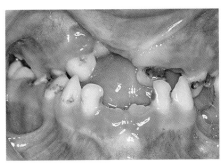

Fig. 16.11 The dental effects of frequent medication in a child with a cleft of the lip and palate.

Key Points

Dietary advice:
- restrict sweet foods/drinks to mealtimes
- limit sweetened foods/drinks to three times a day
- keep food and drinks clear of bedtime by about an hour
- carbonated drinks are erosive to teeth
- ask for sugar-free medicines

Fluorides

Many special milk formulae and food supplements, as well as containing non-milk extrinsic sugars in order to boost the child's calorie intake, also in some cases have quite substantial amounts of fluoride. It is wise therefore to check the diet carefully before advocating the use of fluoride supplements for such children.

Where dental caries is potentially a real problem,and in the absence of any other form of systemic fluorides, then the regimen of 0.25 mg from 6 months of age, followed by an increase to 0.5 mg at 2 years of age and then 1.0 mg from 4 years of age is to be advocated. In these circumstances the slight risk of developing mild enamel opacities is outweighed by the benefits of caries prevention. These fluoride supplements can be prescribed by the general dental practitioner, either as drops for the younger child or tablets for the pre-school child. It is likely that some disabled children will never cope with fluoride tablets and have to remain on drops. As long as the parent is given written instructions to overrule the prescribing schedule given for younger children on the label of the bottle, there is no reason why older children should not be prescribed fluoride drops.

The dentist should also advise on the appropriate fluoride toothpaste to be used in conjunction with fluoride supplementation or water fluoridation. Each case should be considered individually with the relative risks and benefits that may occur. Paramount is the consideration of the risk from developing dental caries versus the potential for enamel opacities in the permanent dentition. As a guideline, if the risk from caries is minimal, and if the diet is reasonably well controlled and home oral care is generally good, then it is sensible to suggest the use of a pea-sized amount of toothpaste containing approximately 500–600 p.p.m. fluoride, for the child under 6 years of age, provided that toothpaste can be used successfully. Older children,in the same situation should use a toothpaste containing between 1000 and 1500 p.p.m. fluoride as the risk of enamel opacities on anterior teeth is now considerably reduced and this formulation will provide optimal protection against caries. In the child where the development of dental disease would pose a real hazard to their general health, and where home care in terms of oral hygiene and diet is poorly controlled, then it is advisable to confer maximum protection by advising the use of a toothpaste containing 1000–1500 p.p.m. fluoride even during the pre-school years.

Because of the inability of many disabled children to hold solutions in their mouths or to be able to expectorate, fluoride mouthwashes are contra-indicated, but can be used on a toothbrush (dipped) where toothpaste is not well tolerated.

Key Points

Fluoride advice:
- supplements to give optimal caries protection
- fluoride mouthwash on a toothbrush instead of paste in cases of paste intolerance
- low caries risk   — 500–600 p.p.m. fluoride paste (< 6 years)
                    — 1000–1500 p.p.m. fluoride paste (> 6 years)
                    (pea-sized amount)
- high caries risk 1000–1500 p.p.m. fluoride paste (pea-sized amount) from time of eruption onwards

16.3   PHYSICAL DISABILITY — CEREBRAL PALSY

The commonest physical disabilities the dentist will encounter are *developmental* neuromuscular disorders, for example cerebral palsy, spina bifida, scoliosis, and osteogenesis imperfecta, and *degenerative* neuromuscular disorders for example muscular dystrophy and juvenile forms of arthritis. Included in this general category of physical disability, are children with clefts of the lip and/or palate (Chapter 13) where in up to 19 per cent of cases there will be an associated syndrome.

16.3.1   General considerations

Cerebral palsy occurs in one to two children per 1000 of school age, a figure which has been relatively stable because of the improved quality of survival of premature babies.

It is a group of non-progressive neuromuscular disorders caused by brain damage, which can be pre-, peri-, or post-natal in origin and is classified according to the type of motor defect:

1. Spasticity — impaired ability to control voluntary movements. There is the appearance of severe muscle stiffness and the planned movement of an affected limb results in a hypotonic tendon reflex, especially with rapid movements. Spasticity occurs in about 50 per cent of cases of cerebral palsy.

2. Athetosis — uncontrolled, slow twisting and writhing movements which are frequent and involuntary and occur in over 16 per cent of cases.

3. Rigidity — resistance to passive movement, which may be overcome by sudden action. It is uncommon and the majority of these children are mentally impaired.

4. Ataxia — disturbance of equilibrium as well as difficulty in grasping objects. It is also uncommon.

5. Hypotonia — all muscles are flaccid with decreased function

6. Mixed — combination of the above.

The last 20 years has seen a change in the proportion of the different subtypes, for example, with the decrease in kernicterus (neonatal jaundice), there has been a fall in the athetoid form, but the spastic form, associated with prematurity, has increased. An affected child may be monoplegic with only one limb affected (Fig. 16.12) or have all four limbs affected (quadraplegia). In addition they may be handicapped by other disabilities such as convulsions, intellectual impairment, sensory disorders, emotional disorders, speech and communication defects, and a poorly developed swallowing and cough reflex.

16.3.2 Oral health

The dental features that may be seen in children with cerebral palsy are: increased periodontitis and drug-induced gingival overgrowth; malocclusion (increased prevalence of skeletal class II with anterior open bite) and a tendency to bruxism; tongue thrust and mouth breathing; an increase in caries prevalence and anterior trauma; enamel hypoplasia; increased gag reflex and peri-oral sensitivity; poor oral hygiene; drooling; and decreased parotid flow rate. Although not confined to children with cerebral palsy, gastric reflux is relatively common (Fig. 16.13). There may be an obvious aetiology, for example, a hiatus hernia, but quite often, a cause for the erosion cannot be identified (Chapter 9).

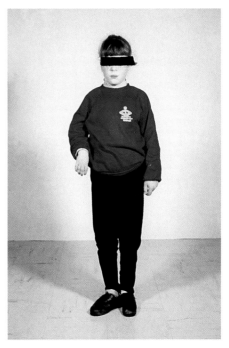

Fig. 16.12 Monoplegia of the right arm in a child with cerebral palsy and a congenital heart defect.

Key Points

Oral features in cerebral palsy:
- gingival hyperplasia
- increased caries prevalence
- malocclusion
- enamel hypoplasia
- increased gag reflex
- dental erosion

16.3.3 Operative procedures

Children who are severely physically disabled will probably be brought to the dental surgery in a wheelchair or be carried. Care is required in the handling of such patients (see 16.4.1 below).

Altered gag and cough reflexes may complicate the delivery of dental care or the provision of prostheses, as well as adding to the patient's anxiety. Plentiful reassurance, good aspiration, and skilled assistance are vital to success in these situations. Impaired ventilation may accompany scoliosis and becomes an even more important consideration if procedures involving a general anaesthetic are contemplated.

Children who spend long periods of time in one position may be predisposed to pressure sores and lengthy procedures in the dental chair without a break are best avoided.

Hypoplastic teeth, can be very sensitive, particularly to extreme cold. They can cause acute discomfort during tooth preparation or ultrasonic scaling (even when they are distant from the operating site), merely from the cold produced by high volume aspiration. The use of a desensitizing varnish like Duraphat fluoride varnish or fissure sealing the symptomatic surface can be helpful if a restoration is not indicated. Hypoplastic enamel does not have the same ordered prism structure as normal enamel and despite acid etching may not provide optimum reten-

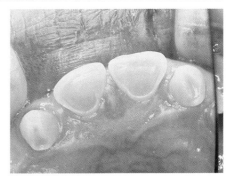

Fig. 16.13 Palatal erosion in a child with cerebral palsy.

tion for conventional resins. In this situation, glass ionomer cements may be a more suitable alternative.

Some less severely disabled children will have little or no mental impairment but a degree of spasticity or rigidity. This may prevent them from co-operating fully with dental procedures, despite their willingness to do so, and they may be helped by nitrous oxide sedation (Chapter 4). Such sedation may also help diminish a heightened gag reflex.

16.3.4   Home care

Oral hygiene

Physical impairment may hinder oral hygiene procedures and for the child who has gingival overgrowth the problem may be compounded. Most children require help with brushing until they are 7 years or older but for the child with physical limitations this may be a permanent commitment. Limited or bizarre muscle movements prevent normal mouth clearing and food is often left impacted in the vault of the palate. This is readily removed with the end of a toothbrush handle or a spoon handle, and carers need to be aware of the potential for this, otherwise food residues may be left in the oral cavity for days. Electric toothbrushes may be helpful for a child with limited dexterity not only because of the relative efficiency of cleaning but also because of the larger size of the handle of most of these brushes.

When normal limb movement is impaired or absent and/or normal speech is not possible the mouth assumes an even greater importance as a means of holding mouth sticks to grasp pens or to operate a variety of equipment. It is vital the dentition is maintained to the highest standard as the successful use of such mouth sticks is reliant on having a good occlusal table for balanced contact (Fig. 16.14).

Children with cerebral palsy, especially where there is accompanying intellectual impairment, will on occasion adopt a habit of self-mutilation by chewing soft tissues around the mouth (Fig. 16.15). This can be triggered by teething, although no cause may be found. It is distressing for the parents as the child is obviously in pain from the ulcerated areas and may refuse all food and drink, but there is little they can do to break the habit. There are a number of solutions to the problem depending on the cause and the severity of the condition. In a child who is erupting primary teeth it may be possible to fit an occlusal splint provided

Fig. 16.14   A modified pen holder for a child with arthrogyphosis.

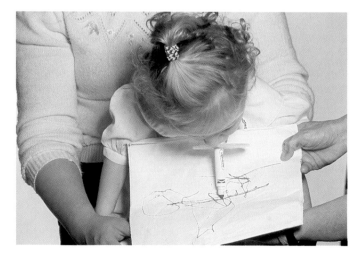

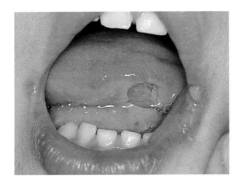

Fig. 16.15 Self-mutilation in a child with cerebral palsy.

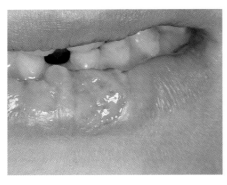

(a)

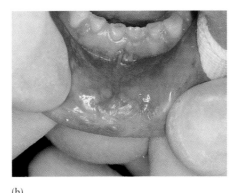

(b)

Fig. 16.16 (a) and (b) Traumatic self-mutilation in a boy with cerebral palsy — before and after the use of a composition 'splint' to protect the traumatized area.

that sufficient teeth are available for retention. Fabrication of the splint may necessitate a short general anasthetic for impression taking. If only anterior primary teeth are present then composition moulded over the offending tooth surfaces as a temporary splint may break the habit and allow healing. (Fig. 16.16a and b). If the problem is more severe and a splint is not feasible, it is sensible to extract the primary teeth involved. In the permanent dentition, rounding off of pointed or sharp tooth surfaces and/or fitting a splint is usually successful.

During the acute phase the use of a topical analgesic such as 0.15 per cent benzydamine hydrochloride ('Difflam') in spray form increases mouth comfort prior to eating and 0.2 per cent chlorhexidine gluconate solution ('Corsodyl') swabbed around the mouth or applied as a gel on a finger promotes more rapid healing in addition to keeping the area clean. Ensuring that the child has plenty of fluids is of paramount importance as small, debilitated children rapidly become dehydrated. It may be helpful to discuss the child's medication with their physician as the prescription of a drug to reduce muscle tonus, which can be an exacerbating factor in this situation, could be considered.

The other area of concern to parents and carers is drooling. For some disabled children this can be excessive and surgery to divert submandibular flow more posteriorly may alleviate the problem. However, this is not always successful and carries the risk of increasing caries prevalence as a result of the greatly diminished salivary volume. Outside the United Kingdom use is made of acrylic training plates that encourage the formation of an oral seal as well as promoting a more active swallowing mechanism so that saliva does not pool in an open mouth (Fig. 16.17). Anecdotal case reports support the use of these plates but there are no studies published which give objective data on their success.

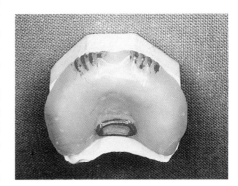

Fig. 16.17 A palatal training plate designed to improve lip and tongue posture.

Diet

Considerations on dietary aspects have been covered in the section on intellectual impairment (16.2.4).

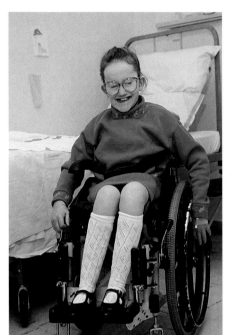

Fig. 16.18 A girl with spina bifida — wheelchair bound.

16.4 PHYSICAL DISABILITY — SPINA BIFIDA

Spina bifida occurs as a result of non-fusion of one or more posterior vertebral arches, with or without protrusion of some or all of the contents of the spinal canal. It may be accompanied by hydrocephalus in up to 95 per cent of cases. It is estimated that in 50–60 per cent of affected children the defect is inherited and that in the remainder, environmental agents may be responsible. In the United Kingdom the incidence is 2.5 per 1000 births and, unlike other malformations, is commoner in females. A quarter of children will also have epilepsy and about a third will have some degree of intellectual impairment.

16.4.1 General considerations

Children with spina bifida will, unless the defect is slight, spend much of their time confined to a wheelchair (Fig. 16.18) and be incontinent. Urinary tract infections are common and the child may be on frequent courses of antibiotics. Hydrocephalus, unless arrested, is treated by the insertion of a shunt (Spitz–Holter valve) to drain fluid from the ventricles into the superior vena cava. It is important to protect this shunt from blockage, (which may arise from a bacteraemia of oral origin), otherwise intracranial pressure will increase causing convulsions. Although opinion is divided on the necessity to cover invasive dental procedures in children with a shunt, those erring on the side of caution will use the same prophylaxis regimen as in cardiac disease (Chapter 15). Children who are confined to a wheelchair for much of the time will need to be treated either in their chair or transferred carefully to the dental chair.

It is possible to use special equipment (Hatrick recliner) to allow a wheelchair to be tipped back into a more conventional semi-supine operating position. This is helpful if the child is too heavy to transfer easily to the dental chair or if the procedure is more easily accomplished for the operator and patient in this position. Shaped body supports, which are essentially modifications of a bean bag, are also available for use in the dental chair for any patient with a physical disability who cannot otherwise be comfortably accommodated. These supports contain a material that allows them to mould to the body shape of the patient and be remoulded for subsequent patients (Fig. 16.19).

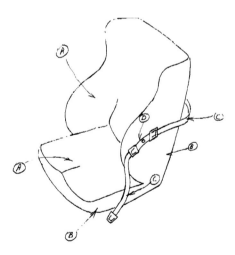

Fig. 16.19 Burnett supports — for remoulding in the dental chair for each individual patient.

16.4.2 Oral health and operative procedures

There is little in the dental literature to suggest that the dental health of children with spina bifida is different from other disabled children. The same principles of treatment apply to these children as to others who are disabled, namely aggressive prevention and early intervention with a radical approach if dental treatment under general anaesthesia is required.

16.4.3 Home care

The issues relevant to spina bifida have been covered in the appropriate sections under intellectual impairment and physical disability.

16.5   PHYSICAL DISABILITY — MUSCULAR DYSTROPHY

Muscular dystrophy is a group of muscle diseases which present as progressive atrophy and weakness of skeletal muscles with resultant disability and deformity. The muscle fibres degenerate and are replaced by fatty and fibrous tissue. The disease is eventually fatal as a result of recurrent respiratory infections. Prevalence rates in children are of the order of four per 100 000 children.

16.5.1   General considerations

The child with muscular dystrophy will initially be mobile but as the disease progresses they will become reliant on a wheelchair. A respirator will be necessary in the later stages of the disease and patients are then confined to home or to long-stay care. There are a number of variants of the disease with different signs and symptoms; males are exclusively affected in the Duchenne type, while facial musculature is always affected in the fascioscapulohumeral type, but rarely in other forms.

16.5.2   Oral health

The dental effects of the disease are numerous and include:

(1) weakness of the facial muscles;
(2) poor oral hygiene secondary to the general inability to provide oral self-care;
(3) increased dental decay;
(4) increased potential for periodontal disease;
(5) malocclusion secondary to decreased facial muscle tone while retaining tongue function;
(6) decreased protective reflexes and reduced ability to swallow or clear secretions from the oropharynx, thus increasing the potential for aspiration.

16.5.3   Operative procedures

Consideration needs to be given to wheelchair transfer techniques and padding as well as the length of appointments (see above). The use of sedation and general anaesthesia may need to be avoided due to the decrease in respiratory function and the risk of post-anaesthetic complications. Frequent recall is important with applications of topical fluorides and antiplaque agents (0.2 per cent chlorhexidine gluconate). There are no contra-indications to dental treatment, with the exception of orthodontics because of the changing muscle forces. As a consequence of tooth movement seen as part of the disease, and the likely development of anterior or posterior open bites, prosthetic appliances may become non-functional.

16.5.4   Home care

Appropriate support and training needs to be given to the parent or carer so that in the later stages of the disease, when contact with dental services may be difficult, adequate plaque control can be maintained. Dental treatment may need to be provided within the home environment, although this will usually be at the stage when the patient has reached adulthood. It is important that every effort is made to optimize oral function and facial appearance and thereby encourage a positive self-image.

16.6   OTHER MUSCULOSKELETAL DISABILITIES

There are a variety of other defects, some degenerative and some developmental, which also affect children; however, these are relatively rare and unlikely to be encountered regularly in practice. For example, osteogenesis imperfecta, juvenile arthritis, and multiple sclerosis. When patients present with such disabilities there may be significant oral signs, for example in rheumatoid arthritis there is an increased incidence of Sjögren's syndrome (autoimmune) and anaemia (secondary to anti-inflammatory and steroid medication). Aggressive prevention is vital to prevent dental disease.

16.7   BLINDNESS AND VISUAL IMPAIRMENT

Visual impairments vary from total blindness to sight limitations of size, colour, distance, and shape. The prevalence is of the order of three per 1000 children.

16.7.1   Oral health

The oral health of children with a visual impairment is no different from the normal population and with good home care this can be maintained. In the United Kingdom many children are educated in boarding schools and their supervision with regard to personal hygiene and diet (restraint from between-meal snacking), often means that their oral health is good.

16.7.2   Operative procedures

Consideration should be given to the design and format of written material available for use by patients who may be visually impaired, for example, instructions for the wearing of orthodontic appliances and diet history sheets. Highly stylized type should be avoided and a mix of upper and lower case should be used. Letters should be at least one-eighth inch high and be on uncoated (non-glare) paper. The best contrast for ease of reading is black type on white or off-white paper.

It is important to assist the visually impaired person according to their individual needs. Patients with a sight defect object to being forcefully guided around by a nurse or dentist enthusiastic to help. Many sight impaired patients will have an increased sensitivity to bright lights and perhaps touch. The former needs caution during use of the operating light and the latter should be utilized to enhance the patients perception of what is being done; for example, being allowed to feel the instruments and the dental chair.

It is not unusual for people to shout at those with a visual impairment. Sight impaired children are not usually deaf as well and should therefore be addressed in a normal voice. It is important to the patient, and not only those with visual impairments, that conversation is addressed to them and not to the person with them — the so-called 'Does he take sugar?' approach. Because vision is impaired and the sense of touch may be heightened, it can be startling suddenly to feel a cold mirror in your mouth without a warning of its coming. A 'tell-then-do' approach is even more important for these children who may be unnerved by contact without forewarning. With these considerations in mind, there are no areas of dental treatment that are unsuitable for the child with a visual impairment provided that they or their parent can maintain an adequate standard of oral hygiene. Insertion of orthodontic appliances may initially be difficult and techniques like flossing take time to master.

16.8 DEAFNESS AND HEARING IMPAIRMENT

Loss of hearing is a disability acquired by many with age. However, some children are born with either partial or total loss of hearing and this can occur in isolation or in combination with other disabilities, for example, rubella syndrome (auditory, visual, intellectual, and cardiac defects). The prevalence is three per 1000 children.

16.8.1 General considerations

Patients who have hearing impairment may be fearful, or even hostile, because they feel they are not going to understand what is being asked of them. The child may not hear what has been said but pretends they have done so to avoid embarrassment. In this situation visual aids assume an even greater importance. It is important for optimizing hearing that all extraneous background noise is removed when communicating with the hearing impaired child. Piped music in the surgery, noise from the reception area as well as internal noises like aspirators and scavenging systems should be reduced or eliminated.

16.8.2 Oral health

There is a paucity of data concerning the oral health of children with hearing impairment. As with visually impaired children, residence away from home in special boarding schools sometimes means that eating patterns are more desirable dentally, with less opportunity for between meal snacking compared to day pupils. Supervision of oral hygiene measures can also be better in institutionalized children and is reflected in their oral hygiene scores, but this is very variable. Like many other disabled children, hearing impaired patients are initially wary of battery operated toothbrushes because of the sensation they produce intra-orally and generally these brushes have not been shown to be better in terms of plaque removal than a well manipulated manual brush.

16.8.3 Operative procedures

Many deaf or hearing impaired children will wear aids (Fig. 16.20) to enable them to pick up more sounds and older children may have become skilled not only in lip reading but also in signing. However, there is now a trend towards discouraging the use of signing and to positively encourage a child to acquire some speech, utilizing any residual vocal potential. For those children who can lip read it is necessary to sit well in front of the child, with good lighting to the operator's face. Masks are therefore to be put to one side and bearded operators should ensure that facial hair does not obscure clear visualization of lip movement! Children wearing hearing devices may be disturbed by the high-pitched noise produced by handpieces and ultrasonic scalers. This may make them less co-operative and less amenable to treatment. Similarly, the conduction of vibrations from the handpiece and burs via bone is more disturbing for the hearing impaired child. After initial communications are complete it may be advisable to suggest that the hearing device is removed or turned off and only re-inserted on completion of the dental treatment in time for final instructions. Very young children often have difficulty keeping the aids in place simply because of the size of the immature pinnae. This is especially so when lying supine in the dental chair.

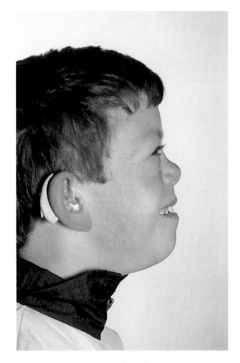

Fig. 16.20 A child with William's syndrome with hearing aids.

16.9 SUMMARY

1. Disabled children present the dental team with the challenge of adapting familiar skills to new situations.

2. To meet this challenge effectively we need to re-examine some of the stereotypes of disability we carry in our own minds.

3. A disability becomes a handicap by virtue of other peoples attitudes, the things we do or do not do, the facilities we do not offer, as well as the physical barriers the environment throws up.

4. Dental health is little different between disabled children and others. What is different is the type of treatment provided, with more missing teeth and fewer filled teeth in disabled populations.

5. Some disabled children have specific oral conditions as a result of their disability, e.g. Down syndrome.

6. A degree of common sense, a willingness to be flexible as well as a working familiarity with the commoner medical conditions and their implications for dental health, are most of what a general dental practitioner requires to provide dental care for the disabled child in his/her community.

16.10 FURTHER READING

Hunter, B. (1987). *Dental care for handicapped patients. Dental practitioner handbook.* Wright, Bristol. (*Compact summary of the practical problems of providing care.*)

Nunn J. H. (1996). Preventing a dental handicap. In *The prevention of dental disease* (ed. J. J. Murray) (3rd edn). Oxford Medical Publications, Oxford. (*A more comprehensive review of the subject.*)

Index

Note: Page numbers in *italic* refer to figures and/or tables